PREVENTIVE AND THERAPEUTIC ROLE OF VITAMINS AS NUTRACEUTICALS

AAP Advances in Nutraceuticals

PREVENTIVE AND THERAPEUTIC ROLE OF VITAMINS AS NUTRACEUTICALS

Edited by

Khemchand R. Surana, MSPharm

Eknath D. Ahire, MSPharm

Raj K. Keservani, PhD, MPharm

Rajesh K. Kesharwani, PhD

APPLE ACADEMIC PRESS

First edition published 2024

Apple Academic Press Inc.
1265 Goldenrod Circle, NE,
Palm Bay, FL 32905 USA

760 Laurentian Drive, Unit 19,
Burlington, ON L7N 0A4, CANADA

CRC Press
2385 NW Executive Center Drive,
Suite 320, Boca Raton FL 33431

4 Park Square, Milton Park,
Abingdon, Oxon, OX14 4RN UK

Library and Archives Canada Cataloguing in Publication

Title: Preventive and therapeutic role of vitamins as nutraceuticals / edited by Khemchand R. Surana, MSPharm, Eknath D. Ahire, MSPharm, Raj K. Keservani, PhD, Rajesh K. Kesharwani, PhD.
Names: Surana, Khemchand R., editor. | Ahire, Eknath D., editor. | Keservani, Raj K., 1981- editor. | Kesharwani, Rajesh Kumar, 1978- editor.
Series: AAP advances in nutraceuticals.
Description: First edition. | Series statement: AAP advances in nutraceuticals | Includes bibliographical references and index.
Identifiers: Canadiana (print) 20230597246 | Canadiana (ebook) 20230597289 | ISBN 9781774914441 (hardcover) | ISBN 9781774914458 (softcover) | ISBN 9781003414025 (ebook)
Subjects: LCSH: Vitamin therapy. | LCSH: Vitamins. | LCSH: Functional foods.
Classification: LCC RM259 .P74 2024 | DDC 615.3/28—dc23

Library of Congress Cataloging-in-Publication Data

CIP data on file with US Library of Congress

ISBN: 978-1-77491-444-1 (hbk)
ISBN: 978-1-77491-445-8 (pbk)
ISBN: 978-1-00341-402-5 (ebk)

About the Book Series: AAP Advances in Nutraceuticals

Series Editor:
Raj K. Keservani, PhD, MPharm
Faculty of B. Pharmacy, CSM Group of Institutions, Allahabad, India

Rajesh K. Kesharwani, PhD
Nehru Gram Bharati (Deemed to be University), Prayagraj, India

Anil K. Sharma, PhD, MPharm
Department of Pharmacy, School of Medical and Allied Sciences,
GD Goenka University, Gurugram, India

In the modern era, mankind has witnessed a paradigm shift with respect to fundamental eating behavior. The lack of physical workouts and busy schedules at offices and in households have promoted the consumption of junk foods, which eventually results in numerous diseases and disorders since the nutritional content from fast food is inadequate. Plumpness and obesity have become a global health threat. The leading causes of death from most developing nations are noncommunicable diseases such as cardiovascular diseases, cancer, arthritis, osteoporosis, and liver toxicity. Patients suffering from such lifestyle ailments are a bit apprehensive towards prolonged use of costly modern therapeutics, which encourages instead the use of alternative approaches for management of such diseases and disorders.

The emerging sector of the nutraceutical industry encompasses products derived from nature, dietary supplements, and functional foods. Nutraceuticals are used for treatment and prevention of a broad range of diseases, such as the common cold, arthritis, sleep-related disorders, cancers, cardiovascular complications, metabolic disorders, and others.

The research on nutraceuticals is increasing day by day, considering the beneficial effects of food or food supplements in the management of diverse diseases. The issue of paramount concern is standardization and establishment of clinical efficacy of nutraceuticals, which is in fact a challenge for researchers around the globe.

This book series aims at realizing the significance of the variety of nutraceuticals for human well-being. The books in the series will also emphasize the role of dieticians and nutritionists for the prescription of judicious eating habits. The key food components such as carbohydrates, proteins, and lipids as well as micronutrients (vitamins, minerals) are demonstrated to maintain good health, obviating the need for medicines. Thus, nutraceuticals that are indeed derived from food ingredients are believed to be potential alternative therapeutics.

Asymptomatic diseases/disorders necessitate proper diagnosis. Stressed circumstances have been reported to cause weight loss. Workplace stress is a key variable in the genesis and propagation of metabolic disorders. The nuances of the underlying mechanisms are still to be deciphered. Poor lifestyle trends have been attributed along with the consumption of junk foods in several such instances. Sugar-rich carbonated beverages, the use of contraband drugs, and the consumption of liquor in excess are assigned as risk factors. This book series will cover advances and applications in addition to providing the basics of nutraceuticals.

The books in this series will be valuable resources for industry professionals to design and develop quality products for end users. In addition, the book series will be fortified by ideas of innovation, concept building, manufacturing aspects, quality control, and regulatory status of nutraceuticals.

Ostensibly, business has seen a rise in the nutraceutical consumption in recent years. Pure, safe, efficacious products are the need of the hour globally. There are a number of books on nutraceuticals in the market, yet these are only a few books presenting certain aspects of nutraceuticals therein. This book series aims to offer a holistic view of this promising strategy, which is picking up pace with time. This book series will be a unique endeavor to bring manufacturing, research and development, and marketing strategies under a single umbrella.

CURRENT BOOKS IN THE SERIES

- **Micronutrients and Macronutrients as Nutraceuticals**
  Editors: Prakash Chandra Gupta, PhD, Sayan Bhattacharyya, MBBS, MD, Nisha Sharma, PhD, MPharm, Rajesh K. Kesharwani, PhD, and Raj K. Keservani, PhD, MPharm

- **Formulations, Regulations, and Challenges of Nutraceuticals**
  Editors: Tingirikari Jagan Mohan Rao, PhD, Rajesh K. Kesharwani, PhD, Raj. K. Keservani, PhD, and Anil K. Sharma, PhD

- **Food Supplements and Dietary Fibers in Health and Disease**
  Editors: Bhushan R. Rane, PhD, MPharm, Raj K. Keservani, PhD, MPharm, Durgesh Singh, DPhil, Nayan A. Gujarathi, PhD, and Ashish S. Jain, PhD
- **Nutraceuticals in Cancer Prevention, Management, and Treatment**
  Editors: Raj K. Keservani, PhD, MPharm Bui Thanh Tung, PhD, Sippy Singh, DPhil, and Rajesh K. Kesharwani, PhD
- **Advances in Flavonoids for Human Health and Prevention of Diseases**
  Editors: Nisha Sharma, PhD, Deepika Saini, PhD, Rajesh K. Kesharwani, PhD, Prakash Chandra Gupta, and Raj. K. Keservani, PhD
- **The Flavonoids: Extraction and Applications**
  Editors: Deepika Saini, PhD, Rajesh K. Kesharwani, PhD, and Raj K. Keservani, PhD, MPharm
- **Immune-Boosting Nutraceuticals for Better Human Health: Novel Applications**
  Editors: Urmila Jarouliya, PhD, Raj K. Keservani, PhD, MPharm Rajesh K. Kesharwani, PhD, Virendra K. Patel, PhD, and Adi D. Bharti
- **Applications of Functional Foods in Disease Prevention**
  Editors: Raj K. Keservani, PhD, MPharm, and Eknath D. Ahire, MSPharm
- **Plant Metabolites and Vegetables as Nutraceuticals**
  Editors: Raj K. Keservani, PhD, MPharm, Bui Thanh Tung, PhD, Rajesh K. Kesharwani, PhD, MPharm, and Eknath D. Ahire
- **Preventive and Therapeutic Role of Vitamins as Nutraceuticals**
  Editors: Khemchand R. Surana, Eknath D. Ahire, Raj K. Keservani, PhD, MPharm, and Rajesh K. Kesharwani, PhD
- **Nutraceuticals and Bone Health**
  Editors: Deepak Sharma, PhD, Madan Mohan Gupta, PhD, Anil K. Sharma, PhD, MPharm, Raj K. Keservani, PhD, MPharm, and Rajesh K. Kesharwani, PhD
- **Flavonoids as Nutraceuticals**
  Editors: Rajesh K. Kesharwani, PhD, MTech, Deepika Saini, PhD, Raj K. Keservani, PhD, MPharm, and Anil Kumar Sharma, PhD
- **Herbals as Nutraceuticals: Their Role in Healthcare**
  Editors: Raj K. Keservani, PhD, MPharm, Rajeshwar Kamal Kant Arya, PhD, and Rajesh K. Kesharwani, PhD

- **Nutraceutical Fruits: Overview and Disease Prevention**
  Editors: Raj K. Keservani, PhD, MPharm
- **Nutrigenomics and Nutraceuticals**
  Editors: Raj K. Keservani, PhD, MPharm, Eknath D. Ahire, Shubham J. Khainar, PhD, Sanjay J. Kshirsagar, PhD, and Rajesh K. Kesharwani, PhD
- **Nutraceuticals in Cardiac Health Management**
  Editors: Raj K. Keservani, PhD, MPharm, Rajesh K. Kesharwani, PhD, Praveen Kumar Jain, PhD, Bhushan R. Rane, PhD, and Nayan A. Gujarathi, PhD
- **Nutraceuticals for the Treatment and Prevention of Sexual Disorders**
  Editors: Raj K. Keservani, PhD, MPharm, Sharangouda J. Patil, PhD, and Ivan Aranha, PhD
- **Nutraceuticals in Obesity Management and Control**
  Editors: Raj K. Keservani, PhD, MPharm, and Alka Lohani, PhD
- **Antioxidants as Nutraceuticals**
  Editors: Nayan A. Gujarathi, PhD, Raj K. Keservani, PhD, MPharm, Rajesh K. Kesharwani, PhD, Bhushan R. Rane, PhD, and Yogeeta Sameer Goyal, PhD
- **The Nature of Nutraceuticals: History, Properties, Sources, and Nanotechnology**
  Editors: Rajesh K. Kesharwani, PhD, Prashant Kumar, PhD, and Raj K. Keservani, PhD, MPharm
- **Nutraceuticals in Insomnia and Sleep Problems**
  Editors: Raj K. Keservani, PhD, MPharm, Sayan Bhattacharyya, PhD, and Rajesh K. Kesharwani, PhD
- **Nutraceuticals in Respiratory and Pulmonary Diseases**
  Editors: Deepika Saini, PhD, Rajesh K. Kesharwani, PhD, and Raj K. Keservani, PhD, MPharm
- **Nutraceuticals in Arthritis and Psoriasis**
  Editors: Meenakshi Jaiswal, PhD, Raj K. Keservani, PhD, MPharm Rajesh K. Kesharwani, PhD, and Swati G. Talele, PhD

About the Editors

Khemchand R. Surana, MSPharm
Assistant Professor, Department of Pharmaceutical Chemistry, Shreeshakti Shaikshanik Sanstha Divine College of Pharmacy, Satana, Nashik, Maharashtra, India

Khemchand R. Surana, MSPharm, is presently working as Assistant Professor in the Department of Pharmaceutical Chemistry at Shreeshakti Shaikshanik Sanstha Divine College of Pharmacy, Satana, Nashik, India. He earned his master's degree (MSPharm) in medicinal chemistry at the National Institute of Pharmaceutical Education and Research, Ahmadabad (NIPER-A), India. He has attended several national and international conferences and workshops. He has published more than 35 publications, which include reviews, research articles, and book chapters in national and international publications. He has also published nine books on pharmacy. His research work involved synthesis of novel anti-inflammatory agent via C-H activation mechanism and coumarin-based anti-inflammatory agents as well as benzophenone scaffold. His areas of interest include computer-aided drug design and synthesis, biological activity, evaluation, and nutraceuticals.

Eknath D. Ahire, MSPharm
Assistant Professor, Department of Pharmaceutics, MET's, Institute of Pharmacy, Bhujbal Knowledge City, Adgaon, Nashik, Maharashtra, India

Eknath D. Ahire, MSPharrm, is currently working as an Assistant Professor in the Department of Pharmaceutics at MET's, Institute of Pharmacy, Bhujbal Knowledge City, Adgaon, Nashik, affiliated to Savitribai Phule Pune University, Pune. He has obtained his graduation (BPharm) degree from Savitribai Phule Pune University. He obtained his master's degree (MSPharm) in pharmaceutics from the National Institute of Pharmaceutical Education and Research-Ahmedabad (NIPER-A). Currently, he is enrolled as a PhD Scholar with Savitribai Phule, Pune University, (MH), and India. He has been awarded NFST (RGNF) PhD Research Scholar fellowship by the Government of India. He is working for QCS Labs LLP, Mumbai, as

Inspector for Nigeria's regulatory market pre-shipment inspection under Earn and Learn scheme. He has a total of five years of experience, working as Formulation Scientist II at Torrent Research Centre – Gandhinagar, Gujrat, as well as four years of academic experience. He is working as Reviewer for several reputed international journals like, *Pharmaceutical Development and Technology* (Taylor and Francis), *International Journal of Applied Nanotechnology Research (IJANR)* (IGI Global), and *Exploration of Immunology Journal.* He is an Editorial Board Member at *Acta Scientific and Community Acquired Infection*, an open access journal. He is a life member of the Association of Pharmaceutical Teachers of India (APTI). He has more than 30 publications (Research, Review, and Book chapters) published in different national and international well-reputed and indexed journals with six textbooks. He has participated in and attended several national and international conferences and workshops. He has worked on nanotechnology-based novel drug delivery systems, nutraceuticals, and immunology.

Raj K. Keservani, PhD, MPharm
Associate Professor, Faculty of B. Pharmacy, CSM Group of Institutions, Prayagraj, Uttar Pradesh, India

Raj K. Keservani, PhD, MPharm, is working as Associate Professor in the Faculty of B. Pharmacy at the CSM Group of Institutions, Prayagraj, India. He has more than 12 years of academic (teaching) experience from various institutes of India in pharmaceutical education. He has supervised more than 25 undergraduate students for their research work. He has published over 30 peer-reviewed papers in the field of pharmaceutical sciences in national and international journals, six patents, over 70 book chapters, three co-authored books, and over 40 edited books. He is also active as a reviewer for several international scientific journals. His research interests include nutraceutical and functional foods, novel drug delivery systems (NDDS), transdermal drug delivery/drug delivery, health science, cancer biology, and neurobiology. Dr. Keservani graduated with a pharmacy degree from the Department of Pharmacy, Kumaun University, Nainital, Uttarakhand, India. He received his Master of Pharmacy (MPharm) (specialization in pharmaceutics) from the School of Pharmaceutical Sciences, Rajiv Gandhi Proudyogiki Vishwavidyalaya, Bhopal, India. He earned his PhD degree from IKG Punjab Technical University, Jalandhar, Punjab, India. Dr. Keservani is a life member of the Society of Pharmaceutical Education and Research (SPER).

Rajesh K. Kesharwani, PhD

Associate Professor, Department of Computer Application, Nehru Gram Bharati (Deemed to be University), Prayagraj, Uttar Pradesh, India

Rajesh K. Kesharwani, PhD, MTech, is working as Associate Professor, Department of Computer Application, Nehru Gram Bharati (Deemed to be University), Prayagraj, India. He has more than 11 years of research and nine years of teaching experience at various institutes of India, imparting bioinformatics and biotechnology education. He has received several awards, including the NASI-Swarna Jayanti Puruskar by The National Academy of Sciences of India. He has supervised one PhD and more than 20 undergraduate and graduate students for their research work. Dr. Kesharwani has authored over 49 peer-reviewed articles, 20 book chapters, and 14 edited books with international publishers. He has been a member of many scientific communities as well as a reviewer for many international journals. He has presented many papers at various national and international conferences. Dr. Kesharwani received his PhD from the Indian Institute of Information Technology, Allahabad, and worked at NIT Warangal for two semesters. He has been a recipient of a Ministry of Human Resource Development (India) Fellowship and a Senior Research Fellowship from the Indian Council of Medical Research, India. His research fields of interest are medical informatics, protein structure and function prediction, computer-aided drug designing, structural biology, drug delivery, cancer biology, nanobiotechnology, and biomedical sciences.

Contents

Contributors

Pankaj R. Aher
Department of Pharmaceutical Chemistry, Loknete Dr. J. D. Pawar College of Pharmacy, Manur, Kalwan, Nashik, Maharashtra, India

Sayali P. Aher
Department of Pharmacology, R.C. Patel Institute of Pharmaceutical Education and Research, Shirpur, Maharashtra, India

Eknath D. Ahire
Department of Pharmaceutics, MET's Institute of Pharmacy, Bhujbal Knowledge City, Adgaon, Nashik, Maharashtra, India

Supriya R. Bhamare
Department of Pharmaceutical Chemistry, Sir Dr. M.S. Gosavi College of Pharmaceutical Education and Research, Nashik, Maharashtra, India

Chandrakant G. Bonde
School of Pharmacy and Technology Management, Mukesh Patel Technology Park, Babulde, Shirpur, Dhule, Maharashtra, India

Ganesh U. Chaturbhuj
Department of Pharmaceutical Sciences and Technology, Institute of Chemical Technology (ICT), Mumbai, Maharashtra, India

Ramesh A. Herole
Department of Pharmaceutical Chemistry, K. K. Wagh Institute of Pharmacy, Chandori, Niphad, Nashik, Maharashtra, India

Shivraj P. Jadhav
Department of Pharmaceutics, Shreeshakti Shaikshanik Sanstha, Divine College of Pharmacy, Satana, Nashik, Maharashtra, India

Pankaj G. Jain
Department of Pharmacology, R.C. Patel Institute of Pharmaceutical Education and Research, Shirpur, Maharashtra, India

Vandana N. Jain
Department of Pharmacognosy, Oriental Education Society College of Pharmacy, Navi Mumbai, Maharashtra, India

Raj K. Keservani
Faculty of B. Pharmacy, CSM Group of Institutions, Prayagraj, Uttar Pradesh, India

Aditi M. Kokande
Department of Pharmaceutical Chemistry, Oriental Education Society College of Pharmacy, Navi Mumbai, Maharashtra, India

Snehal S. Kolpe
Department of Pharmaceutical Chemistry, M.G.V's Samajshri Prashant Dada Hiray, College of Pharmacy, Malegaon, Nashik, Maharashtra, India

Sanjay J. Kshirsagar
Department of Pharmaceutics, MET's Institute of Pharmacy, Bhujbal Knowledge City, Adgaon, Nashik, Maharashtra, India

Tushar N. Lokhande
Department of Pharmaceutical Chemistry, Maharashtra Educational Society's H. K. College of Pharmacy, Oshiwara, Jogeshwari (W), Maharashtra, India

Sunil K. Mahajan
Department of Pharmaceutical Chemistry, M.G.V's Samajshri Prashant Dada Hiray, College of Pharmacy, Malegaon, Nashik, Maharashtra, India

Vaishali N. Pardeshi
Department of Pharmaceutical Chemistry, Mahatma Gandhi Vidyamandir's Pharmacy College, Panchavati, Nashik, Maharashtra, India

Abhijeet G. Parkhe
Research Associate, In Vivo Pharmacology Department, Glenmark Pharmaceutical Ltd., Navi Mumbai, Maharashtra, India

Afsar S. Pathan
Department of Pharmacology, R.C. Patel Institute of Pharmaceutical Education and Research, Shirpur, Maharashtra, India

Dhananjay M. Patil
Department of Pharmaceutics, Shreeshakti Shaikshanik Sanstha, Divine College of Pharmacy, Satana, Nashik, Maharashtra, India

Manoj S. Patil
Department of Pharmacology, R.C. Patel Institute of Pharmaceutical Education and Research, Shirpur, Maharashtra, India

Snehal D. Pawar
Department of Pharmaceutical Chemistry, M.G.V's Samajshri Prashant Dada Hiray, College of Pharmacy, Malegaon, Nashik, Maharashtra, India

Ashwini V. Shelke
Department of Pharmaceutical Chemistry, Mahatma Gandhi Vidyamandir's Pharmacy College, Panchavati, Nashik, Maharashtra, India

Subhash S. Shinde
Department of Pharmaceutical Chemistry, Mahatma Gandhi Vidyamandir's Pharmacy College, Panchavati, Nashik, Maharashtra, India

Deepak D. Sonawane
Department of Pharmaceutics, Shreeshakti Shaikshanik Sanstha, Divine College of Pharmacy, Satana, Nashik, Maharashtra, India

Vijayraj N. Sonawane
Department of Pharmaceutical Chemistry, Shreeshakti Shaikshanik Sanstha, Divine College of Pharmacy, Satana, Nashik, Maharashtra, India

Khemchand R. Surana
Department of Pharmaceutical Chemistry, Shreeshakti Shaikshanik Sanstha, Divine College of Pharmacy, Satana, Nashik, Maharashtra, India

Santosh R. Tambe
Department of Pharmaceutical Chemistry, M.G.V's Samajshri Prashant Dada Hiray, College of Pharmacy, Malegaon, Nashik, Maharashtra, India

Yogita B. Thombare
Department of Pharmaceutical Chemistry, Mahatma Gandhi Vidyamandir's Pharmacy College, Panchavati, Nashik, Maharashtra, India

Komal S. Valve
Department of Pharmaceutical Chemistry, Mahatma Gandhi Vidyamandir's Pharmacy College, Panchavati, Nashik, Maharashtra, India

Kshitij S. Varma
Department of Pharmaceutical Chemistry, Mahatma Gandhi Vidyamandir's Pharmacy College, Panchavati, Nashik, Maharashtra, India

Abbreviations

5-LOX	5-lipoxygenase
7-DHC	7-dehydrocholesterol
AA	ascorbic acid
AD	Alzheimer disease
ALS	amyotrophic lateral sclerosis
API	active pharmaceutical ingredient
ARDS	acute respiration distress syndrome
ART	antiretroviral treatment
ATBC	alpha-tocopherol, beta-carotene
ATR	all-trans-retinol
ATT	antituberculosis therapy
AU	alopecia universalis
CAGR	compound annual growth rate
CARET	carotene and retinol efficacy trial
COVID-19	coronavirus disease 2019
COX	cyclo-oxygenase
CRP	C-reactive protein
DMB	dimethyl benzimidazole
DNA	deoxyribonucleic acid
EFSA	European Food Safety Authority
FAD	flavin adenine dinucleotide
FDA	Food and Drug Administration
FIM	foundation for innovation in medicine
FMN	flavin mononucleotide
FT3	free triiodothyronine
FT4	free thyroxine
HCC	hepatocellular carcinoma
HD	Huntington disease
HIV	human immunodeficiency virus
HPV	human papilloma virus
ICU	intensive care unit
IL-6	interleukin-6
IL-8	interleukin-8
LTBI	latent tuberculosis infection
MAIT	mucosal invariant T cells
MCM	methylmalonyl-CoA mutase
MDA	malondialdehyde

MERS	middle east respiratory syndrome
MetH	methionine synthase
MRSA	methicillin-resistant Staphylococcus aureus
MS	multiple sclerosis
MTB	mycobacteria
MVM	multivitamin/mineral
NAD	nicotinamide adenine dinucleotide
NADP	nicotinamide adenine dinucleotide phosphate
NAFLD	non-alcoholic fatty liver disease
NO	nitric oxide
NSAIDs	nonsteroidal anti-inflammatory drugs
OSAS	obstructive sleep apnea syndrome
OTC	over-the-counter
PD	Parkinson's disease
PL	pyridoxal
PLP	pyridoxal phosphate
PM	pyridoxamine
PMP	pyridoxamine phosphate
PN	pyridoxine
PNP	pyridoxine phosphate
PNPO	pyridoxamine phosphate oxidase
PPAR	proliferator-activated receptor
PR	pathogenesis-related
PUD	peptic ulcer disease
RAEs	retinol activity equivalents
RBC	red blood cells
RBP	retinol-binding protein
RDA	recommended daily amount
RNA	ribonucleic acid
ROS	reactive oxygen species
SAM	S-adenosyl methionine
SARS	serious respiratory syndrome
TB	tuberculosis
TNF	tumor necrosis factor
UV	ultraviolet
UVB	ultraviolet B
UVR	UVB radiation
VB5	vitamin B5
VDRs	vitamin D receptors
VEGF	vascular endothelial growth factor

Preface

Nutraceuticals are components of food that have health benefits in addition to their food value. These can be in the form of nutritional supplements or other added elements that are meant to improve health. They include foods fortified with vitamins, minerals, probiotics, and fiber, like juices and cereals as well as nutrient-dense components such as fruits and vegetables. Nutraceuticals, are known by many names such as, medical foods, designer foods, phytochemicals, functional foods, and nutritional supplements and include commonplace items like “bio” yogurts and fortified breakfast cereals, as well as vitamins, herbal cures, and genetically modified meals and supplements. In this book, we have attempted to synthesize the role of numerous vitamins in various human diseases and disorders.

Vitamins, supplements and otherwise, can be used to help you get more of the nutrients you need.

This book will have a significant impact on filling any gaps in your food routine and improving overall health. We are confident that this book will provide readers with the most up-to-date information on vitamins.

This book, Preventive and Therapeutic Role of Vitamins as Nutraceuticals, is divided into 15 chapters with four sections, each of which describes recent breakthroughs in vitamins and their ability to prevent diseases.

- **Part I: Role of Vitamins in Chronic Diseases**

  Chapter 1, Vitamins as Nutraceuticals in Cancer, written by Tushar N. Lokhande and his associates, emphasizes the impact of different vitamins on cancer patients and their potential role as nutraceuticals in treating cancer through their antitumor and antioxidant activity.

  Vaishali N. Pardeshi et al. offer a quick summary of the known benefits of Vitamin-B complex, Vitamin C, Vitamin D, Vitamin E, and Vitamin K in the context of TB treatment and control, in Chapter 2, Vitamins as Nutraceuticals for Tuberculosis. Chapter 3, Vitamins as Nutraceuticals for HIV and AIDS, written by Khemchand R. Surana and his colleagues, looks at how these vitamins improve the immunity of patients (HIV and AIDS) and related facts and figures from literature.

Chapter 4, Vitamins as Nutraceuticals for Peptic Ulcer, written by Pankaj G. Jain and associates, focuses on all vitamins effective in the treatment of peptic ulcer.

- **Part II: Vitamins in the Management of Infectious Diseases**

Chapter 5 briefly explains vitamins as nutraceuticals for viral infection, as reflected by the title, Vitamins as Nutraceuticals for Viral Infection, written by Snehal D. Pawar and her coworker.

Chapter 6, Vitamins as Nutraceuticals for Microbial Infections, written by Ashwini V. Shelke et al., reports on how vitamins could be useful in treating some microbial diseases, and how they can be administered as nutraceuticals.

Khemchand R. Surana and his associates thoroughly elaborate on the proof surrounding vitamins, including the prophylaxis dietary supplements and COVID-19 treatment in Chapter 7, Vitamins as Nutraceuticals for COVID-19.

- **Part III: Functional Activity of Vitamins in Brain Health and Obesity Management**

The essential function of vitamins in the management, prevention, or delay of hypertension and its related problems, as well as its ability to regulate blood pressure, has received substantial support from clinical trials reported by Kshitij S. Varma et al. in Chapter 8, Vitamins as Nutraceuticals for Hypertension.

Abhijeet G. Parkhe et al. wrote Chapter 9, Vitamins as Nutraceuticals for Neurodegenerative Disease, and covers each major vitamin with food sources that play a role in neurodegenerative diseases and, in some cases, how it adversely affects human health.

Pankaj R. Aher and his coworker briefly discuss the role of vitamins in weight loss and obesity in Chapter 10, Vitamins as Nutraceuticals for Weight Loss and Obesity.

- **Part IV: Nutritional Function of Vitamins**

Vitamins B1, B2, and B12 play an important role in normal vision. All these vitamins can be obtained from different nutraceuticals, as discussed by Shivraj P. Jadhav et al. in Chapter 11, Vitamins as a Nutraceutical for

Blindness. Low vitamin levels have been linked to androgenic alopecia and alopecia areata (patchy hair loss), in addition to its treatment by vitamins discussed by Kshitij S. Varma et al. in Chapter 12, Vitamins as Nutraceuticals for Baldness.

Chapter 13, Vitamins as Nutraceuticals for Skin Care, written by Khemchand R. Surana and his associates, discusses some nutraceutical products present in the market which are prepared in combination with vitamins.

Chapter 14, Overview and Recent Advances of Vitamins, written by Khemchand R. Surana et al. briefly discusses about vitamins and recent advances in the study of vitamins.

Vitamins are important meal ingredients that offer dietary blessings in addition to medicinal effects. This is due to the presence of energetic compounds, including carotenoids, collagen hydrolysate, and nutritional fibers as discussed in Chapter 15, Vitamins as Nutraceuticals for Human Nutrition, written by Vijayraj N. Sonawane and his colleagues.

PART I

Role of Vitamins in Chronic Diseases

CHAPTER 1

Vitamins as Nutraceuticals in Cancer

TUSHAR N. LOKHANDE,[1] KOMAL S. VALVE,[2] SUBHASH S. SHINDE,[2] KHEMCHAND R. SURANA,[3] and GANESH U. CHATURBHUJ[4]

[1]*Department of Pharmaceutical Chemistry, Maharashtra Educational Society's H. K. College of Pharmacy, Oshiwara, Jogeshwari (W), Maharashtra, India*

[2]*Department of Pharmaceutical Chemistry, Mahatma Gandhi Vidyamandir's Pharmacy College, Panchavati, Nashik, Maharashtra, India*

[3]*Department of Pharmaceutical Chemistry, Shreeshakti Shaikshanik Sanstha, Divine College of Pharmacy, Satana, Nashik, Maharashtra, India*

[4]*Department of Pharmaceutical Sciences and Technology, Institute of Chemical Technology (ICT), Mumbai, Maharashtra, India*

ABSTRACT

Cancer is a disease characterized by the development of abnormal cells that divide uncontrollably and have the ability to infiltrate and destroy normal body tissue. Cancer has a high proclivity for spreading throughout the body. Cancer is the world's second biggest cause of death, but advances in cancer screening, therapy, and prevention are increasing survival rates for many types of cancer. There are four main types of cancer: Carcinomas, Sarcomas, Leukemia, and Lymphomas. Vitamins are the compounds that the body requires for appropriate growth and development. Several clinical trials have been carried out in recent years to establish the role of vitamins in the treatment or prevention of cancer. Because of their contentious role in cancer, taking vitamins for treatment or the prevalence of cancer is still prescribed. Vitamins have been shown in epidemiological research to have anticancer

Preventive and Therapeutic Role of Vitamins as Nutraceuticals. Khemchand R. Surana, Eknath D. Ahire, Raj K. Keservani, & Rajesh K. Kesharwani (Eds.)

properties. Furthermore, a growing body of experimental evidence clearly supports their anticancer activity *in-vitro* and *in-vivo*, even if the actuation mechanism is not totally understood. Understanding the role of vitamins in cancer would be beneficial to prevent or treat cancer. We emphasized the impact of different vitamins on cancer patients and their potential role as nutraceuticals in treating cancer through their antitumor and antioxidant activity.

1.1 INTRODUCTION

Cancer is a major health problem whose mortality levels are increasing day by day every year. Scientists tried to develop a variety of cancer-preventative and treatment options. Anti-tumoral therapies like surgery. The most common treatments include chemotherapy, and radiation. But still, it is necessary to develop new innovative approaches in the effective treatment and prevention of cancer. Vitamins are used as chemoprotective agents along with anticancer drugs (Smith-Warner et al., 2000). Vitamins are the natural organic compounds which are essential part of regular diet for various biochemical and physiological processes occurs in the body. There are two sorts of vitamins – fat soluble (A, D, E, and K) and water-soluble (C and B complex). Vitamins are required in small quantities, to full-fill the requirement of vitamins, people can consume food enrich with vitamin or in the form of functional foods (Keservani et al., 2010a, b, 2017, 2020) as nutraceuticals while some vitamins are extracted from natural sources. Health benefits of vitamins are, as immune booster, decrease blood pressure, cardiovascular disease prevention, and cancer risk reduction (Kazanci et al., 2001; Surana, 2021a–c). Classification of vitamins (Figure 1.1), with them at a glance information is given in Figure 1.1 and Table 1.1.

1.1.1 VITAMIN A

Vitamin A is a fat-soluble vitamin. Pro-vitamin A and produced vitamin A are both found in the food. Preformed vitamin A examples are retinol and retinyl ester. Provitamin A is carotenoid pigments (Dong et al., 2009). Vitamin A has active forms retinoic acid and retinal. Vitamin A metabolized intracellularly into retinal and retinoic acid. Preformed vitamin A is obtained from animal sources while plant sources provide pro-vitamin A. The liver is a storehouse for vitamin A. It is stored in the form of retinyl esters. Vitamin A sources are

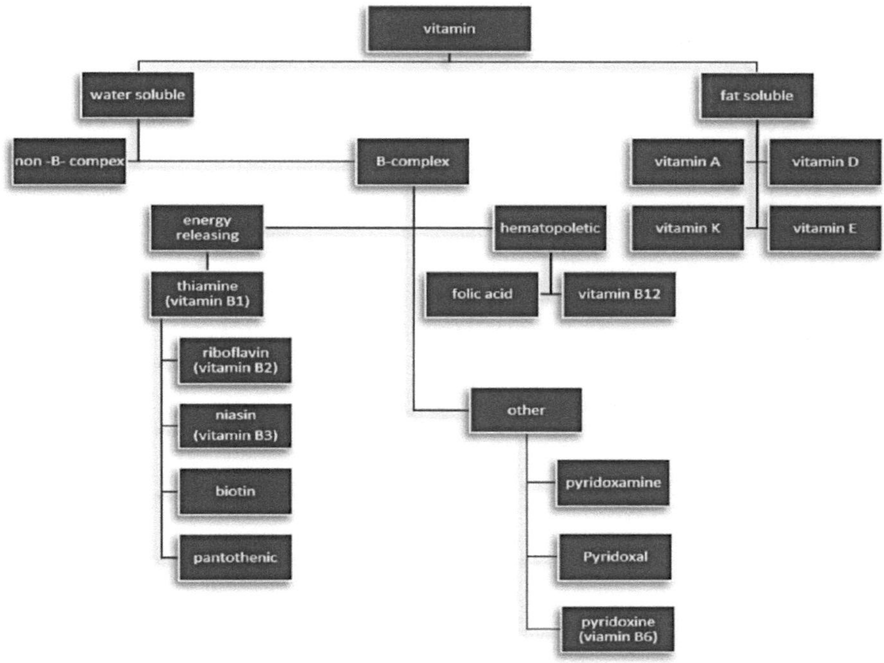

FIGURE 1.1 Classification of vitamins.

Cod liver oil, Beef liver, Carrot, Sweet potato, Black-eyed peas, Spinach, Broccoli, and Sweet red pepper (Basu et al., 2007).

1.1.1.1 VITAMIN A ROLE IN CANCER PREVENTION

Vitamin A is involved in cell growth and differentiation modulation. Retinoid and antioxidants prevent or delay the occurrence of cancer in the upper or lower airways. Retinoid are used to reverse the progression of cancer cells. β-Carotene is one of the few carotenoids with pro-vitamin A activity, and it is the carotenoid that converts to retinol, the quickest in the human body (Gu et al., 2008). Carotene's purported cancer-preventive qualities could be represented by a variety of ways. A hypothesis has been established that -carotene may be beneficial at the tissue level via local conversion to retinol (Kanai et al., 2010).

TABLE 1.1 Vitamins at Glance

Chemical Name	Source	Basic Ring	Biological Role	Deficiency Causes	Toxicity	References
Vitamin A	Carrot, mangoes, papaya	β-ionone ring	Cell development and differentiation are regulated by Vitamin A.	Night blindness	Headache, nausea	Strzałka et al. (2003)
Vitamin D	Synthesize from 7-dehydrocholesterol	Steroid	Bone mineralization is improved.	Osteomalacia	Vitamin D aids bone calcification.	Thorne & Campbell (2008)
Vitamin C	Citrus fruits	Mono-saccharides	Bone formation	Scurvy	Kidney stones, gout	Moreno et al. (2005)
Vitamin B1	Food grains	Pyrimidine ring and a thiazole ring held via way of means of a methylene bridge.	In the HMP shunt mechanism, transketolase is TPP dependent. Pyruvate dehydrogenase is an enzyme that catalyzes the irreversible conversion of pyruvate into acetyl coenzyme A (oxidative carboxylation). TPP plays a crucial part in nerve transmission. Coenzymes play a role in glucose and branched-chain amino acid metabolism.	Beri-Beri, polyneuritis, and Wernicke-Korsakoff syndrome.	–	Holt et al. (2002)
Vitamin B2	Liver, dried yeast.	Isoalloxazine ring attached to D-ribitol by a nitrogen atom.	FAD and FMN are coenzymes that are connected to enzymes involved in carbohydrate, lipid, protein, and purine metabolism, as well as the electron transport chain.	Glossitis, cheilosis	–	Deeb et al. (2007)

TABLE 1.1 *(Continued)*

Chemical Name	Source	Basic Ring	Biological Role	Deficiency Causes	Toxicity	References
Vitamin B9	Yeast, eggs, green vegetables.	Components pteridine ring	The folic acid coenzyme THF is engaged in the one-carbon metabolism.	Hemolytic anemias	–	Brigelius-Flohé & Traber (1999)
Vitamin B12	Milk, eggs	The corrin ring has four pyrrole units, just like a porphyrin.	Methymalonyl CoA is isomerized to succinyl CoA. Methionine is made from homocysteine.	Pernicious anemia	–	Weber et al. (2002)
Vitamin K	Bacteria in the GIT naturally make vitamin K.	Naphthoquinone	Methymalonyl CoA is isomerized to succinyl CoA. Methionine is made from homocysteine.	The time it takes for blood to clot is lengthened.	In large doses of vitamin K, red blood cell break-down and liver damage may ensue.	van Poppel & van den Berg (1997)
Vitamin P	Lemons, grapefruits	–	Cataracts can be prevented and treated using this supplement.	Easy bruising	–	Malafa & Neitzel (2000)

1.1.1.2 MECHANISM

Retinoid can prevent carcinogenesis by stimulating gap junction hyperplasia and hypertrophy. Gap Junction is an intercellular membrane structure that connects adjacent epithelial cells. During carcinogenesis, most gap junctions disappear. Gap junctions play central role in regulating tissue organization and growth control (Jiang & Ames, 2003).

1.1.2 VITAMIN D

Vitamin D are the fat soluble prehormones, substances which body can turn into hormone are called prehormones. Vitamin D is categorized into two forms. Vitamin D2 or ergocalciferol and Vitamin D3 or cholecalciferol. Vitamin D2 obtained from plants while vitamin D3 is obtained from sunlight. Both forms of vitamin D are converted to 25-OH vitamin D in the liver, travels into the kidney. Kidney converts them into calcitriol. It is the active form of vitamin D (Jiang et al., 2008.). Much experimental evidence suggested that vitamin D has a possible association with cancer risk. Vitamin D contains a number of properties that may help to prevent or delay the onset of cancer (Moreno et al., 2005). Activities shown by vitamin D are Promoting cell differentiation, Inhibits growth of cancer cell, stimulate cell death, Reduces tumor blood vessel production (Serbinova et al., 1991). Vitamin D has piqued people's interest in cancer prevention, especially when it comes to breast, colorectal, and prostate cancers (Packer et al., 2001). Vitamin D3 has been depicted to decrease the occurrence of human breast Cancer, prostate cancer, and colon cancers and induces apoptosis and cell cycle arrest of various cancer cell types. Vitamin D3 stimulates colon carcinoma cell differentiation through induction of E-cadherin expression and inhibition of β-catenin signaling (Gysin, Azzi, & Visarius, 2002). Vitamin D anticancer properties via immune system regulation are mostly for the prevention of tumor formation rather than the treatment of existing tumors. Every day, millions of normal cells convert into cancer cells in each of us, yet the overwhelming majority of them are discovered early by cytolytic T cells and removed as a result. So, vitamin D stimulation of cytolytic T cells is an effective method for cancer prevention. In conclusion, one of the primary activities of vitamin D is to modulate cells of the immune system, both innate and adaptive, which influences cancer cell differentiation, proliferation, and death through a variety of methods. As a result, vitamin D's anticancer properties are well-known (Sun et al., 2009; Mo & Elson, 1999).

1.1.3 VITAMIN E

Vitamin E has 8 forms:

- α-, β-, γ-, δ-tocopherol;
- α-, β-, γ-, δ-tocotrienol.

These all are antioxidants and lipophilic. α-tocopherol is the most popular form. Because it is the main type of vitamin E. Deficiency of α-tocopherol leads to ataxia, increased risk of atherosclerosis, and possibly immune dysfunction (Srivastava & Gupta, 2006).

1.1.4 α-TOCOPHEROL

Tocotrienols and tocopherols both show antitumor effects, and it seems that tocotrienols has a higher biological activity than tocopherols (Jiang, 2014). Figure 1.2 represents vitamin E rich foods.

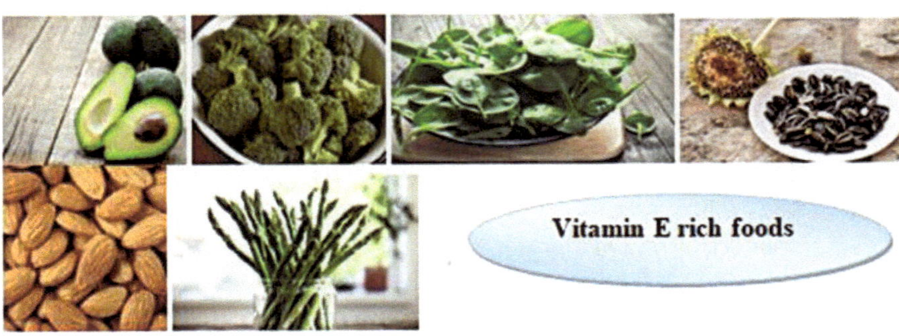

FIGURE 1.2 Vitamin E rich foods.

1.1.4.1 ROLE

Three large intervention studies have found that α-Tocopherol reduces cancer risk. In abnormal populations, supplementation of even low-dose α-Tocopherol and/or its combinations with other nutrients would be enough to defeat the increased risk of cancer (Blaszczak et al., 2019). α-Tocopheryl succinate is a redox-inactive derivative of vitamin E, is a stronger inducer of apoptosis than α-Tocopherol in cell-based studies. α-TOS is a potent antitumor agent. α-TOS and α-Tocopherol inhibits tumor growth by 80 and 35%, respectively. α-TOS shows anti-proliferative activity, it also has pro-apoptotic activity. It has greater ability to prevent cancer as compared to α-Tocopherol (Luk et al., 2011). Most of the studies have reported that α-TOS defeat the growth of tumors induced from breast cancer cells (Naidu, 2003), lung cancer cells (Watson & Preedy, 2008), prostate cancer cells (Akhilender, 2003), squamous cell carcinoma of the head and neck, bladder cancer cells (Du et al., 2010).

1.1.5 γ-TOCOPHEROL

γ-Tocopherol has unique activities that are potentially important for cancer prevention and therapy. γ-Tocopherol exhibit anti-inflammatory effects (unlike α-Tocopherol) by inhibition of cyclooxygenase (COX)-catalyzed formation of prostaglandin E2 (PGE2) in LPS-treated macrophages and IL-1β activated epithelial cells as well as in carrageenan-induced inflammation model in rats. In this model, γ-Tocopherol inhibited 5-lipoxygenase (5-LOX)-catalyzed formation of Leukotriene B_4 and TNFα (Stephenson et al., 2013). Recent studies have found that 13-carboxychromanol, which is a metabolized form of vitamin E and is eliminated through feces, is a much more good inhibitor of COX-1, COX-2, and 5-LOX than the unmetabolized form of vitamin E (Vollbracht et al., 2011; Monti et al., 2012).

1.1.6 ANTITUMOR EFFECT OF VITAMIN E ON CANCER CELLS

1.1.6.1 ANTIOXIDANT ACTIVITY

In-vitro studies show antioxidant activity of vitamin E derivatives in the following manner: α-tocopherol >β-tocopherol >γ-tocopherol>δ-tocopherol.

α-tocopherol acts as an antioxidant in greater potency, while δ-tocopherol, showed the weakest potency, when organic solution is used to measure their potency (Frei, England, & Ames, 1989). Some studies have shown that the tocotrienols had a higher anti-oxidative potency than the tocopherols (Bánhegyi et al., 2014). There are various reasons for higher antioxidant activity of alpha-tocotrienol compared with alpha-tocopherol: (i) membrane bilayers of alpha tocopherol have more uniform distribution; (ii) lipids in membranes are more disorganized; (iii) collisions with radicals are more effective; and (iv) a higher chromanoxyl radical recycling activity and a recycling activity that coincides with lipid peroxidation inhibition (Chen et al., 2005; Singh et al., 2017).

1.1.6.2 INHIBITION OF CELL CYCLES

In the human prostate cancer cell line DU-145, γ-tocopherol was found to suppress cell cycle progression by lowering cyclin D1 and cyclin E levels (Chen et al., 2007). In human gastric adenocarcinoma cells and murine melanoma cells, γ-tocotrienol treatment caused a G1 phase arrest (Hotta et al., 2007). TRF also caused a G0/G1 phase arrest and sub-G1 accumulation in three different cell lines of human prostate cancer cells (Kakizaki et al., 2007; Surana et al., 2018).

1.1.6.3 NOVEL ANTICANCER EFFECTS

It has been demonstrated that prostate cancer stem cells are eliminated, with tocotrienol down-regulating the expression of prostate cancer stem cell markers (CD133 and CD44) in androgen-independent prostate cancer cell lines. Since it is well-known that cancer stem cells contribute to chemoresistance, the combined use of an anticancer drug and γ-tocotrienol might be potent enough to achieve complete remission (Yoshida et al., 2011). It was recently revealed that the high activity of telomerase is essential for immortalization and tumorigenesis. Despite numerous cell divisions, cancer cells frequently prevent cell death by preserving their telomeres. This is possible because cancer cells activate the telomerase enzyme, which adds genetic units to telomeres to prevent them from shortening to the point of cell death. This is called telomerase activity. Treatment with 5 μM of δ-tocotrienol and 10 μM of β-tocotrienol for 24 h significantly suppressed the telomerase activity. On the contrary, the tocopherols showed only a very weak telomerase inhibition (Mizuta et al., 2006).

1.1.7 VITAMIN C

Vitamin C is a water-soluble antioxidant. At high concentrations, it acts as a pro-oxidant. As a result, it's linked to cancer avoidance, progression, and treatment. Studies show that cancers of the lungs and the breast can be prevented by vitamin C intake. High-dose of vitamin can be used potential anticancer (Reinke, 2019). Vitamin Co-administered intravenously in cancer patients was considered safe with minimum side effects. Vitamin C is given by intravenous route in high doses in cancer patient improves the quality of life with improved physical and mental health. High dose of the vitamin C inhibits the tumors growth in pancreatic, liver (O'Byrne et al., 2008), prostate (Schellack et al., 2016), ovarian cancer sarcoma and malignant mesothelioma (Frei et al., 1989), but Vitamin C in high doses sometimes shows adverse effects such as fatigue, nausea, vomiting, pain, and appetite loss. Vitamin C works with vitamin E as an antioxidant, and it neutralizes free radicals within the body. An antioxidant minimizes the oxidation process and repairs damaged body cells. Studies conclude that vitamin C may lessen the possibility of certain cancers, heart disease, and cataracts. Consuming vitamin C-rich foods is a good way to increase this vitamin in the body. While many common plant foods are rich with vitamin C, Citrus fruits are the best sources of vitamin C, for example, a kiwi fruit, grapes, and sweet red pepper (Brenner & Stevens, 2012). The effects of vitamin C on cancer progression depends on route of administration and expression and categorization of vitamin C transporters. According to data obtained from preclinical studies, in pancreatic cancer, Vitamin C reduces tumor growth rates and improves survival when administered alone or in conjunction with gemcitabine, according to clinical studies, with reduced primary tumor sizes and improved performance status (Chen, 2005, 2007).

1.1.8 VITAMIN K

Vitamin K is a fat-soluble vitamin very important for protein formation within the body, such as the coagulation factors (II, VIII, IX, X, C protein and S protein), osteocalcin (a bone-forming protein). This vitamin contains the naphthoquinone ring as well as variety of side chain of different compositions, lengths, and saturation. Mainly naturally occurring vitamin k are of two types K_1 (Phylloquinone) and K_2 (Menaquinone) where K_2 is further subdivided into MK-*n* depending upon the amount of units of isoprene. Sources of vitamin k are the protein K_1 is mostly present in leafy vegetables, olive oil, and soyabean oil, whereas K_2 is found in fermented foods like curd, cheese, butter, egg yolks, and fermented soybeans (Bellows et al., 2012).

Vitamin K_2 inhibits cancer cell lines from humans, including hepatoma lines and treat myelodysplastic syndrome. The two clinical trials conducted which show that vitamin K_2 45 mg/day reduces the development of hepatocellular carcinoma (HCC). It can reduce the re-occurrence of the tumor after the treatment of HCC (De Vet, 1989).

1.2 VITAMIN B COMPLEX

The B-complex vitamins are soluble in water and get easily eliminated through renal excretion. B-complex contains thiamine (vitamin B1), Riboflavin (Vitamin B2), niacin (vitamin B3), pantothenic acid, also called vitamin B5,

Pyridoxine (Vitamin B6), biotin (Vitamin B7), Folic acid (Vitamin B9) and cobalamin (Vitamin B12) (Chen et al., 2010). Inositol, Para-amino benzoic acids, and Choline are included by some authors in this group. B-complexes act as cofactors or coenzymes for the metabolism functions occurred in the body. This plays an important role in the formation and normal functioning of RBC (Pálmer et al., 2001).

1.3 THIAMINE (VITAMIN B_1)

It is a water-soluble vitamin. It is quite unstable. It destroys with heat and in alkaline environment. Its active forms are Thiamine pyrophosphate and Thiamine tri-phosphate. It is easily absorbed in the small intestine. It combined with the intestinal mucosal cells and transported through the portal vein into the general circulation. It is primarily discovered in liver, heart, brain, and muscle tissue. It is a coenzyme involved in the metabolism of proteins, carbohydrates, and lipids, as well as the synthesis of ribose deficiency of vitamin B1 causes beri-beri and Wernicke's syndrome (Carlberg & Velleuer, 2021).

Sources of vitamin B1 are cereals, meats, and legumes. The richest sources are brewer's yeast, lean pork, liver beef, dried peas and beans, nuts, and whole wheat and enriched cereals and breads (Jain et al., 2017).

1.3.1 RIBOFLAVIN B_2

It is relatively stable and acts as a coenzyme. Its active forms are Flavin mononucleotide (FMN) or Flavin dinucleotide (FAD). Before it can be absorbed, it is phosphorylated in the digestive tract, and any excess B2 is eliminated in the urine. It acts as the hydrogen carrier and assists in carbohydrate, protein, and fats metabolism, and it also oxidizes most drugs. Drug vitamin deficiency of B2 causes hypermotility of the gastrointestinal tract, Angular stomatitis, and Glossitis (Dowling & Wald, 1960). Sources of B2 are milk, lean meat, cheese, eggs, and leafy green vegetables.

1.3.2 NIACIN B_3

It is a B-complex nutrient and very stable. Its active forms are nicotinamide adenine dinucleotide and NAD-phosphate (NADP). It's a peculiar vitamin and may be made in the body via tryptophan. It is absorbed in the upper section of the small intestine, and it is stored sparingly in the liver, heart, kidney, and brain before being eliminated in the urine. In cellular respiration, glucose metabolism, and fat synthesis, It acts as a catalyst for absorbing and releasing hydrogen. A deficiency of B3 causes Pellagra (Muschitz et al., 2015).

Sources of B3 are yeast, meat legumes, liver, peanuts, whole cereals, and food which are rich in tryptophan, such as animal protein and vegetable protein (Bieri et al., 1983).

1.3.3 PANTOTHENIC ACID B5

Vitamin B5 is involved in the release of energy from the catabolism of proteins, carbohydrates, and lipids. It initiates the Krebs cycle and releases ATP. It is the starting substance for the biosynthesis of cholesterol and other sterols, a component of hemoglobin deficiency that causes fatigue, sleep disturbances, abdominal stress, paresthesia cramming in legs, and impaired coordination (McCourt et al., 2006).

Sources of vitamin B5 are yeasts, animal tissue such as liver and eggs, whole grain cereals and legumes, milk, fruits, broccoli, cauliflower, and potatoes (Rivlin & Pinto, 2001).

1.3.4 PYRIDOXINE B_6

It is a white crystalline compound and water-soluble. It helps in the formation of red blood cells, and it helps in the metabolism of fatty acids and amino acids, and deficiency in nerve tissue function causes weakness, nervousness, and insomnia (Jain et al., 2017).

Sources of B6 are liver, muscle meat yeast, Legumes whole grain, cereals, wheat germ, and wheat bran (Risch & Risch, 2019).

1.3.4.1 ROLE OF B-COMPLEX IN THE TREATMENT OF CANCER

Water soluble vitamins include vitamins B2, B1, B6, B9, B12, and folate. The majority of studies on their roles in treatment are limited and conflicting, with some showing anticancer efficacy and others showing little activity or co-carcinogenic action. Multiple vitamins (for example, vitamins B1, B2, B6, and B12 in tablets as food supplements for six years) were used in nutrition intervention trials in Linxian (China), But there was no substantial difference in decreasing occurrences of esophageal dysplasia in the patients (Eitsuka et al., 2006). Folic acid, also known as leucovorin, was discovered to reduce the negative effects of 5-FU in individuals with advanced colorectal cancer (Vermeer, 1990; Rudy et al., 1944).

1.4 CONCLUSION

Most of the studies have been done about the role of nutritional ingredients in terms of avoiding cancer. From the various study, it is clear that nutritional recommendation for cancer prevention requires knowledge about the causes of cancer. Vitamins have a crucial part in cancer prevention in a variety of ways. Studies show that many of these can be prevented by dietary components that influence the cellular environment. Epidemiological, preclinical, and Clinical evidence backs up the claim that vitamins like vitamin D and vitamin A have a significant protective effect against cellular change that leads to cancer, whereas vitamins B, C, E, and K show modest anticancer activity. In the early stages of cancer, new potent analogs and combinations of vitamins may be used to accomplish the potential benefits of vitamins in the avoidance and treatment of cancer. The roles of vitamins in cancer in terms of synergistic, antagonistic, and potentiating effects against cancer still need more study.

ACKNOWLEDGMENTS

We thank the Mahatma Gandhi Vidyamandir's Pharmacy College, Panchavati, Nashik, Maharashtra, India, for their constant support and providing all facilities to complete this work. Also, many thanks to all the known and unknowns who helped us right from the writing till the publishing of this chapter.

KEYWORDS

- **antitumor**
- **cancer**
- **cell cycles**
- **novel anticancer effects**
- **nutraceuticals**
- **pantothenic acid**
- **thiamine**
- **vitamins**

REFERENCES

Akhilender, N. K., (2003). Vitamin C in human health and disease is still a mystery? An overview. *Nutrition Journal.*

Bánhegyi, G., Benedetti, A., Margittai, É., Marcolongo, P., Fulceri, R., Németh, C. E., & Szarka, A., (2014). Subcellular compartmentation of ascorbate and its variation in disease states. *Biochimica et Biophysica Acta (BBA)-Molecular Cell Research, 1843*(9), 1909–1916.

Basu, A., Grossie, B., Bennett, M., Mills, N., & Imrhan, V., (2007). Alpha-Tocopheryl succinate (α-TOS) modulates human prostate LNCaP xenograft growth and gene expression in BALB/c nude mice fed two levels of dietary soybean oil. *European Journal of Nutrition, 46*(1), 34–43.

Bellows, L., Moore, R., Anderson, J., & Young, L., (2012). Water-soluble vitamins: B-complex and vitamin C. *Food and Nutrition Series.* Health; no. 9.312.

Bieri, J. G., Corash, L., & Hubbard, V. S., (1983). Medical uses of vitamin E. *New England Journal of Medicine, 308*(18), 1063–1071.

Blaszczak, W., Barczak, W., Masternak, J., Kopczyński, P., Zhitkovich, A., & Rubiś, B., (2019). Vitamin C as a modulator of the response to cancer therapy. *Molecules, 24*(3), 453.

Brenner, G. M., & Stevens, C. W., (2012). *Pharmacology E-Book: With Student Consult Online Access.* Elsevier Health Sciences.

Brigelius-Flohé, R., & Traber, M. G., (1999). Vitamin E: Function and metabolism. *The FASEB Journal, 13*(10), 1145–1155.

Carlberg, C., & Velleuer, E., (2021). Vitamin D and the risk for cancer: A molecular analysis. *Biochemical Pharmacology*, 114735.

Chen, P., Hu, P., Xie, D., Qin, Y., Wang, F., & Wang, H., (2010). Meta-analysis of vitamin D, calcium and the prevention of breast cancer. *Breast Cancer Research and Treatment, 121*(2), 469–477.

Chen, Q., Espey, M. G., Krishna, M. C., Mitchell, J. B., Corpe, C. P., Buettner, G. R., Shacter, E., & Levine, M., (2005). Pharmacologic ascorbic acid concentrations selectively kill cancer cells: Action as a pro-drug to deliver hydrogen peroxide to tissues. *Proceedings of the National Academy of Sciences, 102*(38), 13604–13609.

Chen, Q., Espey, M. G., Sun, A. Y., Lee, J. H., Krishna, M. C., Shacter, E., Choyke, P. L., et al., (2007). Ascorbate in pharmacologic concentrations selectively generates ascorbate radical and hydrogen peroxide in extracellular fluid *in vivo. Proceedings of the National Academy of Sciences, 104*(21), 8749–8754.

De Vet, H. C., (1989). The puzzling role of vitamin A in cancer prevention. *Anticancer Research, 9*(1), 145–151.

Deeb, K. K., Trump, D. L., & Johnson, C. S., (2007). Vitamin D signalling pathways in cancer: Potential for anticancer therapeutics. *Nature Reviews Cancer, 7*(9), 684–700.

Dong, L. F., Freeman, R., Liu, J., Zobalova, R., Marin-Hernandez, A., Stantic, M., Rohlena, J., et al., (2009). Suppression of tumor growth *in vivo* by the mitocan α-tocopheryl succinate requires respiratory complex II. *Clinical Cancer Research, 15*(5), 1593–1600.

Dowling, J. E., & Wald, G., (1960). The biological function of vitamin A acid. *Proceedings of the National Academy of Sciences of the United States of America, 46*(5), 587.

Du, J., Martin, S. M., Levine, M., Wagner, B. A., Buettner, G. R., Wang, S. H., Taghiyev, A. F., et al., (2010). Mechanisms of ascorbate-induced cytotoxicity in pancreatic cancer. *Clinical Cancer Research, 16*(2), 509–520.

Eitsuka, T., Nakagawa, K., & Miyazawa, T., (2006). Down-regulation of telomerase activity in DLD-1 human colorectal adenocarcinoma cells by tocotrienol. *Biochemical and Biophysical Research Communications*, *348*(1), 170–175.

Frei, B., England, L., & Ames, B. N., (1989). Ascorbate is an outstanding antioxidant in human blood plasma. *Proceedings of the National Academy of Sciences*, *86*(16), 6377–6381.

Gu, X., Song, X., Dong, Y., Cai, H., Walters, E., Zhang, R., Pang, X., et al., (2008). Vitamin E succinate induces ceramide-mediated apoptosis in head and neck squamous cell carcinoma *in vitro* and *in vivo*. *Clinical Cancer Research*, *14*(6), 1840–1848.

Gysin, R., Azzi, A., & Visarius, T., (2002). γ-Tocopherol inhibits human cancer cell cycle progression and cell proliferation by down-regulation of cyclins. *The FASEB Journal*, *16*(14), 1952–1954.

Holt, P. R., Arber, N., Halmos, B., Forde, K., Kissileff, H., McGlynn, K. A., Moss, S. F., et al., (2002). Colonic epithelial cell proliferation decreases with increasing levels of serum 25-hydroxy vitamin D. *Cancer Epidemiology and Prevention Biomarkers*, *11*(1), 113–119.

Hotta, N., Ayada, M., Sato, K., Ishikawa, T., Okumura, A., Matsumoto, E., Ohashi, T., & Kakumu, S., (2007). Effect of vitamin K2 on the recurrence in patients with hepatocellular carcinoma. *Hepato-Gastroenterology*, *54*(79), 2073–2077.

Jain, A., Tiwari, A., Verma, A., & Jain, S. K., (2017). Vitamins for cancer prevention and treatment: An insight. *Current Molecular Medicine*, *17*(5), 321–340.

Jiang, Q., & Ames, B. N., (2003). γ-Tocopherol, but not α-tocopherol, decreases proinflammatory eicosanoids and inflammation damage in rats. *The FASEB Journal*, *17*(8), 816–822.

Jiang, Q., (2014). Natural forms of vitamin E: Metabolism, antioxidant, and anti-inflammatory activities and their role in disease prevention and therapy. *Free Radical Biology and Medicine*, *72*, 76–90.

Jiang, Q., Yin, X., Lill, M. A., Danielson, M. L., Freiser, H., & Huang, J., (2008). Long-chain carboxychromanols, metabolites of vitamin E, are potent inhibitors of cyclooxygenases. *Proceedings of the National Academy of Sciences*, *105*(51), 20464–20469.

Kakizaki, S., Sohara, N., Sato, K., Suzuki, H., Yanagisawa, M., Nakajima, H., Takagi, H., et al., (2007). Preventive effects of vitamin K on recurrent disease in patients with hepatocellular carcinoma arising from hepatitis C viral infection. *Journal of Gastroenterology and Hepatology*, *22*(4), 518–522.

Kanai, K., Kikuchi, E., Mikami, S., Suzuki, E., Uchida, Y., Kodaira, K., Miyajima, A., et al., (2010). Vitamin E succinate induced apoptosis and enhanced chemosensitivity to paclitaxel in human bladder cancer cells *in vitro* and *in vivo*. *Cancer Science*, *101*(1), 216–223.

Kazanci, N., Toyran, N., Haris, P. I., & Severcan, F., (2001). Vitamin D 2 at high and low concentrations exert opposing effects on molecular order and dynamics of dipalmitoyl phosphatidylcholine membranes. *Spectroscopy*, *15*(2), 47–55.

Keservani, R. K., Kesharwani, R. K., Sharma, A. K., Vyas, N., & Chadoker, A., (2010b). Nutritional supplements: An overview. *International Journal of Current Pharmaceutical Review and Research*, *1*(1), 59–75.

Keservani, R. K., Kesharwani, R. K., Vyas, N., Jain, S., Raghuvanshi, R., & Sharma, A. K., (2010a). Nutraceutical and functional food as future food: A review. *Der Pharmacia Lettre*, *2*(1), 106–116.

Keservani, R. K., Sharma, A. K., & Kesharwani, R. K., (2017). An overview and therapeutic applications of nutraceutical and functional foods. *Recent Advances in Drug Delivery Technology*, 160–201. ISBN:9781522507543.

Keservani, R. K., Sharma, A. K., & Kesharwani, R. K., (2020). *Nutraceuticals and Dietary Supplements: Applications in Health Improvement and Disease Management*. CRC Press. ISBN: 9781771888738.

Knapp, H., Knothe, G., Kodali, D., List, G. R., Makowski, J. V., McKeon, T., Moreau, R., et al. (2013). *AOCS Mission Statement*.

Luk, S. U., Yap, W. N., Chiu, Y. T., Lee, D. T., Ma, S., Lee, T. K. W., Vasireddy, R. S., et al., (2011). Gamma-tocotrienol as an effective agent in targeting prostate cancer stem cell-like population. *International Journal of Cancer*, *128*(9), 2182–2191.

Malafa, M. P., & Neitzel, L. T., (2000). Vitamin E succinate promotes breast cancer tumor dormancy. *Journal of Surgical Research*, *93*(1), 163–170.

McCourt, J. A., Nixon, P. F., & Duggleby, R. G., (2006). Thiamin nutrition and catalysis-induced instability of thiamin diphosphate. *British Journal of Nutrition*, *96*(4), 636–638.

Mizuta, T., Ozaki, I., Eguchi, Y., Yasutake, T., Kawazoe, S., Fujimoto, K., & Yamamoto, K., (2006). The effect of menatetrenone, a vitamin K2 analog, on disease recurrence and survival in patients with hepatocellular carcinoma after curative treatment: A pilot study. *Cancer*, *106*(4), 867–872.

Mo, H., & Elson, C. E., (1999). Apoptosis and cell-cycle arrest in human and murine tumor cells are initiated by isoprenoids. *The Journal of Nutrition*, *129*(4), 804–813.

Monti, D. A., Mitchell, E., Bazzan, A. J., Littman, S., Zabrecky, G., Yeo, C. J., Pillai, M. V., et al., (2012). Phase I evaluation of intravenous ascorbic acid in combination with gemcitabine and erlotinib in patients with metastatic pancreatic cancer. *PloS One*, *7*(1), e29794.

Moreno, J., Krishnan, A. V., & Feldman, D., (2005). Molecular mechanisms mediating the anti-proliferative effects of vitamin D in prostate cancer. *The Journal of Steroid Biochemistry and Molecular Biology*, *97*(1, 2), 31–36.

Muschitz, C., Kocijan, R., Stütz, V., Kaider, A., Muschitz, G. K., Resch, H., & Kapiotis, S., (2015). Vitamin D levels and comorbidities in ambulatory and hospitalized patients in Austria. *Wiener Klinische Wochenschrift*, *127*(17), 675–684.

Naidu, K. A., (2003). Vitamin C in human health and disease is still a mystery? An overview. *Nutrition Journal*, *2*(1), 1–10.

O'Byrne, P. J., Patry, A., & Carnegie, J. A., (2008). The development of interactive online learning tools for the study of anatomy. *Medical Teacher*, *30*(8), e260–e271.

Packer, L., Weber, S. U., & Rimbach, G., (2001). Molecular aspects of α-tocotrienol antioxidant action and cell signaling. *The Journal of Nutrition*, *131*(2), 369S–373S.

Pálmer, H. G., González-Sancho, J. M., Espada, J., Berciano, M. T., Puig, I., Baulida, J., Quintanilla, M., et al., (2001). Vitamin D3 promotes the differentiation of colon carcinoma cells by the induction of E-cadherin and the inhibition of β-catenin signaling. *The Journal of Cell Biology*, *154*(2), 369–388.

Reinke, N. B., (2019). Promoting student engagement and academic achievement in first-year anatomy and physiology courses. *Advances in Physiology Education*, *43*(4), 443–450.

Risch, C., & Risch, L., (2019). Nutritiver vitamin-B12-mangel. *Pipette*, 18.

Rivlin, R. S., & Pinto, J. T., (2001). Riboflavin (vitamin B2). *Handbook of Vitamins* (pp. 255–273). New York: Marcel Dekker.

Rudy, A., BEASER, S. B., & Seligman, A. M., (1944). Vitamin therapy in increased capillary fragility of diabetes mellitus. *Archives of Internal Medicine*, *73*(1), 23–28.

Schellack, G., Harirari, P., & Schellack, N., (2016). B-complex vitamin deficiency and supplementation. *SA Pharmaceutical JOURNAL*, *83*(4), 14–19.

Serbinova, E., Kagan, V., Han, D., & Packer, L., (1991). Free radical recycling and intramembrane mobility in the antioxidant properties of alpha-tocopherol and alpha-tocotrienol. *Free Radical Biology and Medicine, 10*(5), 263–275.

Singh, P., Kesharwani, R. K., & Keservani, R. K., (2017). Antioxidants and vitamins: Roles in cellular function and metabolism. In: *Sustained Energy for Enhanced Human Functions and Activity* (pp. 385–407). Academic Press. ISBN:9780128054130.

Smith-Warner, S. A., Elmer, P. J., Tharp, T. M., Fosdick, L., Randall, B., Gross, M., Wood, J., & Potter, J. D., (2000). Increasing vegetable and fruit intake: Randomized intervention and monitoring in an at-risk population. *Cancer Epidemiology and Prevention Biomarkers, 9*(3), 307–317.

Srivastava, J. K., & Gupta, S., (2006). Tocotrienol-rich fraction of palm oil induces cell cycle arrest and apoptosis selectively in human prostate cancer cells. *Biochemical and Biophysical Research Communications, 346*(2), 447–453.

Stephenson, C. M., Levin, R. D., Spector, T., & Lis, C. G., (2013). Phase I clinical trial to evaluate the safety, tolerability, and pharmacokinetics of high-dose intravenous ascorbic acid in patients with advanced cancer. *Cancer Chemotherapy and Pharmacology, 72*(1), 139–146.

Strzałka, K., Kostecka-Gugała, A., & Latowski, D., (2003). Carotenoids and environmental stress in plants: Significance of carotenoid-mediated modulation of membrane physical properties. *Russian Journal of Plant Physiology, 50*(2), 168–173.

Sun, W., Xu, W., Liu, H., Liu, J., Wang, Q., Zhou, J., Dong, F., & Chen, B., (2009). γ-Tocotrienol induces mitochondria-mediated apoptosis in human gastric adenocarcinoma SGC-7901 cells. *The Journal of Nutritional Biochemistry, 20*(4), 276–284.

Surana, K. R., Ahire, E. D., Sonawane, V. N., & Talele, S. G., (2021). Biomolecular and molecular docking: A modern tool in drug discovery and virtual screening of natural products. In: *Applied Pharmaceutical Practice and Nutraceuticals* (pp. 209–223). Apple Academic Press.

Surana, K. R., Ahire, E. D., Sonawane, V. N., Talele, S. G., & Talele, G. S., (2021). Molecular modeling: Novel techniques in food and nutrition development. *Natural Food Products and Waste Recovery: Healthy Foods, Nutrition Design, and Extraction of Valuable Compounds*, 17.

Surana, K. R., Ahire, E. D., Sonawane, V. N., Talele, S. G., & Talele, G. S., (2021). Informatics and methods in nutrition design and development. *Natural Food Products and Waste Recovery: Healthy Foods, Nutrition Design, and Extraction of Valuable Compounds*, 33.

Surana, K., Chaudhary, B., Diwaker, M., & Sharma, S., (2018). Benzophenone: A ubiquitous scaffold in medicinal chemistry. *MedChemComm, 9*(11), 1803–1817.

Thorne, J., & Campbell, M. J., (2008). The vitamin D receptor in cancer: Symposium on 'diet and cancer.' *Proceedings of the Nutrition Society, 67*(2), 115–127.

Traber, M. G., & Atkinson, J., (2007). Vitamin E, antioxidant and nothing more. *Free Radical Biology and Medicine, 43*(1), 4–15.

Vermeer, C., (1990). Gamma-carboxyglutamate-containing proteins and the vitamin K-dependent carboxylase. *Biochemical Journal, 266*(3), 625.

Vollbracht, C., Schneider, B., Leendert, V., Weiss, G., Auerbach, L., & Beuth, J., (2011). Intravenous vitamin C administration improves quality of life in breast cancer patients during chemo-/radiotherapy and aftercare: Results of a retrospective, multicenter, epidemiological cohort study in Germany. *In Vivo, 25*(6), 983–990.

Watson, R. R., & Preedy, V. R., (2008). *Tocotrienols: Vitamin E Beyond Tocopherols*. CRC press.

Weber, T., Lu, M., Andera, L., Lahm, H., Gellert, N., Fariss, M. W., Korinek, V., et al., (2002). Vitamin E succinate is a potent novel antineoplastic agent with high selectivity and cooperativity with tumor necrosis factor-related apoptosis-inducing ligand (Apo2 ligand) *in vivo*. *Clinical Cancer Research, 8*(3), 863–869.

Yoshida, H., Shiratori, Y., Kudo, M., Shiina, S., Mizuta, T., Kojiro, M., Yamamoto, K., et al., (2011). Effect of vitamin K2 on the recurrence of hepatocellular carcinoma. *Hepatology, 54*(2), 532–540.

CHAPTER 2

Vitamins as Nutraceuticals for Tuberculosis

VAISHALI N. PARDESHI,[1] TUSHAR N. LOKHANDE,[2]
KHEMCHAND R. SURANA,[3] ASHWINI V. SHELKE,[1] and
YOGITA B. THOMBARE[1]

[1]*Department of Pharmaceutical Chemistry, Mahatma Gandhi Vidyamandir's Pharmacy College, Panchavati, Nashik, Maharashtra, India*

[2]*Department of Pharmaceutical Chemistry, Maharashtra Educational Society's H. K. College of Pharmacy, Oshiwara, Jogeshwari (W), Maharashtra, India*

[3]*Department of Pharmaceutical Chemistry, Shreeshakti Shaikshanik Sanstha, Divine College of Pharmacy, Satana, Nashik, Maharashtra, India*

ABSTRACT

Tuberculosis (TB) is still a significant public health issue across the world, especially with the advent of multidrug-resistant TB. The incapacity of humans to manage this illness derives from the fact that formerly successful TB vaccinations and treatments are no longer effective. As a result, researchers are looking for novel anti-tuberculosis drugs and adjuvant treatments. Vitamins are being studied again for their involvement in pathogenesis and anti-mycobacterial effects. Vitamins like biotin and thiamin are necessary for Mycobacterium TB to form an infection. Vitamins like Vitamin C and Vitamin D, on the contrary, have been demonstrated to have anti-mycobacterial effects. Innovative techniques must be designed to battle *M. tuberculosis*, keeping the effectiveness of the drug in mind. Vitamins

Preventive and Therapeutic Role of Vitamins as Nutraceuticals. Khemchand R. Surana, Eknath D. Ahire, Raj K. Keservani, & Rajesh K. Kesharwani (Eds.)

may show to be effective agents for altering *M. tuberculosis*' life cycle and biology. Pyridoxine (vitamin B6) is recommended by the WHO when isoniazid at a high dose is used. Vitamin C sterilizes drug-susceptible, MDR, and MTB that is extensively drug-resistant cultures, preventing the formation of persistent drug users; vitamin D inhibits mycobacterium multiplication *in vitro*; and vitamin E has a prospective function in TB management due to its link to oxidative equilibrium. We present here a brief overview of the available knowledge on Vitamin-B complex, Vitamin C, Vitamin D, Vitamin E, and Vitamin K keeping TB treatment and control in perspective.

2.1 INTRODUCTION

Tuberculosis (TB) has been with us since ancient times and has caused more deaths than any other infectious disease over the last 200 years (Siddiqi et al., 2005; Ali et al., 2016). Evidence of tuberculosis has been found in 9,000-year-old mummies. There are conflicting concepts at the time of the beginning of Mycobacterium tuberculosis (*M. tuberculosis*) as a human pathogen, with two recent theories proposing 6,000 to 70,000 years ago. The later evidence proposed that lids first transmitted the disease to humans (Ahmad et al., 2011; Ramsay et al., 2009, 2001; Surana, 2021a).

Tuberculosis (TB) is a granulomatous infection that is one of the world's leading causes of mortality (Bonnet et al., 2008; Surana, 2021b). In fact, 10 million people contract tuberculosis each year, with 1.5 million dying from the disease. In 2012, 8.6 million new active cases of tuberculosis were expected worldwide, with 1.3 million fatalities; therefore, for every 4 s, there is one new TB case, and for every minute, more than two TB deaths are occurring (Boehme et al., 2011). The 80% of all TB cases notice in 22 high-burden countries, where India and China alone share nearly 40% (26 and 12%, respectively).

Due to reduced systemic levels of immunomodulatory vitamins, people are more prone to be malnourished (Liu et al., 2018; Van Lettow et al., 2004). The major risk factors are nearly all infectious diseases, specifically tuberculosis, caused due to malnutrition and undernutrition (Chandra, 2004; Hood, 2013). Vitamins are organic bio-molecules that must be gained from food, whereas vitamin D can be synthesized after exposure to sunlight in the human body (Range et al., 2005). Vitamins have a significant part in healthy activities, such as pro-oxidant, anti-oxidant, anti-inflammatory, and metabolic processes; they are crucial both in latent tuberculosis infection (LTBI) and active tuberculosis, and for patients of all ages (Grobler et al., 2016;

Range et al., 2006). Vitamins have been examined for their anti-tubercular properties since the pre-antibiotic period, but until today there is no definitive evidence for vitamin supplementation to treat the disease or the infection (Di Gennaro et al., 2020; Marotta et al., 2018). The aim of this chapter is to concentrate on nourishment supplementation as a prophylactic measure in those at associated augmented risk of mycobacteria (MTB) infection and active TB (Surana, 2021c).

2.2 ROLE OF VITAMINS

2.2.1 VITAMIN A

Vitamin A is obtained from the diet in the form of all-trans-retinol (ATR), retinol esters, or β-carotene. It's a lipid-soluble vitamin from the retinoic acid family. It's made up of four isoprenoid units that are joined at the head and tail. The vitamin A in various forms is provitamin A carotenoids (beta-carotene, alpha-carotene, and beta-cryptoxanthin) and preformed vitamin A (Christian & West, 1998; Lloyd et al., 1989; Rwangabwoba et al., 1998).

Various studies found association between vitamin A deficiency and a variety of infectious diseases, schistosomiasis, malaria, tuberculosis, leprosy, rheumatic fever, diarrheal, respiratory diseases, and otitis media (Contreras et al., 2017; Hanukah et al., 1997; Mugusi et al., 2003; Wiid et al., 2004). Vitamin A has a role in antibody production, as well as T- and B-lymphocyte activity and macrophage activity (Wheelwright et al., 2014).

Several studies proved the role of vitamin A and its metabolites in the development of tuberculosis (Ramachandran et al., 2004; Karyadi et al., 2002). Retinol, the circulating form of Vitamin A, has low amounts and enhances susceptibility to illness, resulting in a 10-fold greater risk of tuberculosis. High dosages of vitamin A promote antibacterial activity in *M. tuberculosis*-infected macrophages. In *M. tuberculosis*-infected macrophages, high doses of vitamin A stimulate antimicrobial action (Visser et al., 2010; Wheelwright et al., 2014).

The supplement of zinc with vitamin A enhances the effect of antituberculosis treatment and the survival with pulmonary TB in patients shows sputum culture conversion after mineral supplementation (Pakasi, 2009; Ruimy et al., 2019). This may be the explanation for a strong association between vitamin A deficiency and wasting observed in patients with TB. Therefore, supplementation with VA may not be beneficial in TB without correction of the zinc deficiency.

2.2.2 VITAMIN B COMPLEX

The thiamine (vitamin B1), Riboflavin (B2), Niacin (B3), Pantothenic acid (B5), Pyridoxine (B6), Biotin (B7), Folic acid (B9), and Cobalamins (B12) are the B-complex vitamins.

2.2.2.1 VITAMIN B1 (THIAMINE)

Vitamin B1 (Thiamine) is an essential micronutrient act as a metabolic enzyme in its active form, i.e., thiamin diphosphate is required for amino acid and carbohydrate. By modifying the peroxisome proliferator-activated receptor (PPAR), which promotes significant microbicidal action, vitamin B1 boosted tumor necrosis factor (TNF) and interleukin-6 (IL-6) production (Harale et al., 2021). Vitamin B1 boosts PPAR, which integrates mitochondrial respiration and lipid metabolism. Metabolic processes and inflammatory signaling are controlled by vitamin B1 (Hu et al., 2018). In addition, MTB deficiencies cause thiamin salvage mechanisms, building thiamine biosynthetic processes and pleasing therapeutic targets. The gene responsible for thiamin phosphate production is *M. tuberculosis* thiamin phosphate synthase; investigators used bioinformatics to search for therapeutic targets in TB thiamin phosphate synthase, which is phosphorylated to the end product, thiamin pyrophosphate in mycobacteria.

2.2.2.2 VITAMIN B2 (RIBOFLAVIN)

Riboflavin (vitamin B2) is a direct forerunner of the redox enzyme cofactors flavin mononucleotide (FMN) and flavin adenine dinucleotide (FAD), which are required for a variety of cellular functions. The biosynthesis route for riboflavin is thought to be a significant supply of therapeutic targets for broad-spectrum antibiotics. The role of riboflavin in the treatment of tuberculosis has been discovered since 1962 by Huempfner, who showed no adding value of riboflavin added to isoniazid. Some researchers observe a lower lifetime hazard of developing active tuberculosis associated with mucosal invariant T cells (MAIT) from riboflavin precursor metabolites, which shows the cumulative safety in the early phase of mycobacterial infections (Ruimy et al., 2019).

In fact, flavin mononucleotide (FMN) ribose which is bound to synthetic riboflavin analogs, may repress the adjacent riboflavin synthetic genes expression, and this could have resulted in the inhibition of *M. tuberculosis* growth (Xiong et al., 2020). This could be dependent upon the endogenous biosynthesis of riboflavin since *M. tuberculosis* lacks riboflavin transporter. Therefore, riboflavin biosynthetic enzymes might be potential anti-TB drug targets. Elucidation of the role of these enzymes in the M. tuberculosis survival or virulence might validate its drug target value.

2.2.2.3 VITAMIN B5 (PANTOTHENIC ACID)

The significance of vitamin B5 as an adjuvant treatment for tuberculosis has gradually become highly essential in treatment because of the processes by which vitamins affect immunity and their effects. Vitamin B5 (VB5) can promote epithelial cells to express inflammatory cytokines, causing pro-inflammatory and antibacterial effects in TB patients (Beggs & Jenne, 1967; He et al., 2018).

2.2.2.4 VITAMIN B6 (PYRIDOXINE)

Vitamin B6 (pyridoxine) is a vitamin that is water soluble and essential for healthy cell function (Dick et al., 2010). It aids in metabolism, blood cell formation, and cell health. The antioxidant capabilities of vitamin B6, which include the scavenging capacity for reactive oxygen species (ROS), are well-known (Matxain et al., 2009). Pyridoxal 5-phosphate (PLP), which is generated by a heteromeric PLP synthase, is the bioactive form of vitamin B6, which is produced by a heteromeric PLP synthase made up of Pdx1 and Pdx2. Vitamin B6 (pyridoxine) concomitantly with isoniazid (INH) therapy is necessary to prevent the development of peripheral neuropathy.

2.2.2.5 VITAMIN B7 (BIOTIN)

Pyridoxal 5-phosphate (PLP) that is generated through a heteromeric PLP synthase is the bioactive shape of nutrition B6. It cannot be synthesized through human cells; however, it's far produced through microorganisms withinside the body, and its miles are found in several foods (Khare et al., 2011).

M. tuberculosis requires vitamin B7 (biotin) as a cofactor required for enzymes acyl CoA carboxylase and pyruvate carboxylase, which can be worried in fatty acid synthesis and anaplerosis. There is a want of de novo biotin synthesis in *M. tuberculosis* as it lacks biotin transporters, as confirmed through genetic research. In the human host's serum, the biotin attentiveness is insufficient to satisfy the microorganism's necessities.

The biotin synthesis enzymes BioF, BioA, BioD, and BioB require pimeloyl-CoA as a precursor. The enzymes BioF, BioA, and BioB are required for *M. tuberculosis* virulence and pathogenicity. As a result, we are able to see enzymes that can synthesize biotin as exciting healing goals for novel antibiotics in *M. tuberculosis* because it calls for biotin synthesis (Bose et al., 2017). The biotin (for the development and pathogenicity of *M. tuberculosis*) should be an important target for antituberculous therapy, which synthesis genes, as biotin is an essential substrate for MTB evolution and virulence.

2.2.2.6 VITAMIN B12 (COBALAMIN)

Vitamin B12 has one of the most multifarious structures embracing a centrally chelated cobalt ion held in place by a lower axial base having a tetrapyrrole framework, dimethyl benzimidazole, and an upper ligand that determines the B12 form (Gebremicael et al., 2019). Only the prokaryotes biosynthesize the vit B12 and mandates substantial genetic investment (Boritsch et al., 2014). The collective precursor for de novo biosynthesis of Ado-Cbl of several tetrapyrrolic cofactors from uroporphyrinogen III comprising heme requires over 25 enzyme-catalyzed reactions (Gopinath et al., 2013).

The potential for de novo biosynthesis of diet B12 (VB12) in *M. tuberculosis* is associated corrinoids are scavenged with the aid of using the bacillus the usage of an ATP-binding cassette (Di Gennaro et al., 2018). They partake an impact on Vit B12 degrees in diseased human beings because of the unsure numbers of bacterial tuberculosis; the mycobacterial pathogens generated or ingested Vit B12 may also have a nearby impact on human granulomatous lesions with the aid of using the metabolic environment (Sancho-Vaello et al., 2020; Young et al., 2015). The MTB regulates its core metabolic operations according to B12 accessibility by the gaining of B12 via endogenous or through uptake from the environment. The frequency of tuberculosis in vegetarians was very less in patients as compared to varied diets. There is one more captivating assumption that may be applicable. In *M. tuberculosis*, Mycocerosic acid and methylmalonic acid are two cell wall components that are required for its formation. The rise in methylmalonic acid concentrations causes *M. tuberculosis* to multiply and methylmalonic acid. The multiplication of *M. tuberculosis* is due to the increase in concentrations of methylmalonic acid, which exit in vitamin B12 (Rekha et al., 2015; Toosi et al., 2008). The concentration of Vitamin B12 in the blood is used as a biomarker in the identification of active tuberculosis with and without HIV infection, according to a recent study.

2.2.3 VITAMIN C

Because humans cannot produce Vitamin C due to a mutation in the enzyme-coding gene, the enzyme gluconolactone oxidase, it must be taken as a dietary supplement (Combs et al., 2016). Vitamin C protects the body from mycobacterial infection-induced reactive oxygen and nitrogen intermediates (Nishikimi et al., 1996). It has a role in collagen formation, iron transport, and as a physiological antioxidant. It also boosts T-cell response and drives enhanced leukocyte migration to the infection site (Field et al., 2002). Linus Pauling suggested 1–3 g of Vitamin C per day for the prevention of the common cold and influenza in 1976. According to a number of research, vitamin C can help prevent and cure tuberculosis when taken orally. TB infection has also been connected to vitamin C deficiency (Andosca et al., 1948). Nutrition status was linked to the possibility of contracting TB in research, including 1,100 people who were first identified as nontuberculous. Throughout the course of the study, 28 people contracted tuberculosis, and it was discovered that they had low Vitamin C levels (Getz et al., 1951). Vitamin C has also been proven to be a trigger for the induction of dormancy in Mycobacterium TB. Vitamin C activates the DevR (DosR) regulon, which is important for bacterial dormancy (Taneja et al., 2010). A study that looked for synergistic effects of Vitamin C when combined with rifampicin and isoniazid came up with some intriguing findings. When cultivated in the presence of Vitamin C and rifampicin at inadequate MIC, the colony-forming units of wild-type H37Rv strains, as well as drug-resistant bacteria, were reduced. When Vitamin C was tested in combination with isoniazid, it reduced CFU in both wild-type and drug-resistant bacteria. When in comparison to the wild kind H37Rv, the isoniazid-Vitamin C synergy had a lesser impact on resistant strains (Khameneh et al., 2016). Narwadiya et al. discovered a link between vitamin C content and medicinal plant anti-TB capabilities (Narwadiya et al., 2011). In the presence of oxygen, vitamin C lowers ferric to ferrous ion, which produces superoxide, hydrogen peroxide, and hydroxyl radicals via the Fenton and Haber–Weiss reactions (Mishra et al., 2015). These radical moieties subsequently damage *M. tuberculosis* DNA and lipids, causing growth inhibition. Vitamin C is expected to lower the amount of guanosine 5′-diphosphate 3′-diphosphate (ppGpp), a chemical involved in *M. tuberculosis* growth control and stress response (Syal, 2017) used Vitamin C supplementation in their trials and found some promising benefits that warrant further exploration.

2.2.4 VITAMIN D

Vitamin D is widely recognized for its involvement in regulating calcium homeostasis and bone mineral density in humans. It comes in two forms: ergocalciferol (Vitamin D2) and cholecalciferol (Vitamin D3). Vitamins can be gained through diet or by exposing the skin to sunlight (ultraviolet B [UVB] radiation). However, its potential as a disease-fighting agent is being reconsidered (Selvaraj et al., 2015). Vitamin D insufficiency and susceptibility to tuberculosis have been linked in studies. Since 1651, when vitamin insufficiency was first identified, it was first linked to TB signs and symptoms. Later, heliotherapy became a standard treatment for tuberculosis patients and was used in sanatoria. Furthermore, Stead et al. discovered ethnic disparities in the prevalence of tuberculosis, which were linked to levels of 25-hydroxyvitamin D (Stead et al., 1990; Salahuddin et al., 2013). Ralph et al. and Daley et al., on the contrary, found no significant improvement in the culture conversion rate in Vitamin D-treated individuals. It's debatable if culture conversion rate can be used as a criterion for researching the effects of vitamin D administration. While studying the effects of Vitamin D supplementation, relapse prevention or tissue damage restriction may show to be useful measures (Cegielski et al., 2015). Vitamin D levels in people have been shown to depend on the situation, the season, and latitude, and this has been linked to the development of tuberculosis. TB notifications increased by 24.1% during the summers, according to Birmingham research using data from 9,739 individuals over a 28-year period. Vitamin D levels were depleted throughout the winter months due to a lack of sunlight, which resulted in a spike in tuberculosis cases during the summer season (Koh, 2013). In South Africa, similar research was undertaken, and the findings followed the same trend (Martineau, 2013). Vitamin D concentration in humans is influenced by a number of variables, including human biosynthesis, pigmentation, latitude, dietary supplementation, obesity, heredity, and illness condition. Vitamin D insufficiency [50 nmol/l 25(OH)D] is a worldwide concern, with severe deficiency occurring in locations such as the Middle East and South Asia, which may increase vulnerability to numerous illnesses (Edwards et al., 2014).

2.2.5 VITAMIN E

Vitamin E is distinguished by a long isoprenoid side. It is a robust antioxidant, supports membrane integrity, and inhibits platelet aggregation. It is attached at the 2 positions of a 6-chromanol ring, which gives unique biochemical properties: it is a potent antioxidant, supports membrane integrity, and inhibits platelet aggregation. Vitamin E has been demonstrated to provide a variety of health advantages, including anti-infection defense. Vitamin E boosts the body's defenses, improves humoral and cell immune responses, and increases phagocytic activities, among other things (Rizvi et al., 2014). Vitamin E is an extremely effective antioxidant that neutralizes free radicals and protects the structural components of cell membranes from oxidation (Burton et al., 1983), and it's also involved in T-cell differentiation and proliferation, as well as infection prevention.

When researching the link between Vitamin E and tuberculosis, it's important to keep in mind a contentious pathophysiological component: On the one hand, phagocytic immunity is an important part of the host's response to tuberculosis; oxidative stress is a common reaction to *M. tuberculosis*. This counteractive reaction is triggered by a concentration-dependent trigger: *M. tuberculosis* only produces DNA damage-responsive genes when ROS levels are low, hence this method does not defend against oxidative stress at high levels (Pizzol et al., 2017).

The nutritional state of TB patients has been reported to have VE levels (along with other antioxidants like VA) are lower, anti-oxidase, and beta-carotene) than that of non-TB patients (Dou et al., 2013). The VE level was tested before and after the start of antituberculosis therapy (ATT): unacceptable levels were detected, but no rise was associated with the start of ATT (Iddir et al., 2020; Lamsal et al., 2007). In TB, researchers discovered negative associations between VE (and therefore vitamin C and A) and oxidative stress, as well as nitrosative stress indicators such as nitric oxide, carbonyl protein, and lipid peroxidation. Following six months of antitubercular therapy, the abnormalities were reversed in individuals who recovered well; however, the worry had not totally vanished (Dalvi et al., 2013). When it comes to protection, empowerment, VE has been reported to help enhance the levels of immunoglobulins and T-cell types that fight tuberculosis (Hussain et al., 2019).

Certain studies have looked into the *in vivo* relationship between Vitamin E and ATT. Pretreatment of albino rabbits with high doses of tocopherol (100 mg/kg) may protect them from hepatotoxicity caused by Isoniazid and Rifampicin (Tayal & Kalra, 2007). Vitamin E and Vitamin C were found to have a favorable effect on sperm quality, hematological damage, and brain damage induced by anti-tuberculous medications in rats (Abdel-Azeem et al., 2013).

Nonetheless, the second research comes to no findings regarding this, suggesting that the sole advantage of vitamin supplementation may be tied to weight gain rather than a direct positive TB result, as well as other infectious disorders, including surgical site infection and pneumonia (Di Gennaro, 2020).

2.2.6 VITAMIN K

Antituberculous agents produced vitamin K insufficiency, which was studied in clinical patients and animals. A significant rise in plasma PIVKA-II and a drop in thrombo-test value were found when antituberculous medicines were administered to patients who were on a whole elemental diet due to small intestine dysfunction. Despite the success or failure of antituberculous agents, these alterations were promptly normalized by vitamin K treatment. Four drugs (ethambutol, isoniazid, paraaminosalicylate, and rifampicin) were tested in rat trials (Van Steenbergen et al., 1995) to see how they affected prothrombin time. Only rifampicin prolonged prothrombin time among these drugs. The length of time this effect lasted was determined by the medication dosages and duration of administration. A rise in plasma PIVKA-II was detected additionally to the hypoprothrombinemia, and both alterations were corrected after 24 hours of vitamin K therapy. These findings show that rifampicin inhibits vitamin K epoxide reductase, preventing vitamin K re-use and resulting in vitamin K insufficiency in individuals on a whole elemental diet (Ishii et al., 1997).

2.3 CONCLUSION

According to our research, there is a substantial relationship between vitamins A, B, C, D, K, and E and tuberculosis. This appears to be linked to their anti-inflammatory properties, poor nutritional status, which is associated with hypovitaminosis on the one hand and a higher chance of developing tuberculosis (TB) on the other, as well as vitamin action that may have a direct relationship with *M. tuberculosis*.

In the case of tuberculosis, supplementing with numerous micronutrients (including zinc) rather than just Vitamin A may be more effective. In the lack of proof that Vitamin A supplementation alone has a therapeutic impact, therapies that incorporate both Vitamin A and zinc may be a better alternative.

When excessive-dose isoniazid is used, Pyridoxine (vitamin B6) is recommended, in addition to in people with diabetes, uremia, HIV infection, seizure disorders, alcohol addiction, malnutrition, or peripheral neuropathy. Vitamin B6 ought to additionally take delivery of two pregnant and post-partum women, in addition to solely breastfed newborns, while taking Isoniazid (A everyday dose of pyridoxine is 10–25 mg/day while administered prophylactically to keep away from neuropathy in Isoniazid sufferers).

Each day consumption of Vitamin C in a regular human food plan is substantially beneath the ranges required for maximal movement *in vitro* towards MTB; human sufferers have obtained megadose of Vitamin C, ensuing in excessive Vitamin C plasma concentrations (as much as 49 mM), that have been proved to be safe. As a result, destiny randomized scientific trials to higher apprehend if Vitamin C is a method of reaching quicker sputum smear-poor conversion, which could imply a quicker discount withinside the mycobacterial burden, and if it may shorten TB treatment, decreasing the incidences of each drug resistance improvement and sickness relapse, may be very interesting. In the case of Vitamin D, given the inexpensive cost of the medicine and the evidence of *in vitro* efficacy but questionable *in vivo* outcomes, it would be advantageous to assess Vitamin D in all patients with TB, as well as people at risk of acquiring active TB, and prescribe Vitamin D supplementation. However, more clinical trials are needed to uncover any confounding variables *in vivo* and to assess the potential use of Vitamin D in the prevention and treatment of tuberculosis, as well as doses and the best mode of delivery.

Furthermore, because of its link to oxidative equilibrium, Vitamin E has shown promise in the treatment of tuberculosis. This assertion is backed up by laboratory data. Vitamin E administration therefore protects against TB development in household contacts, ATT-related organ damage, and extra-pulmonary TB indirect complications including kidney stone formation. Vitamin E, like any other vitamin, can have negative side effects if used in excess. Thus, it shouldn't be avoided continuously. More investigation is required to determine which patients might benefit the most. Positive sputum time conversion is not the subject of any investigations. Vitamin supplementation in tuberculosis patients is suggested and encouraged in our study. Indeed, their usage may enhance results by assisting with nutrition as well as interacting directly or indirectly with MTB. To back up these claims, further studies with a larger sample size are required.

ACKNOWLEDGMENTS

We thank the Mahatma Gandhi Vidyamandir's Pharmacy College, Panchavati, Nashik, Maharashtra, India, for their constant support and providing all facilities to complete this work. Also, many thanks to all the known and unknowns who helped us right from the writing till the publishing of this chapter.

KEYWORDS

- **mycobacterium tuberculosis**
- **pantothenic acid**
- **riboflavin**
- **thiamine**
- **vitamin B-complex**
- **vitamin C**
- **vitamin D**
- **vitamin E**
- **vitamin K**

REFERENCES

Abdel-Azeem, A. S., Hegazy, A. M., Ibrahim, K. S., Farrag, A. R. H., & El-Sayed, E. M., (2013). Hepatoprotective, antioxidant, and ameliorative effects of ginger (*Zingiber officinale* Roscoe) and vitamin E in acetaminophen-treated rats. *Journal of Dietary Supplements*, *10*(3), 195–209.

Ahmad, S., (2011). Pathogenesis, immunology, and diagnosis of latent *Mycobacterium tuberculosis* infection. *Clin. Dev. Immunol.*, 814943.

Ai, J. W., et al., (2016). Updates on the risk factors for latent tuberculosis reactivation and their management. *Emerging Microbes & Infections, 5*, e10.

Beggs, W. H., & Jenne, J. W., (1967). Mechanism for the pyridoxal neutralization of isoniazid action on *Mycobacterium tuberculosis*. *J. Bacteriol., 94*, 793–797.

Boehme, C. C., Nicol, M. P., Nabeta, P., Michael, J. S., Gotuzzo, E., Tahirli, R., et al., (2011). Feasibility, diagnostic accuracy, and effectiveness of decentralized use of the Xpert MTB/RIF test for diagnosis of tuberculosis and multidrug resistance: A multicenter implementation study. *Lancet, 377*(9776), 1495–1505.

Bonnet, M., Ramsay, A., Githui, W., Gagnidze, L., Varaine, F., & Guerin, P. J., (2008). Bleach sedimentation: An opportunity to optimize smear microscopy for tuberculosis diagnosis in settings of high prevalence of HIV. *Clin. Infect Dis., 46*(11), 1710–1716.

Boritsch, E. C., Supply, P., Honoré, N., Seemann, T., Stinear, T., & Brosch, R., (2014). A glimpse into the past and predictions for the future: The molecular evolution of the tuberculosis agent. *Mol. Microbiol., 93*, 835–852.

Bose, M., Tyagi, G., Singh, P., & Varma-Basil, M., (2017). Role of vitamins B, C, and D in the fight against tuberculosis. *Int. J. Mycobacteriology, 6*, 328.

Burton, G. W., Joyce, A., & Ingold, K. U., (1983). Is vitamin E the only lipid-soluble, chain-breaking antioxidant in human blood plasma and erythrocyte membranes? *Archives of Biochemistry and Biophysics, 221*(1), 281–290.

Cegielski, P., & Vernon, A., (2015). Tuberculosis and vitamin D: What's the rest of the story? *The Lancet. Infectious Diseases, 15*(5), 489.

Chandra, R. K., (2004). Nutrient supplementation as an adjunct therapy in pulmonary tuberculosis. *Int. J. Vitam. Nutr. Res., 74*, 144–146.

Christian, P., & West, K. P. Jr., (1998). Interactions between zinc and vitamin A: An update. *Am. J. Clin. Nutr., 68*(Suppl. 2), 435S–441S.

Combs, Jr. G. F., & McClung, J. P., (2016). *The Vitamins: Fundamental Aspects in Nutrition and Health*. Academic Press.

Contreras, C., et al., (2017). Impact of vitamin A and carotenoids on the risk of tuberculosis progression. *Clin. Infect. Dis., 65*, 900–909.

Daley, P., Jagannathan, V., John, K. R., Sarojini, J., Latha, A., Vieth, R., Suzana, S., et al., (2015). Adjunctive vitamin D for treatment of active tuberculosis in India: A randomized, double-blind, placebo-controlled trial. *The Lancet Infectious Diseases, 15*(5), 528–534.

Dalvi, S. M., Patil, V. W., Ramraje, N. N., Phadtare, J. M., & Gujarathi, S. U., (2013). Nitric oxide, carbonyl protein, lipid peroxidation, and correlation between antioxidant vitamins in different categories of pulmonary and extrapulmonary tuberculosis. *The Malaysian Journal of Medical Sciences: MJMS, 20*(1), 21.

Di Gennaro, F., Gualano, G., Timelli, L., Vittozzi, P., Di Bari, V., Libertone, R., Cerva, C., Pinnarelli, L., Nisii, C., Ianniello, S., et al., (2021). Increase in tuberculosis diagnostic delay during first wave of the COVID-19 pandemic: Data from an Italian infectious disease referral hospital. *Antibiotics, 10*, 272.

Di Gennaro, F., Marotta, C., Pisani, L., Veronese, N., Pisani, V., Lippolis, V., Pellizer, G., et al., (2020). Maternal cesarean section infection (MACSI) in Sierra Leone: A case–control study. *Epidemiology & Infection, 148*.

Di Gennaro, F., Pisani, L., Veronese, N., Pizzol, D., Lippolis, V., Saracino, A., Monno, L., Huson, M. A., Copetti, R., Putoto, G., et al., (2018). Potential diagnostic properties of chest ultrasound in thoracic tuberculosis—A systematic review. *Int. J. Environ. Res. Public Health, 15*, 2235.

Di Gennaro, F., Vittozzi, P., Gualano, G., Musso, M., Mosti, S., Mencarini, P., Pareo, C., Di Caro, A., Schininà, V., Girardi, E., et al., (2020). Active pulmonary tuberculosis in elderly patients: A 2016–2019 retrospective analysis from an Italian referral hospital. *Antibiotics, 9*, 489.

Dick, T., Manjunatha, U., Kappes, B., & Gengenbacher, M., (2010). Vitamin B6 biosynthesis is essential for the survival and virulence of *Mycobacterium tuberculosis. Mol. Microbiol., 78*, 980–988.

Dou, Y., Liang, H., Wang, Q., & Ma, A., (2013). Vitamin A, vitamin E and beta-carotene nutritional status and anti-oxidase level analysis among tuberculosis patients. *Wei Sheng Yanjiu= Journal of Hygiene Research, 42*(3), 364–368.

Edwards, M. H., Cole, Z. A., Harvey, N. C., & Cooper, C., (2014). The global epidemiology of vitamin D status. *J. Aging Res. Clin. Prac., 3*(3), 148–158.

Facchini, L., Venturini, E., Galli, L., De Martino, M., & Chiappini, E., (2015). Vitamin D and tuberculosis: A review on a hot topic. *J. Chemother., 27*, 128–138.

Field, C. J., Johnson, I. R., & Schley, P. D., (2002). Nutrients and their role in host resistance to infection. *Journal of Leukocyte Biology, 71*(1), 16–32.

Gebremicael, G., Alemayehu, M., Sileshi, M., Geto, Z., Gebreegziabxier, A., Tefera, H., Ashenafi, N., et al., (2019). The serum concentration of vitamin B12 as a biomarker of therapeutic response in tuberculosis patients with and without human immunodeficiency virus (HIV) infection. *Int. J. Gen. Med., 12*, 353–361.

Getz, H. R., Long, E. R., & Henderson, H. J., (1951). A study of the relation of nutrition to the development of tuberculosis, influence of ascorbic acid and vitamin A. *American Review of Tuberculosis, 64*(4), 381–393.

Gopinath, K., Moosa, A., Mizrahi, V., & Warner, D. F., (2013). Vitamin B12 metabolism in *Mycobacterium tuberculosis. Futur. Microbiol., 8*, 1405–1418.

Grobler, L., Nagpal, S., Sudarsanam, T. D., & Sinclair, D., (2016). Nutritional supplements for people being treated for active tuberculosis. *Cochrane Database Syst Rev.*, CD006086.

Hanekom, W. A., Potgieter, S., Hughes, E., Malan, H., Kessow, G., & Hussey, G. D., (1997). Vitamin A status and therapy in childhood pulmonary tuberculosis. *J. Pediatr., 131*, 925–927.

Harare, B., Kidwai, S., Ojha, D., Singh, M., Chouhan, D. K., Singh, R., Khedkar, V., & Rode, A. B., (2021). Synthesis and evaluation of antimycobacterial activity of riboflavin derivatives. *Bioorganic Med. Chem. Lett., 48*, 128236.

Harauchi, T., TAKANO, K., MATSUURA, M., & YOSHIZAKI, T., (1986). Liver and plasma levels of des carboxy prothrombin (PIVKA II) in vitamin K deficiency in rats. *The Japanese Journal of Pharmacology, 40*(4), 491–499.

He, W., Hu, S., Du, X., Wen, Q., Zhong, X. P., Zhou, X., Zhou, C. Y., Xiong, W., Gao, Y., Zhang, S., et al., (2018). Vitamin B5 reduces bacterial growth by regulating innate immunity and adaptive immunity in mice infected with *Mycobacterium tuberculosis. Front. Immunol., 9*, 365.

Hood, M. L., (2013). A narrative review of recent progress in understanding the relationship between tuberculosis and protein energy malnutrition. *Eur. J. Clin. Nutr., 67*, 1122–1128.

Hu, S., He, W., Du, X., Huang, Y., Fu, Y., Yang, Y., Hu, C., Li, S., Wang, Q., Wen, Q., et al., (2018). Vitamin B1 Helps to limit *Mycobacterium tuberculosis* growth by regulating innate immunity in a peroxisome proliferator-activated receptor–dependent manner. *Front. Immunol., 9*, 1778.

Hussain, M. I., Ahmed, W., Nasir, M., Mushtaq, M. H., Sheikh, A. A., Shaheen, A. Y., & Mahmood, A. (2019). Immune boosting role of vitamin E against pulmonary tuberculosis. *Pakistan Journal of Pharmaceutical Sciences*, *36*(1SI), 269–277.

Iddir, M., Brito, A., Dingeo, G., Fernandez, D. C. S. S., Samouda, H., La Frano, M. R., & Bohn, T., (2020). Strengthening the immune system and reducing inflammation and oxidative stress through diet and nutrition: Considerations during the COVID-19 crisis. *Nutrients*, *12*(6), 1562.

Ishii, F., Iizuka, B., Nakanishi, T., Nagasako, K., & Hayashi, N., (1997). Vitamin K deficiency syndrome is caused by anti-tuberculous agents. *Nihon Shokakibyo Gakkai Zasshi= The Japanese Journal of Gastroenterology*, *94*(6), 389–397.

Karyadi, E., West, C. E., Schultink, W., Nelwan, R. H. H., Gross, R., Amin, Z., Dolmans, W. M. V., et al., (2002). A double-blind, placebo-controlled study of vitamin A and zinc supplementation in persons with tuberculosis in Indonesia: Effects on clinical response and nutritional status. *Am. J. Clin. Nutr.*, *75*, 720–727.

Khare, G., Kar, R., & Tyagi, A. K., (2011). Identification of inhibitors against *Mycobacterium tuberculosis* thiamin phosphate synthase, an important target for the development of anti-TB drugs. *PLoS One*, *6*, e22441.

Koh, G. C., Hawthorne, G., Turner, A. M., Kunst, H., & Dedicoat, M. (2013). Tuberculosis incidence correlates with sunshine: An ecological 28-year time series study. *PloS One*, *8*(3), e57752.

Lamsal, M., Gautam, N., Bhatta, N., Toora, B. D., Bhattacharya, S. K., & Baral, N., (2007). Evaluation of lipid peroxidation product, nitrite, and antioxidant levels in newly diagnosed and two months follow-up patients with pulmonary tuberculosis. *Southeast Asian Journal of Tropical Medicine and Public Health*, *38*(4), 695.

Liu, Z., Ren, Z., Zhang, J., Chuang, C. C., Kandaswamy, E., Zhou, T., & Zuo, L. (2018). Role of ROS and nutritional antioxidants in human diseases. *Front. Physiol.*, *9*, 477.

Lloyd-Puryear, M., Humphrey, J. H., West, K. P., Aniol, K., Mahoney, F., Mahoney, J., & Keenum, D. G., (1989). Vitamin A deficiency and anemia among Micronesian children. *Nutr. Res.*, *9*, 1007–1016.

Mandl, J., Szarka, A., & Bánhegyi, G., (2009). Vitamin C: Update on physiology and pharmacology. *Br. J. Pharmacol.*, *157*, 1097–1110.

Marotta, C., Di Gennaro, F., Pizzol, D., Madeira, G., Monno, L., Saracino, A., Putoto, G., et al., (2018). At-risk child clinic (ARCC): 3 Years of health activities in support of the most vulnerable children in Beira, Mozambique. *Int. J. Environ. Res. Public Health*, *15*, 1350.

Martineau, A. R., Nhamoyebonde, S., Oni, T., Rangaka, M. X., Marais, S., Bangani, N., Tsekela, R., et al., (2011). Reciprocal seasonal variation in vitamin D status and tuberculosis notifications in Cape Town, South Africa. *Proceedings of the National Academy of Sciences*, *108*(47), 19013–19017.

Matxain, J. M., Padro, D., Ristila, M., Strid, A., & Eriksson, L. A., (2009). Evidence of high _OH radical quenching efficiency BY vitamin B6. *J. Phys. Chem. B.*, *113*, 9629–9632.

Mishra, A., & Sarkar, D. (2015). Qualitative and quantitative proteomic analysis of vitamin C induced changes in *Mycobacterium smegmatis*. *Front Microbiol.*, *6,* 1–10

Mugusi, F. M., Rusizoka, O., Habib, N., & Fawzi, W., (2003). Vitamin A status of patients presenting with pulmonary tuberculosis and asymptomatic HIV-infected individuals, Dar es Salaam, Tanzania. *Int. J. Tuberc. Lung Dis.*, *7*, 804–807.

Narwadiya, S. C., Sahare, K. N., Tumane, P. M., Dhumne, U. L., & Meshram, V. G., (2011). *In vitro* anti-tuberculosis effect of vitamin C contents of medicinal plants. *Asian J. Exp. Biol. Sci.*, *2*(151154), 22.

Nishikimi, M., & Yagi, K., (1996). Biochemistry and molecular biology of ascorbic acid biosynthesis. *Subcellular Biochemistry*, 17–39.

Pakasi, T. A., (2009). *Zinc and Vitamin A Supplementation in Tuberculosis* (p. 1–142). A study in East Nusa Tenggara, Indonesia. Ph.D. Thesis, Radboud University, Nijmegen, The Netherlands.

Pizzol, D., Di Gennaro, F., Chhaganlal, K. D., Fabrizio, C., Monno, L., Putoto, G., & Saracino, A., (2017). Prevalence of diabetes mellitus in newly diagnosed pulmonary tuberculosis in Beira, Mozambique. *African Health Sciences*, *17*(3), 773–779.

Ralph, A. P., Waramori, G., Pontororing, G. J., Kenangalem, E., Wiguna, A., Tjitra, E., Lolong, D. B., et al., (2013). L-arginine and vitamin D adjunctive therapies in pulmonary tuberculosis: A randomized, double-blind, placebo-controlled trial. *PloS One*, *8*(8), e70032.

Ramachandran, G., Santha, T., Garg, R., Baskaran, D., Iliayas, S. A., Venkatesan, P., Fathima, R., & Narayanan, P. R., (2004). Vitamin A levels in sputum-positive pulmonary tuberculosis patients in comparison with household contacts and healthy 'normals.' *Int. J. Tuberc. Lung Dis.*, *8*, 1130–1133.

Ramsay, A., Yassin, M. A., Cambanis, A., Hirao, S., Almotawa, A., Gammo, M., et al., (2009). Front-loading sputum microscopy services: An opportunity to optimize smear-based case detection of tuberculosis in high prevalence countries. *J Trop Med.*, 1–6.

Range, N., Andersen, A. B., Magnussen, P., Mugomela, A., & Friis, H., (2005). The effect of micronutrient supplementation on treatment outcome in patients with pulmonary tuberculosis: A randomized controlled trial in Mwanza, Tanzania. *Trop Med. Int. Health, 10*, 826–832.

Range, N., Changalucha, J., Krarup, H., Magnussen, P., Andersen, B., & Friis, H., (2006). The effect of multi-vitamin/mineral supplementation on mortality during treatment of pulmonary tuberculosis: A randomized two-by-two factorial trial in Mwanza, Tanzania. *Br. J. Nutr.*, *95*, 762–770.

Rekha, R. S., Jagadeeswara, R. M., Min, W., Rubhana, R., Peter, B., Susanna, B., Gudmundur, H., & Birgitta, A., (2015). Phenylbutyrate induces LL-37-dependent autophagy and intracellular killing of *Mycobacterium tuberculosis* in human macrophages. *Autophagy, 11*, 1688–1699.

Rizvi, S., Raza, S. T., Faizal, A. A. A., Abbas, S., & Mahdi, F., (2014). The role of vitamin E in human health and some diseases. *Sultan Qaboos University Medical Journal*, *14*(2), e157.

Ruimy, C. M., Youssef, G. B., Lambert, M., & Tourret, M., (2019). Mucosal-associated invariant T cell levels are reduced in the peripheral blood and lungs of children with active pulmonary tuberculosis. *Front. Immunol.*, *10*, 206.

Rwangabwoba, J. M., Fischman, H., & Semba, R. D., (1998). Serum vitamin A levels during tuberculosis and human immunodeficiency virus infection. *Int. J. Tuberc. Lung Dis.*, *2*, 771–773.

Salahuddin, N., Ali, F., Hasan, Z., Rao, N., Aqeel, M., & Mahmood, F., (2013). Vitamin D accelerates clinical recovery from tuberculosis: Results of the succinct study [supplementary cholecalciferol in recovery from tuberculosis]. A randomized, placebo-controlled, clinical trial of vitamin D supplementation in patients with pulmonary tuberculosis. *BMC Infectious Diseases*, *13*(1), 1–11.

Sancho-Vaello, E., Gil-Carton, D., François, P., Bonetti, E. J., Kreir, M., Pothula, K. R., & Zeth, K., (2020). The structure of the antimicrobial human cathelicidin LL-37 shows oligomerization and channel formation in the presence of membrane mimics. *Sci. Rep., 10*, 17356.

Selvaraj, P., Harishankar, M., & Afsal, K., (2015). Vitamin D: Immuno-modulation and tuberculosis treatment. *Canadian Journal of Physiology and Pharmacology, 93*(5), 377–384.

Siddiqi, K., Lambert, M. L., & Walley, J., (2005). Clinical diagnosis of smear-negative pulmonary tuberculosis in low-income countries: The current evidence. *Lancet Infect Dis., 3*(5), 288–296.

Soh, A. Z., Chee, C. B. E., Wang, Y. T., Yuan, J. M., & Koh, W. P., (2017). Dietary intake of antioxidant vitamins and carotenoids and risk of developing active tuberculosis in a prospective population-based cohort study. *Am. J. Epidemiol., 186*, 491–500.

Stead, W. W., Senner, J. W., Reddick, W. T., & Lofgren, J. P., (1990). Racial differences in susceptibility to infection by *Mycobacterium tuberculosis*. *New England Journal of Medicine, 322*(7), 422–427.

Surana, K. R., Ahire, E. D., Sonawane, V. N., & Talele, S. G., (2021). Biomolecular and molecular docking: A modern tool in drug discovery and virtual screening of natural products. In: *Applied Pharmaceutical Practice and Nutraceuticals* (pp. 209–223). Apple Academic Press.

Surana, K. R., Ahire, E. D., Sonawane, V. N., Talele, S. G., & Talele, G. S., (2021). Informatics and methods in nutrition design and development. *Natural Food Products and Waste Recovery: Healthy Foods, Nutrition Design, and Extraction of Valuable Compounds*, 33.

Surana, K. R., Ahire, E. D., Sonawane, V. N., Talele, S. G., & Talele, G. S., (2021). Molecular modeling: Novel techniques in food and nutrition development. *Natural Food Products and Waste Recovery: Healthy Foods, Nutrition Design, and Extraction of Valuable Compounds*, 17.

Surana, K. R., Ahire, E. D., Sonawane, V. N., Talele, S. G., & Talele, G. S., (2021). Informatics and methods in nutrition design and development. *Natural Food Products and Waste Recovery: Healthy Foods, Nutrition Design, and Extraction of Valuable Compounds*, 33.

Syal, K., Bhardwaj, N., & Chatterji, D., (2017). Vitamin C targets (p) ppGpp synthesis leading to stalling of long-term survival and biofilm formation in *Mycobacterium smegmatis*. *FEMS Microbiology Letters, 364*(1), 282.

Taneja, N. K., Dhingra, S., Mittal, A., Naresh, M., & Tyagi, J. S., (2010). *Mycobacterium tuberculosis* transcriptional adaptation, growth arrest, and dormancy phenotype development are triggered by vitamin C. *PloS One, 5*(5), e10860.

Tayal, V., Kalra, B. S., Agarwal, S., Khurana, N., & Gupta, U., (2007). *Hepatoprotective Effect of Tocopherol Against Isoniazid and Rifampicin Induced Hepatotoxicity in Albino Rabbits., 45*, 1031–1036.

Toosi, T. D., Shahi, F., Afshari, A., Roushan, N., & Kermanshahi, M., (2008). Neuropathy caused by B12 deficiency in a patient with ileal tuberculosis: A case report. *J. Med. Case Rep., 2*, 90.

Van, L. M., Harries, A. D., Kumwenda, J. J., Zijlstra, E. E., Clark, T. D., Taha, T. E., & Semba, R. D., (2004). Micronutrient malnutrition and wasting in adults with pulmonary tuberculosis with and without HIV co-infection in Malawi. *BMC Infect. Dis., 4*, 61.

Van, S. W., & Vermylen, J., (1995). Reversible hypoprothrombinemia in a patient with primary biliary cirrhosis treated with rifampicin. *American Journal of Gastroenterology, 90*(9). Springer Nature.

Visser, E. M., Grewal, H. M., Swart, E. C., Dhansay, M. A., Walzl, G., Swanevelder, S., Lombard, C., & Maartens, G., (2010). The effect of vitamin A and zinc supplementation on treatment outcomes in pulmonary tuberculosis: A randomized controlled trial. *Am. J. Clin. Nutr., 93*, 93–100.

Wheelwright, M., Kim, E. W., Inkeles, M. S., De Leon, A., Pellegrini, M., Krutzik, S. R., & Liu, P. T., (2014). All-trans retinoic acid–triggered antimicrobial activity against *Mycobacterium tuberculosis* is dependent on NPC2. *J. Immunol., 192*, 2280–2290.

Wiid, I., Seaman, T., Hoal, E. G., Benade, A. J., & Van, H. P. D., (2004). Total antioxidant levels are low during active TB and rise with anti-tuberculosis therapy. *IUBMB Life, 56*, 101–106.

Xiong, K., Wang, J., Zhang, J., Hao, H., Wang, Q., Cai, J., & Ma, A., (2020). Association of dietary micronutrient intake with pulmonary tuberculosis treatment failure rate: A cohort study. *Nutrients, 12*, 2491.

Young, D. B., Comas, I., & De Carvalho, L. P., (2015). Phylogenetic analysis of vitamin B12-related metabolism in *Mycobacterium tuberculosis*. *Front. Mol. Biosci., 2*, 6.

CHAPTER 3

Vitamins as Nutraceuticals for HIV and AIDS

ABHIJEET G. PARKHE,[1] KHEMCHAND R. SURANA,[2] EKNATH D. AHIRE,[3] RAJ K. KESERVANI,[4] and SUNIL K. MAHAJAN[5]

[1]*In-Vivo Pharmacology Department, Glenmark Pharmaceutical Ltd., Navi Mumbai, Maharashtra, India*

[2]*Department of Pharmaceutical Chemistry, Shreeshakti Shaikshanik Sanstha, Divine College of Pharmacy, Satana, Nashik, Maharashtra, India*

[3]*Department of Pharmaceutics, METs, Institute of Pharmacy, BKC, Adgaon, Nashik, Maharashtra, India*

[4]*Faculty of B. Pharmacy, CSM Group of Institutions, Prayagraj, Uttar Pradesh, India*

[5]*Department of Pharmaceutical Chemistry, M.G.V's Samajshri Prashant Dada Hiray, College of Pharmacy, Malegaon, Nashik, Maharashtra, India*

ABSTRACT

Human immunodeficiency virus (HIV) is a viral infection spread by multiple agents through multiple routes. The virus is a small group of microorganisms that causes mild to severe infections among human and animal races. In some infections, some are curable with existing medicines, and for some, medicines are yet to discover. Unfortunately, in the case of HIV infection, curable medicines do not exist, but symptomatic relief and life expectancy increase with quality of life. There is antiretroviral treatment (ART) which is available for the control of this infection, but if we shift focus on the modern medicines, side effects go on elevated with the escalating dose. These side

Preventive and Therapeutic Role of Vitamins as Nutraceuticals. Khemchand R. Surana, Eknath D. Ahire, Raj K. Keservani, & Rajesh K. Kesharwani (Eds.)

effects can be lowered, and nutritional supplements can play a vital role in immunity modulation, thereby improving immunity for the fight against the virus. HIV infection basically damages the immune system and their cells like WBC. The body has different lines of defense and barriers. Each barrier has its unique function. This compromised the immunity of patients responsible for catching other severe infections too. Low immunity may cause other opportunistic infections as well. As discussed earlier, there is no proper medicine and cure for AIDS exists, but it could be treated with ART medicines. Fortunately, researchers have recently shed light on the nutraceuticals used in AIDS patients, and adding further, they may improve quality of life with an increase in life expectancy. The report suggests that a study conducted on the HIV-infected adult population reveals that multivitamins therapy before ART significantly improves overall clinical outcomes and also boosts immunity to fight against HIV infection and other opportunistic infections. This chapter focuses on the HIV patient's immunity boosting with the help of multivitamin therapy. Also, we will take a look at how these vitamins improve the immunity of patients and related facts and figures from the literature.

3.1 INTRODUCTION

AIDS has been tabooed for several years in the economically backward regions of the world. In 2007 it was estimated that around 33 million people were living with this disease, and due to the development of modern medicines and drugs quality of life is improving rapidly in the world. There are several theories have been published, but one of them is very factual and impressive and follows science (Piot et al., 2001). Researchers are found that some patients with HIV infection are taking multivitamins daily, and surprisingly who do not take multivitamins supplements and have an infection are likely to get a severe form of the disease too early. Vitamin D, A, E &C were found to be playing a major role by effectively supporting patient immunity and further increasing immunity to take care of disease. Scientists have reported that immune health plays a major role in defending against HIV and supporting immunity with multivitamins supplements, which contain several vitamins and other nutrients (Ruxrungtham et al., 2004). Vitamin C, Vitamin E, Vitamin B1, Vitamin B2, Vitamin B6, Vitamin B12, and folate play a major role in the same. Again, it is uncertain how much these multivitamins one should take to get the desired effect, and doctors' follow-up must be taken by the patient to achieve the desired effect. Researchers are working on the proper estimation of the dose of each vitamin and vitamin in the combination for treating HIV infection as supplementary. Researchers concluded from the study that multivitamins (Vitamin B complex, C and E) daily therapy for 18 months improves immunity, including CD4 cells count (which drops very much in the HIV infection), increases weight, and improves quality of life (Türmen, 2003). Further, they added individual vitamins dose 18 mg of niacin, 70 mg of C, 1.4 mg of B1, 1.4 mg of B2, 1.9 mg of B6, 2.6 mcg of B12, 10 mg of E, and 0.4 mg of folic acid. Figure 3.1 depicts that multivitamin therapy in the right proportion in the right quantity with a combination of ART treatment is beneficial in reducing viral load and thereby restricting disease progression. Table 3.1 summarizes vitamins present in the multivitamin therapy with their food source and used in the viral infection. Figure 3.2 depicts multivitamin supplementary therapy in HIV-infected patients (Gilbert et al., 2007).

In this chapter, several important vitamins are covered, which has proven their value in the past and helped in improving HIV patient's lifestyle significantly (Nair & Maseeh, 2012). Here we also focused on the selective fat-soluble and water-soluble vitamins, which play an important role in the treatment of HIV patients. The researcher also summarizes each vitamin dose and their role individual role in HIV treatment (Visser et al., 2017). As per present data in the literature, it is suggested that HIV-infected patient treatment could be planned, such as HAART therapy in combination with multivitamin supplementary therapy (Isanaka et al., 2012). Figure 3.1 and Table 3.1 represents Vitamins/nutritional treatment for ART-naïve HIV-infected child. This chapter mainly shares light on how malnutrition affects HIV-infected children and how secondary opportunistic infections can be caught by the host (de Oliveira Falco & da Silveira, 2015).

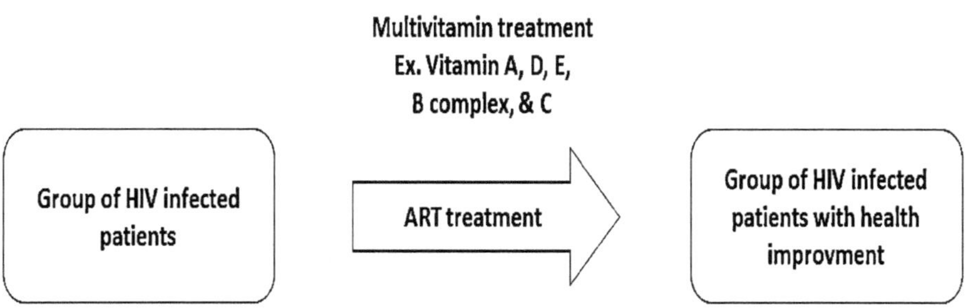

FIGURE 3.1 ART and multivitamin combination improve the health of HIV-infected patients.

TABLE 3.1 Vitamins-Rich Foods for the Management of HIV and AIDS

Sl. No.	Vitamin	Food Source	Disease	References
1.	Vitamin A	Fish, meat, and dairy products.	Human immunodeficiency virus infection	Mehta & Fawzi (2007); Makinde et al. (2017)
2.	Vitamin D	Fatty fish, dairy products, orange juice, cereals, beef liver, cheese, and egg yolks.	Human immunodeficiency virus infection.	Lake & Adams (2011); Villamor (2006); Chun et al. (2015)
3.	Vitamin E	Sunflower seeds, almonds, mango, avocado, and peanuts	Human immunodeficiency virus infection.	Allard et al. (1998); Rizvi et al. (2014); Wang & Watson (1994)
4.	Vitamin B1	Peas, fresh fruits, nuts, and wholegrain breads.	Human immunodeficiency virus infection.	Aris (2003); Thornalley (2005)
5.	Vitamin B2	Milk and dairy products and dark-green vegetables.	Human immunodeficiency virus infection.	Veilleux et al. (1995); Wamono et al. (2011)
6.	Vitamin B6	Fish, potatoes, vegetables, and fruit.	Human immunodeficiency virus infection.	Rail & Meydani (1993); Kesel et al. (1999)
7.	Vitamin B12	Fish, meat, milk, eggs, and cheese	Human immunodeficiency virus infection.	Gay & Meydani (2001); Rule et al. (1994); Tang et al. (1997)
8.	Vitamin C	Citrus fruit, orange, strawberries, sprouts, broccoli, and potatoes.	Human immunodeficiency virus infection.	Stephensen et al. (2006); Allard et al. (1998); Oliveira et al. (2011)

3.2 FAT SOLUBLE VITAMINS REPORTED IN THE LITERATURE ARE NOT SO COMMONLY USED IN THE TREATMENT OF THE HIV AND AIDS

According to the literature, here are some lists of the fat-soluble vitamins actually studied for the treatment of HIV and AIDS.

3.2.1 VITAMIN A

Vitamin A has been researched well for a long time for its effect against AIDS. It is also screened in HIV-positive children for their effectiveness, and more often, the results are surprising from the therapeutic point of view. It has been shown by researchers that it has a protective role in HIV infection in children and reduces mortality and morbidity significantly. All in all, multivitamin therapy is always preferred over a single vitamin for the patient. Vitamin A supplements for HIV-infected pregnant women and children show no evidence that they solely rescue infected people from HIV, but they reduce most of the causes of morbidity and mortality in the patients (Mehta & Fawzi, 2007). The HIV virus, as such, has no potential to cause cancer, but there are reports which say viruses like human papillomavirus (HPV) & hepatitis B have the potential to cause cancer. Vitamin A or Retinoic acid is the most natural form of the vitamin. Retinoic acid also plays an important role in embryonal cancer (Soprano et al., 2007). HIV infection rate and treatment remains a major challenge for developing countries. Reported literature sheds light on the vitamin A role in the prevention of transmission of HIV infection in children from mothers during pregnancy. The role of vitamin A, as such, is unknown, but researchers hypothesize that it has increased lymphoid cell differentiation (Mehta & Fawzi, 2007).

3.2.2 VITAMIN D

It's been known for a long time that HIV-AIDS patients have vitamin D deficiency. Researchers reported that vitamin D deficiency leads to a compromised antibacterial response in HIV-infected patients (Jiménez-Sousa et al., 2018). Hypovitaminosis D is the term used for such conditions wherein vitamin D deficiency occurs in HIV-infected patients. Normally, vitamin D shows its effect by binding to the vitamin D receptors, and it has direct natural resistance to the HIV-1 pathway. According to the literature, in the HIV-infected person, vitamin D deficiency leads to an increase in the chances of pathogenesis by negatively modulating the adaptive and innate immune systems. Low vitamin D levels can promote inflammation and increase the risk of morbidity in HIV-infected patients, but vitamin D prophylactic supplements can reduce this risk (Cervero et al., 2012; Lake & Adams, 2011).

3.2.3 VITAMIN E

As per recent data, there is an 8–10-fold mortality decrease after ART therapy in HIV patients. These figures indicate how ART therapy is improving life expectancy, indicating patients with HIV infection. In AIDS, patient's mortality has fallen 90-fold. From several studies, it has been found that vitamin E has many beneficial effects on the body, but first of all, it has immunomodulatory action. According to the literature, vitamin E is effective and well-tolerated in HIV-infected patients (Sebastiani et al., 2020). Some researchers speak about vitamin E deficiency in HIV-infected patients in their research. Some scientists focus on highly active antiretroviral therapy, which might have a direct impact on vitamin E concentration in the body. Researchers also found that patients with HAART therapy, especially new drugs, show low alpha-tocopherol concentrations. Therefore, it is suggested that physicians need to monitor vitamin E levels in HIV-infected patients before even starting the HAART regimen (Kaio et al., 2014).

3.3 WATER SOLUBLE VITAMINS REPORTED IN THE LITERATURE ARE COMMONLY USED IN THE TREATMENT OF HIV AND AIDS

According to the literature, here are some lists of the water-soluble vitamins actually studied for the treatment of HIV & AIDS.

3.3.1 VITAMIN B1

Vitamin B1 has established a role in HIV & AIDS. Several articles have been published on the said topic, and many research groups are working on it. It has been found that patients with HIV infection have thiamine deficiency. Vitamin B1 and HIV have been illustrated by many researchers, and thiamine provides a beneficial effect on HIV infection. In this scenario, genetic factors also provide different valuable parameters on the basis of which one can link thiamine's role in HIV pathogenesis. It is interesting to know that at non-genomic levels, thiamine also affects HIV pathogenesis, but the mechanism is yet to be known. Studies also revealed that thiamine levels were found to be low in patients with HIV infection. These mentioned hypotheses are yet to be clear with the help of scientific tools (Tattevin et al., 2006; Cissé et al., 2008; Cognat et al., 2010; Mouly, 1996).

3.3.2 VITAMIN B2 AND B6

Studies have revealed that vitamin B2 and vitamin B6 deficiency leads to humoral and cell-mediated immunity damage. These vitamins play a supporting role in the process of lymphocyte differentiation and maturation. Researchers are on their way to finding out the underlying mechanism for the same thing. Vitamin B2 and vitamin B6 levels in the body should be at the limit to show their immunomodulatory effect on the body, and it has been seen that patients with immunity-related diseases face problems related to low levels of vitamin B2 and vitamin B6 (Bouic et al., 2001). In HIV-infected patients, CD4 T cell levels go down significantly, and immunity weakens within days after HIV infection. Researchers also suggest from their studies that these immunomodulatory studies show good results and suggest having a bright future for treating HIV as a supplementary role to HAART therapy (Rail & Meydani, 1993).

3.3.3 VITAMIN B12

Talking about vitamin deficiency in HIV-infected patients is very common, but it has been reported several times that vitamin B12 plays a major role in HIV patients. Also, it is highly recommended that before starting any therapy for HIV-infected patients must put patients under a vitamin B12 deficiency test because it is reported by several researchers that vitamin B12 deficiency is very common in HIV-infected patients. In one meta-analysis, it has been shown that around 39% of the patient population has vitamin B12 deficiency (Ehrenpreis et al., 1994). In another review, researchers have found out that patients who are on ART therapy potentially have low levels of vitamin B12. On the other hand, some scientists reported that six out of 57 patients have low levels of serum B12 levels in the initial phase of HIV infection. Scientists also reported that after initiation of the ART treatment, serum vitamin B12 levels increase with time (Hepburn et al., 2004). Another group of researchers performed an evaluation of iron, folate, and vitamin B12 in HIV-infected patients, and they reported that only 6% of the patient population found normal corpuscular volumes (Castro & Goldani, 2009; Ahire et al., 2020).

3.3.4 VITAMIN C

Vitamin C is a potent natural anti-oxidant and is found to be in several nutritional Vitamin C is a potent natural anti-oxidant and is found to be in several nutritional supplements which are commercially available. Patients with HIV infection are known to be oxidative stressed persons. Studies have been conducted by a group of researchers where they found that the patients who were on the vitamin supplements had more plasma concentrations as compared to the control group. This group also showed a decrease in viral load than other groups. Study investigators reported that vitamin C and vitamin E have antioxidant activity as a reduction in viral load in the patient has been found (Allard et al., 1998). A group of researchers in 2009 published an article wherein they mentioned total antioxidant capacity as a new early detectable biochemical marker of oxidative stress in HIV-infected patients. Figure 3.2 shows vitamins/nutritional treatment for ART-naïve HIV-infected children. Results of the study suggest that HIV-1 seropositive patients show a marked increase in MDA levels as compared to control group patients, and vitamin C is a potent anti-oxidant that could be used in the future for combating this oxidative stress in HIV-1 seropositive patients (Suresh et al., 2009; Ahire et al., 2020). Figure 3.3 represents multivitamin supplementary therapy in HIV-infected patients.

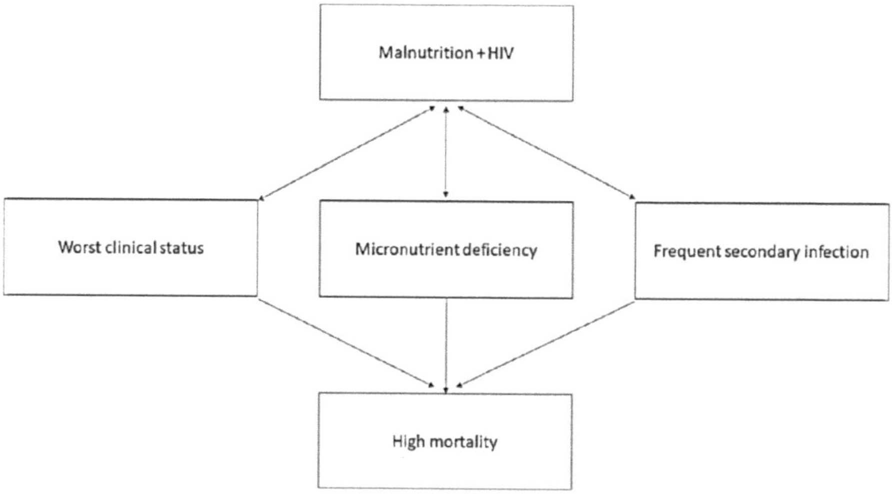

FIGURE 3.2 Vitamins/nutritional treatment for ART-naïve HIV-infected child.

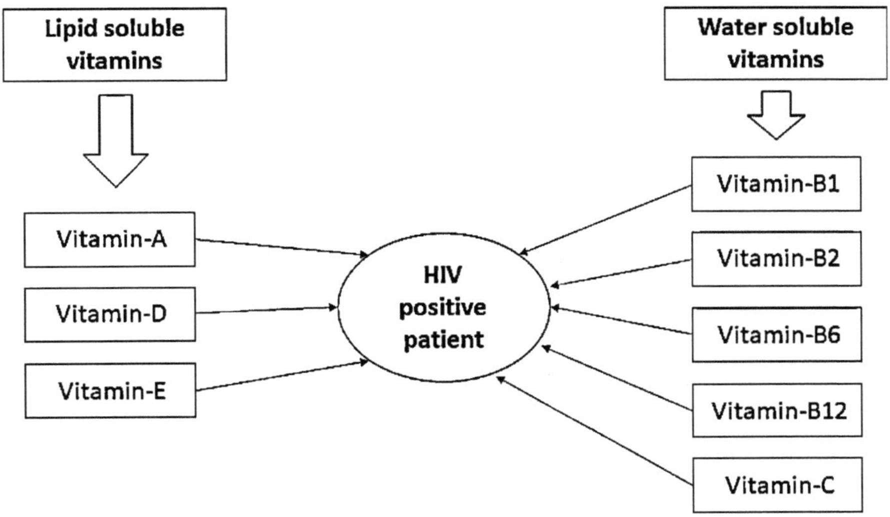

FIGURE 3.3 Multivitamin supplementary therapy in HIV infected patients.

3.4 CONCLUSION

To summarize, multivitamin therapy is the most successful therapy with the HAART treatment. A combination of these is suggested by researchers and scientists around the world for the treatment of HIV-infected patients. Research is in progress for estimating the exact dose of these vitamins to make it cost-effective and reduce related side effects. As HIV patients already have weakened immunity and if treatments have side effects, then for treating those side effects, patients need to take other medicines, but in the current decade, practice has been started to combat HAART treatment side effects by specifically using multivitamin therapy. These therapies are accepted worldwide, and highly effective study shows. In this chapter, we have focused on the HAART therapy and specific vitamin's role and facts available in the literature. Also, we have shed light on the combined use of these two approaches with the help of diagrams. Several vitamin deficiencies have been reported in the HIV-infected patients enlisted in this chapter. Physicians must screen patients for vitamin deficiency and then should start HAART treatment. The future is bright for multivitamin products with traditional treatments. According to some researchers and literature available to date, multivitamin treatments are going to be the gold standard treatment for AIDS in the near future.

ACKNOWLEDGMENTS

We thank Glenmark Pharmaceuticals Ltd. Mumbai, METs, Institute of Pharmacy, Adgaon, Nashik, and Mahatma Gandhi Vidyamandir's Pharmacy College, Panchavati, Nashik, Maharashtra, India, for their constant support and providing all facilities to complete this work. Also, many thanks to all the known and unknowns who helped us right from the writing till the publishing of this chapter.

KEYWORDS

- **fat-soluble vitamins**
- **HAART therapy**
- **HIV and AIDS**
- **nutraceuticals**
- **viral infections**
- **vitamins**
- **water-soluble vitamins**

REFERENCES

Ahire, E. D., Sonawane, V. N., & Surana, K. R., (2020). Role of drug repurposing in current treatment strategies against COVID-19; systemic review. *Pharm. Reson.*, 24–29.

Ahire, E. D., Surana, K. R., Patil, C. D., Shah, H. S., Sonwane, G. B., & Talele, S. G., (2020). Role of omega-3 fatty acids in different neurodegenerative disorders. *Applied Pharmaceutical Science and Microbiology: Novel Green Chemistry Methods and Natural Products*, 173.

Allard, J. P., Aghdassi, E., Chau, J., Tam, C., Kovacs, C. M., Salit, I. E., & Walmsley, S. L., (1998). Effects of vitamin E and C supplementation on oxidative stress and viral load in HIV-infected subjects. *Aids, 12*(13), 1653–1659.

Aris, B., (2003). Maker of vitamin B1-deficient baby milk admits error. *The Lancet, 362*(9397), 1730.

Bouic, P. J. D., Clark, A., Brittle, W., Lamprecht, J. H., Freestone, M., & Liebenberg, R. W., (2001). *Plant Sterol/Sterolin Supplement Use in a Cohort of South African HIV-Infected Patients: Effects on Immunological and Virological Surrogate Markers. 91*(10), 848–850.

Castro, L., & Goldani, L. Z., (2009). Iron, folate, and vitamin B12 parameters in HIV-1 infected patients with anemia in southern Brazil. *Tropical Doctor, 39*(2), 83–85.

Cervero, M., Agud, J. L., García-Lacalle, C., Alcázar, V., Torres, R., Jusdado, J. J., & Moreno, G. S., (2012). Prevalence of vitamin D deficiency and its related risk factor in a Spanish cohort of adult HIV-infected patients: Effects of antiretroviral therapy. *AIDS Research and Human Retroviruses, 28*(9), 963–971.

Chun, R. F., Liu, N. Q., Lee, T., Schall, J. I., Denburg, M. R., Rutstein, R. M., Adams, J. S., et al., (2015). Vitamin D supplementation and antibacterial immune responses in adolescents and young adults with HIV/AIDS. *The Journal of Steroid Biochemistry and Molecular Biology, 148*, 290–297.

Cissé, A. F., Camara, N., Diallo, L. L., Morel, Y., Koné, S., Camara, M. I., Koumbassa, M. L., et al., (2008). Gayet-Wernicke's encephalopathy. A study of 13 cases observed in a refugee population hospitalized at the Conakry teaching hospital. *Bulletin de la Societe de Pathologie Exotique (1990), 101*(5), 402, 403.

Cognat, E., Hainque, E., Mesnage, V., & Levy, R., (2010). Severe dysautonomia revealing Wernicke's encephalopathy. *Revue Neurologique, 167*(3), 250–253.

De Oliveira, F. M., & Da Silveira, E. A., (2015). Nutritional treatment approach for ART-naïve HIV-infected children. In: *Health of HIV Infected People* (pp. 75–93). Academic Press.

Ehrenpreis, E. D., Carlson, S. J., Boorstein, H. L., & Craig, R. M., (1994). Malabsorption and deficiency of vitamin B12 in HIV-infected patients with chronic diarrhea. *Digestive Diseases and Sciences, 39*(10), 2159–2162.

Gay, R., & Meydani, S. N., (2001). The effects of vitamin E, vitamin B6, and vitamin B12 on immune function. *Nutrition in Clinical Care, 4*(4), 188–198.

Gilbert, M. T. P., Rambaut, A., Wlasiuk, G., Spira, T. J., Pitchenik, A. E., & Worobey, M., (2007). The emergence of HIV/AIDS in the Americas and beyond. *Proceedings of the National Academy of Sciences, 104*(47), 18566–18570.

Hepburn, M. J., Dyal, K., Runser, L. A., Barfield, R. L., Hepburn, L. M., & Fraser, S. L., (2004). Low serum vitamin B12 levels in an outpatient HIV-infected population. *International Journal of STD & AIDS, 15*(2), 127–133.

Isanaka, S., Mugusi, F., Hawkins, C., Spiegelman, D., Okuma, J., Aboud, S., Guerino, C., & Fawzi, W. W., (2012). Effect of high-dose vs standard-dose multivitamin supplementation at the initiation of HAART on HIV disease progression and mortality in Tanzania: A randomized controlled trial. *JAMA, 308*(15), 1535–1544.

Jiménez-Sousa, M. Á., Martínez, I., Medrano, L. M., Fernández-Rodríguez, A., & Resino, S., (2018). Vitamin D in human immunodeficiency virus infection: Influence on immunity and disease. *Frontiers in Immunology, 9*, 458.

Kaio, D. J. I., Rondó, P. H. C., Luzia, L. A., Souza, J. M. P., Firmino, A. V., & Santos, S. S., (2014). Vitamin E concentrations in adults with HIV/AIDS on highly active antiretroviral therapy. *Nutrients, 6*(9), 3641–3652.

Kesel, A. J., Sonnenbichler, I., Polborn, K., Gürtler, L., Klinkert, W. E., Modolell, M., Nüssler, A. K., & Oberthür, W., (1999). A new antioxidative vitamin B6 analog modulates pathophysiological cell proliferation and damage. *Bioorganic & Medicinal Chemistry, 7*(2), 359–367.

Lake, J. E., & Adams, J. S., (2011). Vitamin D in HIV-infected patients. *Current HIV/aids Reports, 8*(3), 133–141.

Makinde, O., Rotimi, K., Ikumawoyi, V., Adeyemo, T., & Olayemi, S., (2017). Effect of vitamin A and vitamin C supplementation on oxidative stress in HIV and HIV-TB co-infection at Lagos university teaching hospital (LUTH) Nigeria. *African Health Sciences, 17*(2), 308–314.

Mehta, S., & Fawzi, W., (2007). Effects of vitamins, including vitamin A, on HIV/AIDS patients. *Vitamins & Hormones, 75*, 355–383.
Mouly, S., (1996). Beri-Beri and thiamine deficiency in HIV infection. *Aids, 10*(8), 931.
Nair, R., & Maseeh, A., (2012). Vitamin D: The "sunshine" vitamin. *Journal of Pharmacology & Pharmacotherapeutics, 3*(2), 118.
Oliveira, K. F. D., Cunha, D. F. D., & Weffort, V. R. S., (2011). Analysis of serum and supplemented vitamin C and oxidative stress in HIV-infected children and adolescents. *Jornal De Pediatria, 87*, 517–522.
Piot, P., Bartos, M., Ghys, P. D., Walker, N., & Schwartländer, B., (2001). The global impact of HIV/AIDS. *Nature, 410*(6831), 968–973.
Rail, L. C., & Meydani, S. N., (1993). Vitamin B6 and immune competence. *Nutrition Reviews, 51*(8), 217–225.
Rail, L. C., & Meydani, S. N., (1993). Vitamin B6 and immune competence. *Nutrition Reviews, 51*(8), 217–225.
Rizvi, S., Raza, S. T., Faizal, A. A. A., Abbas, S., & Mahdi, F., (2014). The role of vitamin E in human health and some diseases. *Sultan Qaboos University Medical Journal, 14*(2), e157.
Rule, S. A. J., Hooker, M., Costello, C., Luck, W., & Hoffbrand, A. V., (1994). Serum vitamin B12 and transcobalamin levels in early HIV disease. *American Journal of Hematology, 47*(3), 167–171.
Ruxrungtham, K., Brown, T., & Phanuphak, P., (2004). HIV/AIDS in Asia. *The Lancet, 364*(9428), 69–82.
Sebastiani, G., Saeed, S., Lebouche, B., De Pokomandy, A., Szabo, J., Haraoui, L. P., Routy, J. P., et al., (2020). Vitamin E is an effective treatment for nonalcoholic steatohepatitis in HIV mono-infected patients. *Aids, 34*(2), 237–244.
Soprano, D. R., Teets, B. W., & Soprano, K. J., (2007). Role of retinoic acid in the differentiation of embryonal carcinoma and embryonic stem cells. *Vitamins & Hormones, 75*, 69–95.
Stephensen, C. B., Marquis, G. S., Jacob, R. A., Kruzich, L. A., Douglas, S. D., & Wilson, C. M., (2006). Vitamins C and E in adolescents and young adults with HIV infection. *The American Journal of Clinical Nutrition, 83*(4), 870–879.
Suresh, D. R., Annam, V., Pratibha, K., & Prasad, B. V., (2009). Total antioxidant capacity–a novel early biochemical marker of oxidative stress in HIV-infected individuals. *Journal of Biomedical Science, 16*(1), 1–4.
Tang, A. M., Graham, N. M., Chandra, R. K., & Saah, A. J., (1997). Low serum vitamin B-12 concentrations are associated with faster human immunodeficiency virus type 1 (HIV-1) disease progression. *The Journal of Nutrition, 127*(2), 345–351.
Tattevin, P., Souala, F., Revest, M., Taussig, D., & Michelet, C., (2006). Confusion, memory disorders, and ophthalmoparesis in a patient with AIDS. *The Lancet, 367*(9507), 368.
Thornalley, P. J., (2005). The potential role of thiamine (vitamin B1) in diabetic complications. *Current Diabetes Reviews, 1*(3), 287–298.
Türmen, T., (2003). Gender and HIV/AIDS. *International Journal of Gynecology & Obstetrics, 82*(3), 411–418.
Veilleux, M., Paltiel, O., & Falutz, J., (1995). Sensorimotor neuropathy and abnormal vitamin B12 metabolism in early HIV infection. *Canadian Journal of Neurological Sciences, 22*(1), 43–46.
Villamor, E., (2006). A potential role for vitamin D on HIV infection? *Nutrition Reviews, 64*(5), 226–233.

Visser, M. E., Durao, S., Sinclair, D., Irlam, J. H., & Siegfried, N., (2017). Micronutrient supplementation in adults with HIV infection. *Cochrane Database of Systematic Reviews*, (5).

Wamono, E. B. K., Kaaya, A. N., Wamue, G., Manyama, A., Mwangi, M., & Muyonga, J. H., (2011). Nutrient enhancement of matooke banana for improved nutrient intake of people living with HIV/AIDS in Rakai District, Uganda. *African Journal of Food, Agriculture, Nutrition and Development, 11*(4).

Wang, Y., & Watson, R. R., (1994). Potential therapeutics of vitamin E (tocopherol) in AIDS and HIV. *Drugs, 48*(3), 327–338.

CHAPTER 4

Vitamins as Nutraceuticals for Peptic Ulcer

AFSAR S. PATHAN,[1] MANOJ S. PATIL,[1] PANKAJ G. JAIN,[1] EKNATH D. AHIRE,[2] RAJ K. KESERVANI,[3] and SAYALI P. AHER[1]

[1]*Department of Pharmacology, R.C. Patel Institute of Pharmaceutical Education and Research, Shirpur, Maharashtra, India*

[2]*Department of Pharmaceutics, METs, Institute of Pharmacy, BKC, Affiliated to Savitribai Phule Pune University, Adgaon, Nashik, Maharashtra, India*

[3]*Faculty of B. Pharmacy, CSM Group of Institutions, Prayagraj, Uttar Pradesh, India*

ABSTRACT

A peptic ulcer is the most common disease worldwide. The word peptic ulcer refers to a digestive tract acid peptic injury that results in a mucosal break that reaches the sub-mucosa. A basic paradigm for ulcer disease is the imbalance between the digestive activity of acid and pepsin and the protective mechanisms in place to resist mucosal digestion. Incidence of PUD increases with age, with most ulcers occurring between 25 and 64 years of age; the main pathogenesis behind peptic ulcer is H pylori infection and nonsteroidal anti-inflammatory drugs. Nutraceutical is a product confined or purified from food products that are usually sold in meditative forms, and vitamins are the most famous class of Nutraceuticals. Vitamins having a variety of biological effects and different properties are most useful for counteracting the pathogenesis of peptic ulcers via the antioxidant and anti-inflammatory effects. Due to the side effect of the medicine available in the market world

Preventive and Therapeutic Role of Vitamins as Nutraceuticals. Khemchand R. Surana, Eknath D. Ahire, Raj K. Keservani, & Rajesh K. Kesharwani (Eds.)

moving towards Nutraceuticals, in this chapter, we focus on all insights from peptic ulcer and vitamins.

4.1 INTRODUCTION

Peptic ulcer disease is a word that refers to peptic ulcers that occur in the stomach or duodenum (Lanas & Chan, 2017). Peptic ulcers are caused by acid peptic injury to the digestive tract, follow-on by a mucosal break that reaches the submucosa. Although peptic ulcers are most frequently detected in the stomach or proximal duodenum, they can also arise in the esophagus or Meckel's diverticulum. Recent advancements have resulted in a better knowledge of peptic ulcer pathogenesis. The imbalance between the digestive activity of acid and pepsin and the preventive systems in place to resist mucosal digestion is a core paradigm for ulcer development. Although various irregularities in the regular physiology of the stomach and duodenum have been discovered in ulcer patients, it is still unclear which abnormalities are the most significant. Individuals may have different essential defects or numerous faults may contribute to the common denominator of ulceration (Mertz & Walsh, 1991). Over the last 30 years, the incidence of peptic ulcers has dropped considerably. This is owing to advancements in the pharmaceutical treatment of dyspeptic symptoms and also a better understanding of the etiology. Previously, surgery was a common treatment for chronic peptic ulcer disease (Stewart & Ackroyd, 2011). Historically, it was believed that peptic ulcer disease was caused by a hypersecretory acidic medium compounded with dietary components or tension, but the discovery of *Helicobacter pylori* and the pervasive utilization of nonsteroidal anti-inflammatory drugs (NSAIDs) there in the second half of the 20th century altered this perception of (Miyake et al., 2013).1–3 people with peptic ulcer disease (PUD) are at risk for consequences like gastroduodenal bleeding, perforation, and blockage, and mortality rates are significant among individuals who suffer these complications (Sung, Kuipers & El-Serag, 2009). Peptic ulcer disease (PUD) of the stomach and duodenum was an epidemic in the late 1800s and early 1900s. Because of overcrowding and inadequate sanitation, the frequency of PUD peaked during the period of the industrial revolution, but there were considerable geographical and chronological differences in magnitude (Malfertheiner & Schulz, 2020). PUD is more common as people become older, with the majority of ulcers developing involving the ages of 25 and 64. If correctly examined, the majority of patients with uncomplicated PUD can be successfully treated. Nursing assessment can assist in preventing linked issues in persons who are at risk for and/or have PUD (Dunlap & Patterson, 2019).

4.2 TYPES OF PEPTIC ULCER (BROOKS, 1985)

4.2.1 ON THE BASIS OF LOCATION

1. **Gastric Ulcer:** The development of an ulcer in the stomach, which occurs more frequently in those over the age of 50.
2. **Duodenal Ulcer:** An ulcer develops in the duodenum. They are more common in younger people and are equally dispersed across socioeconomic groups. Acid secretion rates in these patients are higher than usual.

4.2.2 DEPENDING ON SEVERITY

1. **Acute Peptic Ulcer:** These ulcers can affect cells all the downward to the submucosa, leading them to rupture. They might appear as a single lesion or as a cluster of lesions. These cells can be found in a number of different locations throughout the stomach, in addition to the next few millimeters of the duodenum.
2. **Chronic Peptic Ulcer:** These ulcers can spread to the pancreas or liver, as well as to the epithelium and muscular regions of the stomach wall and causing pain and discomfort. In the vast majority of instances, they are found alone in the pyloric antrum of the gut and the duodenum of the small intestine (Gulia & Choudhary, 2011).

4.3 PATHOGENESIS OF PEPTIC ULCER

Putting together all of the factors that cause peptic ulcers make it easier to understand how they work. They all work against each other, but *Helicobacter pylori* are the most frequent cause right now. The pathogenesis of peptic ulcer is finest recognized as a complex situation involving an imbalance between defensive (mucus-bicarbonate layer, prostaglandins, cellular renovation, and blood flow) and aggressive factors (hydrochloric acid, pepsin, ethanol, bile salts, some medications, etc.) (Sivri, 2004). Several environmental and host factors, such as increased stomach acid output or a weakening of the mucosal barrier, contribute to ulcer formation (Malfertheiner, Chan, & McColl, 2009). Our understanding of peptic ulcer disease pathophysiology was centered on abnormalities in stomach acid and pepsin secretion, also the use of acid suppression as a therapy method. In modern peptic ulcer disease, gastric hypersecretion associated with gastrinoma in Zollinger–Ellison syndrome, antral G-cell hyperplasia, a growth in parietal-cell mass, and a physiological mismatch between the antagonistic gastric hormones gastrin and somatostatin remains a significant problem. Additionally, it is well established that cholinergic extreme sensitivity and parasympathetic domination are associated with the activation of not just hydrochloric acid but also pepsin, a sometimes-ignored cofactor in the development of erosive injury to the stomach mucosa (Yuan, Padol, & Hunt, 2006).

In the United States, the most prevalent causes of peptic ulcer disease are *Helicobacter pylori* infection and nonsteroidal anti-inflammatory drug (NSAID) use, accounting for 48% and 24% of the cases, respectively. Certain infections and comorbidities (e.g., CMV, tuberculosis, Crohn's disease, hepatic cirrhosis, chronic renal failure, sarcoidosis, and myeloproliferative disorder) have been associated with an increased chance of developing peptic ulcer disease. Gastroduodenal erosions or ulcers (stress ulcers) can develop as a result of hospitalization, surgery, or hypovolemia, which results in splanchnic hypoperfusion; they might be quiet or present with bleeding or perforation. Smoking raises the hazard of recurrence of ulcers and hinders the healing process (Kron, 2008).

4.3.1 *H. PYLORI*

Peptic ulcer disease is frequent in India, yet there are limited statistics available on the prevalence of the condition. Earlier Indian studies on the prevalence of peptic ulcers were not community-based, and they may have been biased as a result. Furthermore, surveys that rely on symptoms to diagnose peptic ulcers are hampered by the asymptomatic nature of some peptic ulcers. *Helicobacter pylori* (*H. pylori*) is believed to be the principal cause of gastritis and peptic ulcers and a probable cause of stomach cancer (Virendra et al., 2002). According to the World Health Organization, *H. pylori* is still on *H. pylori* is still one of the most pathogens on the planet. Due to increased hygiene and lower transmission in early life, the incidence of *H. pylori* has decreased in developed countries. Because of varied diagnostic procedures and geographical differences, the mean prevalence of *H. pylori* in patients with PPU differs between research. From the prepyloric antrum to the cardia, H pylori colonizes the whole stomach epithelium. The pattern of persistent mucosal inflammation that is produced has an impact on clinical outcomes. In individuals with duodenal ulcers, the infection density and degree of inflammation are greatest in the distal antral region, but the acid-secreting body mucosa is unaffected. Gastric mucosal alterations are usually totally reversible after H pylori eradication. Inflammation affects the body and antral mucosa to a similar extent in gastric ulcers, albeit the severity varies depending on the ulcer's location. Because gastric ulcers are more severe than duodenal ulcers in terms of involvement of the acid-secreting body mucosa, However, a major portion of acid production is always preserved (Malfertheiner, Chan, & McColl, 2009). Mucosal inflammation is caused by *H. pylori* infection. *H. pylori*-related disease is most likely caused by the presence and degree of inflammation. The potential of *H. pylori* strains to generate inflammation varies, and strains that cause severe inflammation are more likely to cause symptomatic disease. Despite the fact that strains differ in virulence, none are avirulent, as every strain can cause inflammation, peptic ulcers, or stomach cancer (Shiotani & Graham, 2002). Infected mucosa in humans has been linked to increased reactive oxygen species (ROS), oxidative DNA damage, and decreased GSH levels. However, no unique *H. pylori* virulence factor has been found to be linked to oxidative stress during *H. pylori* infection. H pylori also use CagA, OipA, and other factors to upregulate interleukin-8 (IL-8) expression in human gastric mucosa *in vivo* and in gastric epithelial cells *in vitro*. Neutrophil activation and infiltration are caused by this cascade of events, which leads to inflammation-related mucosal damage and carcinogenesis. The combination of these factors can cause epithelial cell damage, making gastritis, peptic ulcer disease (PUD), and potentially stomach cancer more likely. However, no study has directly linked *H. pylori* GGT to the creation of reactive oxygen species (ROS), which causes DNA damage and elevation of IL-8 production, culminating in *H. pylori*-mediated gastroduodenal disorders (Gong et al., 2010).

4.3.2 NSAIDS

Because of its analgesic, anti-inflammatory, and antipyretic properties, prescription nonsteroidal anti-inflammatory medications (NSAIDs) are used by more than 30 million individuals globally every day (Melcarne, García-Iglesias, & Calvet, 2016). Since Vane's 1971 discovery that NSAIDs block prostaglandin production, there has been significant evidence that the ulcerogenic impact of an NSAID correlates well with its capacity to suppress prostaglandin synthesis. Endogenous prostaglandins control mucosal blood flow, epithelial cell proliferation, epithelial restoration, mucosal immunocyte activity, mucus and bicarbonate production, and basal acid secretion. Prostaglandin production inhibition likely lowers the stomach mucosal defense against luminal irritants (Kron, 2008). Although inhibition of prostaglandin synthesis is a key element in NSAIDs' ulcerogenic action, it is not the sole one. Mice with faulty gastric prostaglandin production did not develop gastric ulcers on their own. The significance of nitric oxide (NO) in maintaining gastric-mucosal blood flow has received a lot of attention recently. NO has been demonstrated to increase mucosal blood flow, induce mucus secretion, and limit neutrophil adhesion, similar to prostaglandins. NO-releasing NSAIDs have less gastrointestinal harm in animals than their patent medicines, and they even help ulcers recover (Chan & Leung, 2002). The inhibition of COX1 and its role in normal mucosal defense mechanisms (described above), as well as the inhibition of thromboxane A2, which limits platelet function and leads to gastrointestinal bleeding, are the main causes of NSAIDs' harmful gastrointestinal effects. A number of clinical studies have demonstrated that coxibs are linked with fewer ulcers, gastrointestinal bleeding, and ulcer complications than nonselective nonsteroidal anti-inflammatory drugs (NSAIDs) but that this effect is attenuated when taken with low-dose aspirin. Many patients are predicted to transition back to nonselective NSAIDs as a result of the removal of multiple coxibs, with an increase in gastrointestinal bleeding, especially in the elderly (Yuan, Padol, & Hunt, 2006).

4.3.3 MECHANISM OF ACTION

The therapeutic benefits of nonsteroidal anti-inflammatory drugs (NSAIDs) are mediated via the inhibition of prostanoid production. Prostanoid derivatives are formed when arachidonic acid is converted by cyclo-oxygenase (COX) isoenzymes in response to cell damage. COX comes in two different isoforms. COX-1 is found in almost all cells, including endothelial cells, gastrointestinal epithelial cells, and platelets, and it is constantly active. COX-2, on the other hand, is found in only a few tissues and is activated by inflammation. COX-2 is inhibited by NSAIDs, which have anti-inflammatory and analgesic properties. The medicines' stomach and renal toxicity is linked to their suppression of the COX-1 isoform. The inhibition of COX-1 and COX-2 varies depending on the NSAID type (Dini, 2017; Wallace, 2000). Oxidative tissue injury is caused by a combination of COX-dependent and COX-independent processes, which appears to play a key role in the pathophysiology of NSAID-induced stomach damage. Gastric mucosal levels of malondialdehyde (MDA), a result of tissue oxidation, have been reported to rise after NSAID use, supporting this theory. Furthermore, growth factors play a big role in stomach ulcer healing. VEGF (vascular endothelial growth factor) improves ulcer healing by stimulating the development of new microvessels, and indomethacin has been demonstrated to inhibit this process by inhibiting VEGF expression (Fornai et al., 2011).

The mechanisms of action and side effects of the most widely used antiulcer therapy alternatives are discussed in detail in Table 4.1 (Kuna et al., 2019).

TABLE 4.1 Current Antiulcer Treatment and Their Side Effects

Sl. No.	Category	Medicine	Mechanism of Action	Adverse Effect	References
1.	Proton pump inhibitors (PPIs)	Omeprazole, Lansoprazole, Rabeprazole, Esomeprazole, Pantoprazole	Inhibition of the gastric H^+/K^+ -ATPase (proton pump) enzyme system.	Headache, abdominal pain, diarrhea, nausea, vomiting, constipation, flatulence, vitamin B12 deficiency, osteoporosis	Kuna et al. (2019)
2.	H2 receptor blockers	Cimetidine, Famotidine, Nizatidine, Ranitidine	Blocking histamine function at parietal cells' histamine H2 receptors.	Headache, depression, anxiety, dizziness, cardiovascular incidents, thrombocytopenia	Haastrup et al. (2018)
3.	Antacids	Aluminum hydroxide, magnesium hydroxide	Increases stomach pH above four and inhibits pepsin's proteolytic action.	Not specified in terms of frequency: Nausea, vomiting, hypophosphatemia, taste is chalky, constipation	Henry & Langman (1981)
4.	Potassium-competitive acid blocker	Vonoprazan	At the final stage of the acid secretory pathway, inhibits H^+, K^+ -ATPase in gastric parietal cells.	Nasopharyngitis fall, contusion diarrhea, upper respiratory tract inflammation, eczema.	Akazawa, Fukuda, & Fukuda (2016)
5.	Cytoprotective agents	Misoprostol sucralfate	Increase mucus production and blood flow along the gastrointestinal tract's lining.	Constipation, back pain, diarrhea, abdominal pain, headache, constipation	Haastrup et al. (2018)

4.4 VITAMINS

4.4.1 INTRODUCTION

Nutrients are categorized into two major groups, i.e., macronutrients and micronutrients. Nutritional macronutrients are nutrients that our bodies require in significant amounts, whereas micronutrients are nutrients that our bodies require in small quantities. Carbohydrates, proteins (Keservani et al., 2015; Singh et al., 2017b), and lipids are all macronutrients that supply the structural and metabolic components of the human body (Akram et al., 2020a). Micronutrients (vitamins and minerals) are required for normal bodily functioning. Micronutrient requirements are determined by an individual's metabolic functions as well as his or her life cycle. There is no perfect definition for vitamins; they have been characterized as organic chemicals found in minute amounts in biological foodstuffs that are required for regular metabolism and whose absence from the diet causes deficiencies. However, this term is broad and could refer to a variety of molecules generated from the biosynthetic pathways of amino acids, simple sugars, and fatty acids (OSER, 1948). Vitamins are classified on their chemical and physical characteristics, such as their solubility in either water or lipid solvents. Traditional lipid transport systems absorb and transport vitamins that seem to be soluble in lipid solvents (vitamins A, D, E, and K) (Albahrani & Greaves, 2016). The relative solubility coefficients of water-soluble vitamins are key determinants of absorption efficiency. Water-soluble vitamins are typically absorbed by active mechanisms within physiological consumption levels (Akram et al., 2020b).

Vitamins are classified according to their physical characteristic and solubility pattern:

i. Water soluble vitamins;
ii. Water insoluble/fat soluble.

4.4.1.1 WATER SOLUBLE VITAMINS

Vitamins which are soluble in water are referred to as water-soluble vitamins, and the body doesn't store this type of vitamin and easily excretes them from the body, so it is necessary for the body to continue supplementation of water-soluble vitamins in the form of multivitamin tablets of vegetables. During food storage or preparation, water-soluble vitamins are quickly degraded or washed out. Vitamin loss can be reduced by properly storing and preparing meals (Steinberg & Rucker, 2005). Always keep fresh food refrigerated and keep milk and cereals away from intense light to avoid vitamin loss. The vitamin B-complex (Figure 4.1) collection includes thiamin (vitamin B1), riboflavin (vitamin B2), niacin (vitamin B3), vitamin B6 (pyridoxine), folate (folic acid), vitamin B12, biotin, and pantothenic acid, all are water-soluble vitamins. B vitamins may be found in a variety of foods, and their effects can be felt throughout the body. They work as coenzymes, assisting the body in converting food into energy (Chawla & Kvarnberg, 2014). The vital nutritional components choline, inositol, and ascorbic acid are needed in significant amounts in the diet and are frequently referred to as dietary nutrients rather than vitamins.

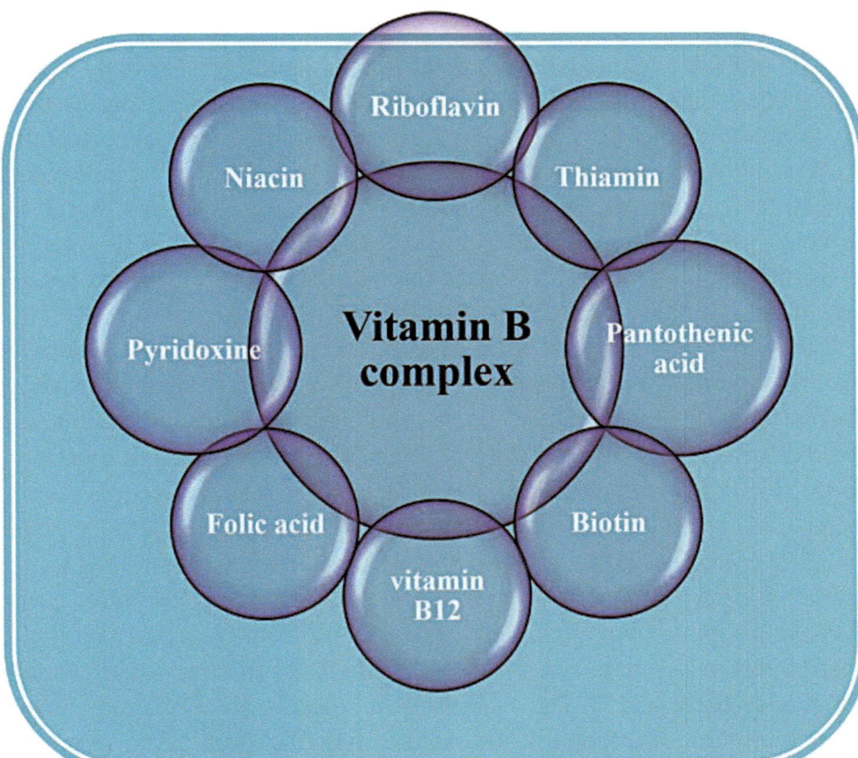

FIGURE 4.1 Vitamin B complex.

4.4.1.1.1 Vitamin C

Vitamin C, commonly known as ascorbic acid (AA), is a vitamin that is required by many multicellular organisms, including humans. Ascorbic acid is a water-soluble vitamin that is abundant in fruits and vegetables, as well as organ meats (e.g., liver and kidney). Scurvy, extensive connective tissue weakening, and capillary fragility are all symptoms of vitamin C deficiency. Vitamin C is involved in a variety of physiological activities in the body (OSER, 1948). It is required for tissue healing in all regions of the body. The production of protein required producing skin, tendons, ligaments, and blood vessels, for mending wounds and generating scar tissue, for restoring cartilage, bones, and teeth, and for assisting in the absorption of iron are all significant functions of vitamin C. Metal nanoparticles can also benefit from it as a reducing and capping agent (Devaki & Raveendran, 2017).

4.4.1.2 FAT SOLUBLE VITAMINS

The fat-soluble vitamins are essential fundamentals for the body's proper functioning. Their deficits have been linked to a variety of diseases. The fat-soluble vitamins A, D, E, and K's recommended daily amount (RDA) are 8,000–1,000 grams per day, 8,000–5,000 grams per day, 8–10 grams per day, and 70–140 grams per day, respectively (Albahrani & Greaves, 2016). Fat-soluble vitamins are classified into four groups: A, D, E, and K. Every one of the fat-soluble vitamins is broken down into a number of groups based on how they are made (Akram et al., 2020b).

Vitamin A has a complex molecular structure that includes 20 carbon materials, a methylcyclohexane ring, a hydroxyl group (retinol), an aldehyde group (retinal), and a carboxylic acid group (retinoic acid). It's a fat-soluble antioxidant vitamin that's yellow in color. Vitamin A comes in a variety of forms, including preformed vitamin A derived from animal sources, retinol, retinoic acid, and retinal, all of which are retinoids (Stevens, 2021). Vitamin A helps epithelial cells in the mucosa keep their membranes intact. The epithelial cells operate as a barrier throughout the body, providing protection against germs. For example, diarrhea can alter the mucosal lining of the gastrointestinal system, resulting in vitamin A insufficiency due to malabsorption (Alpert, 2017). The vitamin A in spinach, broccoli, and carrots is called carotene. Additionally, carotene is found in dark green leafy foods such as spinach as well as Carotene found in dark orange fruits like mangoes, apricots, amaranth, and catalog. It can also be found in milk and cream, eggs, cod liver oil, kidney, tomato juice, and watermelon.

Vitamin D: Vitamin D is a fat-soluble vitamin that is known for its antirachitic properties (treatment of rickets). Vitamin D is also called the "sunshine vitamin" because UV radiation from the sun may convert sterols in the skin to vitamin D. In 1922, McCollum was the first to coin the name vitamin D to describe its antirachitic properties (DeLuca, 2014). Vitamin D is necessary to maintain appropriate calcium and phosphate levels in the blood, which are required for proper bone mineralization, muscular contraction, nerve transmission, and overall cell signaling throughout all cells of the body. Vitamin D deficiency is uncommon since the body produces plenty of it. Hyperparathyroidism is caused by a deficiency in vitamin D in the diet. Hepatic and renal illnesses such as nephrotic syndrome, hepatobiliary syndrome, pancreatic abnormalities, aberrant metabolism, and anticonvulsant medication, among others, cause malabsorption of vitamin D. Due to insufficient calcification of bones, a deficiency may cause rickets (Patwardhan, 1945).

4.4.1.2.1 Vitamin E

The name vitamin E refers to eight fat-soluble elements synthesized in plant organisms and present to varying degrees in fat-rich foods, such as edible oils and seeds, or primarily as tocopherol in fortified foods. Vitamin E has been recognized as a necessary component for reproduction since 1922, but we still don't fully comprehend its physiological effects (Ungurianu et al., 2021). Vitamin E refers to a collection of tocopherols and tocotrienols, the most biologically active of which is a-tocopherol. Because of the high antioxidant characteristics of tocopherol, the role of a-tocopherol in the management of chronic conditions thought to be caused by oxidative stress has been extensively researched, with positive results (Niki & Traber, 2012).

Vitamin K: Vitamin K was found more than half a century ago as an effective antihemorrhagic factor for repairing diet-induced bleeding problems in chickens and also clotting deficiencies induced by obstructive jaundice and other biliary diseases in people. The term "clotting vitamin K" comes from the German word "coagulation vitamin" (McGuffey, 2017). Vitamin K is subclassified into K1 and K2. Vitamin K1 was extracted from alfalfa, while vitamin K2 was extracted from fish meal. Vitamin K1 is mainly found in green leafy vegetables like kale, spinach, and broccoli, but vitamin K2 is mostly found in meat, milk, cheese, and processed soy products like Natto (Booth, 2012). There is limited particular information about vitamin K status and needs in newborns, especially preterm infants, as compared to other fat-soluble vitamins. To prevent newborn hemorrhagic disease, At the moment of delivery, all normal and premature infants in the United States and Canada receive pharmacologic dosages of Vitamin K (Tarango, 2014). Figure 4.2 represents types of vitamins.

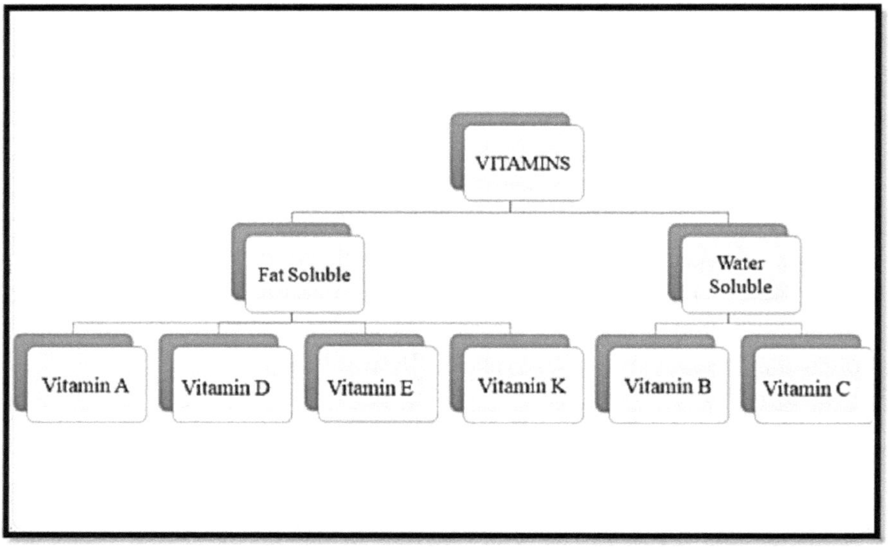

FIGURE 4.2 Types of vitamins.

4.5 VITAMINS AS NUTRACEUTICALS IN THE MANAGEMENT OF PEPTIC ULCER

DeFelice, head of the Foundation for Innovation in Medicine (FIM), coined the term "nutraceutical," which was later defined by Health Canada as "a product confined or purified from food products that is usually sold in medicative forms not usually associated with food and has been indicated to have a biological advantage as well as provide security against chronic disease (Focus, 2017). Nutraceuticals (Keservani et al., 2010a, b, 2017, 2020) include dietary supplements such as minerals, vitamins (Singh et al., 2017a), and antioxidants, as well as probiotics, herbs (Rane et al., 2020a–c), essential oils, and enriched meals and beverages. Reactive oxygen species (ROS) are produced in large quantities in the stomach, with concentrations 1,000 times greater than in other organs or plasma, and they are a major contributor to peptic ulcers" (Aronson, 2017). Exogenous injury to the stomach mucosa, such as damage caused by alcohol or nonsteroidal anti-inflammatory medications, is also aided by the production of reactive oxygen species (ROS; NSAIDs) (Dini, 2017). The most widely used vitamins in peptic ulcer are water-soluble vitamins, i.e., B complex and vitamin C, and some fat-soluble vitamins, like vitamins E and vitamin C, have good anti-inflammatory, antioxidant and other properties that are useful for the management of peptic ulcer. Vitamins are organic molecules which are required in micro-amounts for proper functioning of the organ systems. Their importance in the prevention and recovery of peptic ulcers has already been known. A study in 100 peptic ulcer patients was performed, and results indicated that the administration of Vitamin U (S-methyl methionine), administered as raw cabbage juice, was effective in promoting the rapid healing of uncomplicated peptic ulcers. Earlier, the animals were induced peptic ulcers by deficiencies in vitamins B1 and C (Field & Robinson, 1940). Also, Vitamin C levels are found to be low in the serum of patients suffering from peptic ulcers. Therefore, it has been reported that ascorbic acid supplementation has been found to reduce the bleeding from peptic ulcer and gastric cancer (Mei & Tu, 2018). Vitamin C has also been regarded to have a beneficial effect on the eradication of *H. pylori*, which is the causative organism for peptic ulcers. It is recommended that vitamin A and Vitamin C both serve as useful in the acute as well as recovery phase (Maria, 2014). Also, vitamin C has wound-healing properties, which add up to benefits in peptic ulcers.

4.5.1 VITAMIN A

Vitamin A can be taken as a supplement, although the evidence for this is limited because extremely high doses do not cure, and excessive intake can be hazardous. Vitamin A was administered to 24 patients at a dose of 50 000 units per day, whereas the vitamin was not given to 24 individuals. There was no indication that vitamin A had a favorable effect on the healing of stomach ulcers (Larsson et al., 2007).

4.5.2 VITAMIN C

Vitamin C is a major source of antioxidants and helpful in various diseases, which is cost-effective, and we can take it easily in diet or through supplementation. The main etiology of peptic ulcer is *Helicobacter pylori* and nonsteroidal anti-inflammatory drugs; in both of these conditions, the increased oxidative stress and decreased level of antioxidants. Water soluble vitamins have good antioxidant properties, and that's the reason vitamin C is most important for managing peptic ulcers (Aditi & Graham, 2012). Vitamin C protects the body against the damage caused by free radicals and reactive oxygen species (ROS) produced through normal metabolic processes, by active immune cells, and by exposure to toxins and pollutants

as an antioxidant. Vitamin C may be beneficial to the healing process of an ulcer as well as the ulcer's tendency to bleed. We don't have any direct proof in the case of the former. The role of ascorbic acid in collagen formation in experimental deficiencies and human scurvy, as well as its implications for wound healing, has been well established. As a result, it's possible that vitamin C intake has a role in the recovery of a peptic ulcer. Vitamin C also lowers the level of malondialdehyde inside the skin, which is an oxidative stress marker (Barja et al., 1994). Raw red and green peppers, oranges, grapefruits, kiwifruit, broccoli, strawberries, and Brussels sprouts are the foods with the greatest quantities of vitamin C, and we can add them into our daily diet behalf of other treatments for peptic ulcer. The final conclusion is based on *in vitro* and *in vivo* studies; an *in vitro* investigation revealed that a high dosage of vitamin C inhibited the development of *H. pylori*, indicating that vitamin C has bactericidal properties against *H. pylori*. Furthermore, *in vivo* investigations revealed that dietary vitamin C reduced the *H. pylori* burden (Mei & Tu, 2018). Figure 4.3 demonstrates a systematic illustration of vitamin C mechanism and sources.

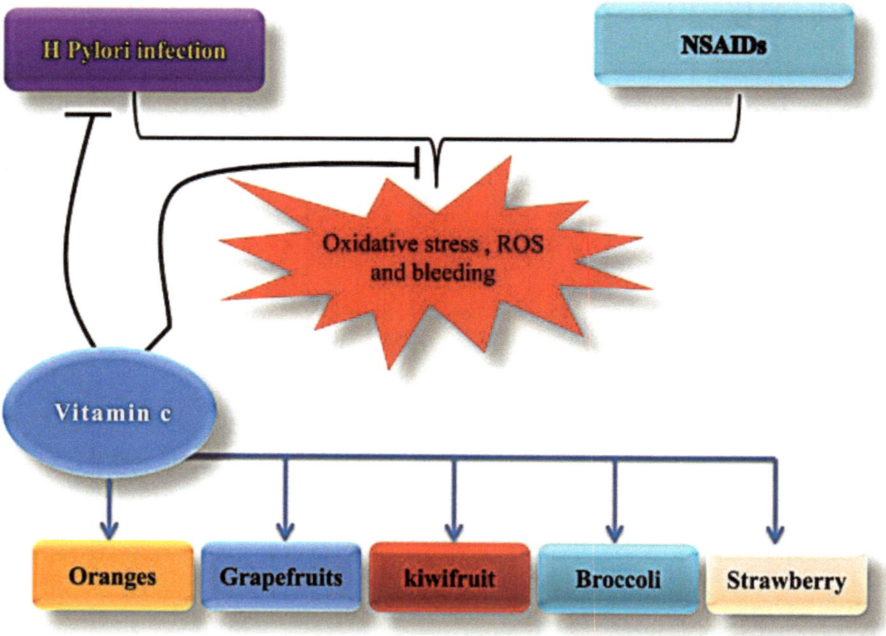

FIGURE 4.3 Systematic illustration of vitamin C mechanism and sources.

4.5.3 *VITAMIN E*

wide variety of NSAID use which can provoke gastric ulcer via different mechanism such as increasing reactive oxygen species, oxidative stress, and also through lipid peroxidation, and for counteract on this all-pathways vitamin E is the most useful asset due to its having, antioxidant, anti-inflammatory, and other activities. Alpha-tocopherol is a naturally antioxidant compound present in various locations and tissue in the body, which is important for radical scavenging activity; vitamin E prevents the radical induce injury via blocking the free radical chain reaction and also reduces the lipid peroxidation (Jaarin, Mtgapor, & Jaafar, 2006). Tocotrienol is a more influential antioxidant than gamma-tocopherol, according to researchers Serbinova and Packer. E concentration derived from palm oil, palmitate, includes around 80% tocotrienols and 20% tocopherols, with the remaining 20% being tocopherols. In this work, the efficiency of palmitate in preventing aspirin-induced stomach lesions in rats was compared to the effectiveness of pure tocopherol in this regard (Nafeeza et al., 2002). Principally via its antioxidant and anti-inflammatory properties ,it provides protection against ulcerogenic factors/agents (Kamisah et al., 2014). Prostaglandin production and secretion are increased as a result of the activation of enzymes in the presence of vitamin E (Yousaf, Ali, & Saeed, 2018).

4.6 CONCLUSIONS

Vitamins are the most promising assets for various disease by counteracting various pathogenesis pathway vitamins are the most powerful antioxidant and anti-inflammatory compound and also possess various biological activities; vitamins are broad categories into Nutraceuticals and functional food, which is easily available with low cost and minimize the risk of another side effect, peptic ulcer is a most common disease caused by *H. pylori* and NSAIDs via the generating ROS, increasing lipid peroxidation and by decreasing the defensive factor. The role of vitamins as a Nutraceutical in peptic ulcer is increasing day by day because vitamins have good counteracting properties to the peptic ulcer with lowering the risk of other effects.

ACKNOWLEDGMENTS

We thank the R.C. Patel Institute of Pharmaceutical Education and Research Shirpur, MH, India, for their constant support and providing all facilities to complete this work. Also, many thanks to all the known and unknowns who helped us right from the writing till the publishing of this chapter.

KEYWORDS

- **antioxidant**
- ***H. pylori***
- **NSAIDs**
- **nutraceuticals**
- **peptic ulcer**
- **vitamins**
- **water-soluble vitamins**

REFERENCES

Aditi, A., & Graham, D. Y., (2012). Vitamin C, gastritis, and gastric disease: A historical review and update. *Digestive Diseases and Sciences, 57*(10), 2504–2515. doi: 10.1007/s10620-012-2203-7.

Akazawa, Y., Fukuda, D., & Fukuda, Y., (2016). Vonoprazan-based therapy for *Helicobacter pylori* eradication: Experience and clinical evidence. *Therapeutic Advances in Gastroenterology, 9*(6), 845–852. doi: 10.1177/1756283X16668093.

Akram, M., et al., (2020a). Vitamins and minerals: Types, sources and their functions. *Functional Foods and Nutraceuticals*, 149–172. doi: 10.1007/978-3-030-42319-3_9.

Albahrani, A. A., & Greaves, R. F., (2016). Fat-soluble vitamins: Clinical indications and current challenges for chromatographic measurement. *The Clinical Biochemist Reviews, 37*(1), 27–47. Available at: http://www.ncbi.nlm.nih.gov/pubmed/27057076%0Ahttp://www.pubmedcentral.nih.gov/articlerender.fcgi?artid=PMC4810759 (accessed on 22 July 2023).

Alpert, P. T., (2017). The role of vitamins and minerals on the immune system. *Home Health Care Management and Practice, 29*(3), 199–202. doi: 10.1177/1084822317713300.

Aronson, J. K., (2017). Defining "nutraceuticals": Neither nutritious nor pharmaceutical. *British Journal of Clinical Pharmacology, 83*(1), 8–19. doi: 10.1111/bcp.12935.

Barja, G., et al., (1994). Dietary vitamin C decreases endogenous protein oxidative damage, malondialdehyde, and lipid peroxidation and maintains fatty acid unsaturation in the guinea pig liver. *Free Radical Biology and Medicine, 17*(2), 105–115. doi: 10.1016/0891-5849(94)90108-2.

Booth, S. L., (2012). Vitamin K: Food composition and dietary intakes. *Food and Nutrition Research, 56*, 1–5. doi: 10.3402/fnr.v56i0.5505.

Brooks, F. P., (1985). The pathophysiology of peptic ulcer disease. *Digestive Diseases and Sciences, 30*(11 Supplement), 15–29. doi: 10.1007/BF01309381.

Chan, F. K. L., & Leung, W. K., (2002). *Peptic-ulcer Disease, 360*, 933–941.

Chawla, J., & Kvarnberg, D., (2014). Hydrosoluble vitamins. *Handbook of Clinical Neurology* (1st edn.). Elsevier B.V. doi: 10.1016/B978-0-7020-4087-0.00059-0.

DeLuca, H. F., (2014). History of the discovery of vitamin D and its active metabolites. *Bonekey Reports, 3*, 1–8. doi: 10.1038/bonekey.2013.213.

Devaki, S. J., & Raveendran, R. L., (2017). Vitamin C: Sources, functions, sensing and analysis. *Vitamin C*. doi: 10.5772/intechopen.70162.

Dini, M. (2017). Peptic ulcer disease and nonsteroidal anti-inflammatory drugs. *Australian Prescriber, 40*(3), 91–93.

Dunlap, J. J., & Patterson, S. (2019). Peptic ulcer disease. *Gastroenterology Nursing, 42*(5), 451–454. doi: 10.1097/SGA.0000000000000478.

Field, B. H., & Robinson, W. D., (1940). Vitamins in peptic ulcer. *Annals of Internal Medicine, 14*(4), 588. doi 10.7326/0003-4819-14-4-588.

Focus, F., (2017). *Nutraceuticals / Functional Foods: An Exploratory Survey on Canada's Potential : Summary Report*, 4179. doi: 10.1300/J133v01n01.

Fornai, M., et al., (2011). Effects of esomeprazole on healing of nonsteroidal anti-inflammatory drug (NSAID)-induced gastric ulcers in the presence of a continued NSAID treatment: Characterization of molecular mechanisms. *Pharmacological Research, 63*(1), 59–67. doi: 10.1016/j.phrs.2010.10.013.

Gong, M., et al., (2010). *Helicobacter pylori* γ-glutamyl transpeptidase is a pathogenic factor in the development of peptic ulcer disease. *Gastroenterology, 139*(2), 564–573. doi: 10.1053/j.gastro.2010.03.050.

Gulia, Y., & Choudhary, M., (2011). *Ewsletter Gulia and Choudhary, 70*, 48–70.

Haastrup, P. F., et al., (2018). Side effects of long-term proton pump inhibitor use: A review. *Basic and Clinical Pharmacology and Toxicology, 123*(2), 114–121. doi: 10.1111/bcpt.13023.

Henry, D. A., & Langman, M. J. S., (1981). Adverse effects of anti-ulcer drugs. *Drugs, 21*(6), 444–459. doi: 10.2165/00003495-198121060-00004.

Jaarin, K., Mtgapor, & Jaafar, F., (2006). Effect of various doses of palm vitamin E and tocopherol on factors affecting gastric lesions in rats. *International Journal of Pharmacology, 2*(1), 98–103. doi: 10.3923/ijp.2006.98.103.

Kamisah, Y., et al., (2014). Vitamin E: A potential therapy for gastric mucosal injury. *Pharmaceutical Biology, 52*(12), 1591–1597. doi: 10.3109/13880209.2014.902082.

Keservani, R. K., Kesharwani, R. K., Sharma, A. K., Vyas, N., & Chadoker, A., (2010b). Nutritional supplements: An overview. *International Journal of Current Pharmaceutical Review and Research, 1*(1), 59–75.

Keservani, R. K., Kesharwani, R. K., Vyas, N., Jain, S., Raghuvanshi, R., & Sharma, A. K., (2010a). Nutraceutical and functional food as future food: A review. *Der Pharmacia Lettre, 2*(1), 106–116.

Keservani, R. K., Sharma, A. K., & Jarouliya, U. (2015). Protein and peptide in drug targeting and its therapeutic approach. *Ars Pharmaceutica (Internet), 56*(3), 165–177.

Keservani, R. K., Sharma, A. K., & Kesharwani, R. K. (2017). An overview and therapeutic applications of nutraceutical and functional foods. *Recent Advances in Drug Delivery Technology*, 160–201. ISBN:9781522507543.

Keservani, R. K., Sharma, A. K., & Kesharwani, R. K. (2020). *Nutraceuticals and Dietary Supplements: Applications in Health Improvement and Disease Management*. CRC Press. ISBN: 9781771888738.

Kron, J., (2008). Peptic ulcer disease. *Journal of Complementary Medicine*, *7*(1), 12–19. doi: 10.1300/j100v01n03_04.

Kuna, L., et al., (2019). Peptic ulcer disease: A brief review of conventional therapy and herbal treatment options. *Journal of Clinical Medicine*, *8*(2). doi: 10.3390/jcm8020179.

Lanas, A., & Chan, F. K. L., (2017). Peptic ulcer disease. *The Lancet*, *390*(10094), 613–624. doi: 10.1016/S0140-6736(16)32404-7.

Larsson, S. C., et al., (2007). Vitamin A, retinol, and carotenoids and the risk of gastric cancer: A prospective cohort study. *American Journal of Clinical Nutrition*, *85*(2), 497–503. doi: 10.1093/ajcn/85.2.497.

Malfertheiner, P., & Schulz, C., (2020). Peptic ulcer: Chapter closed? *Digestive Diseases*, *38*(2), 112–116. doi: 10.1159/000505367.

Malfertheiner, P., Chan, F. K., & McColl, K. E. L., (2009). Peptic ulcer disease. *The Lancet*, *374*(9699), 1449–1461. doi: 10.1016/S0140-6736(09)60938-7.

Maria, S., (2014). *Review Article Nutritional Care in Peptic Ulcer*, *27*(4), 298–302.

McGuffey, R. K. (2017). A 100-year review: Metabolic modifiers in dairy cattle nutrition. *Journal of Dairy Science*, *100*(12), 10113–10142. doi: 10.3168/jds.2017-12987.

Mei, H., & Tu, H., (2018). Vitamin C and *Helicobacter pylori* infection: Current knowledge and future prospects. *Frontiers in Physiology*, *9*(AUG), 1–12. doi: 10.3389/fphys.2018.01103.

Melcarne, L., García-Iglesias, P., & Calvet, X., (2016). Management of NSAID-associated peptic ulcer disease. *Expert Review of Gastroenterology and Hepatology*, *10*(6), 723–733. doi: 10.1586/17474124.2016.1142872.

Mertz, H. R., & Walsh, J. H., (1991). Peptic ulcer pathophysiology. *Medical Clinics of North America*, *75*(4), 799–814. doi: 10.1016/S0025-7125(16)30412-6.

Miyake, K., et al., (2013). Water-soluble vitamin deficiencies in complicated peptic ulcer patients soon after ulcer onset in Japan. *Journal of Nutritional Science and Vitaminology*, *59*(6), 503–508. doi: 10.3177/jnsv.59.503.

Nafeeza, M. I., et al., (2002). Comparative effects of a tocotrienol-rich fraction and tocopherol in aspirin-induced gastric lesions in rats. *Asia Pacific Journal of Clinical Nutrition*, *11*(4), 309–313. doi: 10.1046/j.1440-6047.2002.00298.x.

Niki, E., & Traber, M. G., (2012). History of vitamin E. *Annals of Nutrition and Metabolism*, *61*(3), 207–212. doi: 10.1159/000343106.

Oser, B. L., (1948). The vitamins. *Annual Review of Biochemistry*, *17*, 381–448. doi: 10.1146/annurev.bi.17.070148.002121.

Patwardhan, V. N., (1945). The vitamins. *Medical Digest*, *13*, 297–302. doi: 10.2307/3415286.

Rane, B. R., Bharath, M. S., Patil, R. R., Keservani, R. K., & Jain, A. S. (2020b). Novel approaches in nutraceuticals; Chapter 11. In: Rajesh, K. K., Raj, K. K., & Anil, K. S., (eds.), *Enhancing the Therapeutic Efficacy of Herbal Formulations Through Novel Drug Delivery Systems* (pp. 241–266). IGI Global International Publisher, Pennsylvania, USA. ISBN13: 9781799844532.

Rane, B. R., Patil, A. S., Keservani, R. K., & Jain, A. S., (2020a). Novel approaches in herbal formulation; Chapter 2. In: Rajesh, K. K., Raj, K. K., & Anil, K. S., (eds.), *Enhancing the*

Therapeutic Efficacy of Herbal Formulations Through Novel Drug Delivery Systems (pp. 43–68). IGI Global International Publisher, Pennsylvania, USA. ISBN13: 9781799844532.

Rane, B. R., Tadavi, S. A., & Keservani, R. K., (2020c). Naturopathy; Chapter 12. In: Anil, K. S., Raj, K. K., & Surya, P. G., (eds.), *Herbal Product Development* (pp. 321–347). Apple Academic Press, CRC Press, Taylor & Francis Group. ISBN: 9781771888776.

Shiotani, A., & Graham, D. Y., (2002). Pathogenesis and therapy of gastric and duodenal ulcer disease. *Medical Clinics of North America, 86*(6), 1447–1466. doi: 10.1016/S0025-7125(02)00083-4.

Singh, P., Kesharwani, R. K., & Keservani, R. K., (2017a). Antioxidants and vitamins: Roles in cellular function and metabolism. In: *Sustained Energy for Enhanced Human Functions and Activity* (pp. 385–407). Academic Press. ISBN:9780128054130.

Singh, P., Kesharwani, R. K., & Keservani, R. K., (2017b). Protein, carbohydrates, and fats: Energy metabolism. In: *Sustained Energy for Enhanced Human Functions and Activity* (pp. 103–115). Academic Press. ISBN:9780128054130.

Sivri, B., (2004). Trends in peptic ulcer pharmacotherapy. *Fundamental and Clinical Pharmacology, 18*(1), 23–31. doi: 10.1111/j.1472-8206.2004.00203.x.

Steinberg, F., & Rucker, R. B., (2005). *The Water-Soluble Vitamins*. doi: 10.1201/b15995-12.

Stevens, S. L., (2021). Fat-soluble vitamins. *Nursing Clinics of North America, 56*(1), 33–45. doi: 10.1016/j.cnur.2020.10.003.

Stewart, D. J., & Ackroyd, R., (2011). Peptic ulcers and their complications. *Surgery, 29*(11), 568–574. doi: 10.1016/j.mpsur.2011.08.006.

Sung, J. J. Y., Kuipers, E. J., & El-Serag, H. B., (2009). Systematic review: The global incidence and prevalence of peptic ulcer disease. *Alimentary Pharmacology and Therapeutics, 29*(9), 938–946. doi: 10.1111/j.1365-2036.2009.03960.x.

Tarango, C., (2014). *Disorders of Coagulation in the Neonate, Pathobiology of Human Disease: A Dynamic Encyclopedia of Disease Mechanisms*. Elsevier Inc. doi: 10.1016/B978-0-12-386456-7.07912-0.

Ungurianu, A., et al., (2021). Vitamin e beyond its antioxidant label. *Antioxidants, 10*(5), 1–37. doi: 10.3390/antiox10050634.

Virendra, S., Bandana, T., Chander, K. N., Kartar, S., & Vaiphei, K. (2002). *Helicobacter pylori*: Pathogenesis of gastric injury and epidemiology in India epidemiology of *Helicobacter pylori* and peptic ulcer in India. *Journal of Gastroenterology and Hepatology, 160012*, 659–665.

Wallace, J. L., (2000). How do NSAIDs cause ulcer disease? *Bailliere's Best Practice and Research in Clinical Gastroenterology, 14*(1), 147–159. doi: 10.1053/bega.1999.0065.

Yousaf, A., Ali, S., & Saeed, I. (2018). *Effect of Vitamin E on Indomethacin Induced Gastropathy in Mice Color Page, 22*(3), 291–293.

Yuan, Y., Padol, I. T., & Hunt, R. H., (2006). Peptic ulcer disease today. *Nature Clinical Practice Gastroenterology and Hepatology, 3*(2), 80–89. doi: 10.1038/ncpgasthep0393.

PART II

Vitamins in the Management of Infectious Diseases

CHAPTER 5

Vitamins as Nutraceuticals for Viral Infection

SNEHAL D. PAWAR,[1] SNEHAL S. KOLPE,[1] TUSHAR N. LOKHANDE,[2] KHEMCHAND R. SURANA,[3] SANTOSH R. TAMBE,[1] and CHANDRAKANT G. BONDE[4]

[1]*Department of Pharmaceutical Chemistry, M.G.V's Samajshri Prashant Dada Hiray, College of Pharmacy, Malegaon, Nashik, Maharashtra, India*

[2]*Department of Pharmaceutical Chemistry, Maharashtra Educational Society's H. K. College of Pharmacy, Oshiwara, Jogeshwari (W), Maharashtra, India*

[3]*Department of Pharmaceutical Chemistry, Shreeshakti Shaikshanik Sanstha, Divine College of Pharmacy, Satana, Nashik, Maharashtra, India*

[4]*School of Pharmacy and Technology Management, Mukesh Patel Technology Park, Babulde, Shirpur, Dhule, Maharashtra, India*

ABSTRACT

Vitamins are essential components of life, as they help in the prevention and control of various diseases, also required for normal cell function, growth, and development. Whereas nutraceuticals are substances with physiological benefits which help in the treatment of diseases. Nutraceuticals and pharmaceuticals are different from each other, where pharmaceuticals use drugs in the treatment of diseases, and nutrition that prevents diseases are used in nutraceuticals. Vitamins are used for various health conditions. Here, vitamins as nutraceuticals for viral infection are studied in detail. The present study will briefly help in understanding vitamins as nutraceuticals for viral infection.

Preventive and Therapeutic Role of Vitamins as Nutraceuticals. Khemchand R. Surana, Eknath D. Ahire, Raj K. Keservani, & Rajesh K. Kesharwani (Eds.)

5.1 INTRODUCTION

The term vitamin was coined in 1912 by the Polish biochemist Casimir Funk from "vitamine," a compound word while working at the Lister Institute of Preventive Medicine. They are a group of molecules required for ordinary cell functioning, growth, and development in small amounts (Maria et al., 2020). Vitamins are the classes of molecules that play a crucial role in the metabolism in order to fulfill all the nutritional value of food, and it is sometimes necessary to add those vitamins during processing (Alamgir et al., 2018). Vitamins (Singh et al., 2017a) are catalysts for metabolic reactions which use proteins (Keservani et al., 2015), fats (Singh et al., 2017b), as well as carbohydrates for energy, growth, and cell maintenance (Dickinson et al., 2014). Around 13 required vitamins are there, which are utilized for normal body functioning. Based on solubility, vitamins are characterized in subsections. Table 5.1 represents the names of vitamins with a year of discovery.

5.1.1 CLASSIFICATIONS OF VITAMINS (PARVEEN & SRINIVAS, 2017)

1. **Water Soluble:**
   i. Non-B complex-ascorbic acid (Vitamin C);
   ii. B-complex:
      a. Thiamine (Vitamin B_1);
      b. Riboflavin (Vitamin B_2);
      c. Niacin (Vitamin B_3);
      d. Biotin, pantothenic acid;
      e. Folic acid;
      f. Vitamin B_{12};
      g. Pyridoxine (Vitamin B_6);
      h. Pyridoxal, pyridoxamine.
2. **Fat Soluble:**
   a. Vitamin A;
   b. Vitamin D;
   c. Vitamin E;
   d. Vitamin K.

5.1.2 FUNCTIONS OF VITAMINS

1. One of the main functions of vitamins is to help release the energy found in food.

2. Vitamins help build protein and help your cells multiply.
3. They make collagen, which helps in wound healing, and it also supports blood vessel walls, and promotes strong bones and teeth.
4. They help in keeping the eyes, skin, lungs, digestive tract, and nervous system in proper condition.
5. It provides protection against diseases (Eknath et al., 2020; Nitu et al., 2019; Anup et al., 2021).

5.1.3 DISCOVERY YEAR OF VITAMINS

TABLE 5.1 Name of Vitamins with Year of Discovery (Kogl et al., 1936)

Sl. No.	Name of Vitamin	Name of Scientist	Invention Year
1.	Retinol, retinal, and retinyl esters (Vitamin A)	Thomas Osborne and Lafayette Mendel.	1913
2.	Thiamine (Vitamin B_1)	Casimir Funk	1910
3.	Riboflavin (Vitamin B_2)	D. T. Smith, E. G. Hendrick	1920
4.	Niacin (Vitamin B_3)	Conrad Elvehjem	1937
5.	Pantothenic acid (Vitamin B_5)	Roger J. Williams	1919
6.	Pyridoxine (Vitamin B_6)	Paul Gyorgy	1934
7.	Biotin (Vitamin B_7)	Dean Burk	1936
8.	Folic acid (Vitamin B_9)	Lucy Wills	1933
9.	Cobalamin (Vitamin B_{12})	Filkers	1948
10.	Ascorbic acid (Vitamin C)	James Lind, A. Hoist and T. Froehlich	1920
11.	Calciferol (Vitamin D)	Edward Mellanby	1922
12.	Tocopherol (Vitamin E)	Hertbert Evans and Katherine Bishop	1922
13.	Phylloquinone (Vitamin K_1)	Henrik Dam	1929

Source: Adapted from Kogl et al. (1936)

5.2 NUTRACEUTICALS

Nutraceuticals are a substance that is considered food or part of food that provides medicinal and health benefits resulting in the proper curing of diseases. Nutraceutical products can be considered non-specific biological therapies used to promote general well-being, control symptoms, and prevent malignant processes (Tomislav & Benedette, 2016). The word nutraceuticals came by combining two phrases, "nutrition" and "pharmaceutical," by Stephen L. Defelice, MD8, in 1989 (Jian et al., 2016; Avrelija et al., 2010; Defelice et al., 1995). They are the products other than nutrition which is referred to use as medicine (Hamid et al., 2014).

Nutraceuticals are also considered as "functional foods." The majority of nutraceuticals possess multiple therapeutic properties. The ideology beyond nutraceuticals is to mainly focus on prevention, as stated by Greek physician Hippocrates who is also known as the father of medicine, said that "let food be your medicine." The role of nutraceuticals (Keservani et al., 2010a, b, 2017, 2020) in human nutrition is important areas of study or inspection with Broad implementation for the consumers, healthcare providers, regulators, food producers, and distributors. Because of medicinal importance of food has been discovered for thousands of years, the development of the nutraceutical industry began during the 1980s (Manju et al., 2017).

5.2.1 CATEGORIES OF NUTRACEUTICALS

The precision of nutraceuticals and their related products usually are dependent on the source, their pharmacological conditions, and the chemical composition of products. Mostly, nutraceuticals are grouped into four categories that include dietary supplements, functional food, medicinal food, and pharmaceuticals (Tomislav & Benedette, 2021).

5.2.2 POTENTIAL HEALTH BENEFITS OF NUTRACEUTICALS

Nutraceuticals have captivated appreciable interest due to reasons like potential nutritional, safety, and therapeutic effects over the past many years. These products have a role in the abundance of biological processes, which include antioxidant defenses, cell propagation, gene expression, and protection of mitochondrial integrity. Therefore, nutraceuticals are used for the improvement of health, prevention of diseases that are chronic, postponing the aging process and increasing life anticipation, or just support the functions and integrity of the body. These products are healthy sources for the prevention of life-threatening diseases like diabetes, renal, and GI disorders, as well as different infections (Food & Design, 2021; Surana et al., 2021b).

Examples of nutraceuticals include:

- Carotenoids, such as lycopene;
- Dietary enzymes that are papain and bromelain;
- Hydrolyzed proteins;
- Mineral supplements;
- Phytonutrients, such as resveratrol;
- Prebiotic and probiotic supplements;
- Dietary fiber supplements;

- Vitamin supplements;
- Herbal products.

5.2.3 NUTRACEUTICALS CLASSIFICATION

Classification of nutraceuticals are depicted in Figure 5.1 (Chauhan et al., 2013; Namdeo et al., 2014; Kharb et al., 2004; Rajasekavan et al., 2017).

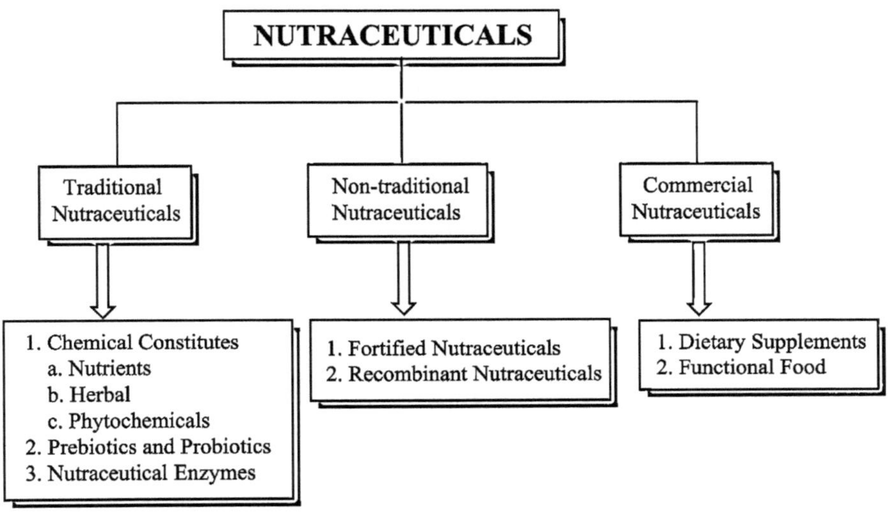

FIGURE 5.1 Classification of nutraceuticals.

5.2.4 NUTRACEUTICALS AND PHARMACEUTICALS

A comparison between nutraceuticals and pharmaceuticals is given in Table 5.2 (Sascha et al., 2016).

TABLE 5.2 Comparison between Nutraceuticals and Pharmaceuticals

Nutraceutical	Pharmaceutical
Inhibition of the diseases takes place	There is treatment if the disease
Long term application	Short-term application or effects
There is weak interaction with target	There is a strong interaction with the target
Low potency	High potency

The shift towards nutraceuticals is due to the following reasons:

- Healthcare costs have been increasing, which is the main concern of consumers.

- Nutraceuticals helps consumer by improving, sustaining the proper functioning of the body.
- People focus on prevention of diseases rather than cure.
- The people that may have chronic disease and they had not got any good results from allopathic medicines started using nutraceuticals.
- People with less income (Olaiya, Soetan, & Esan, 2016; Shilpa et al., 2017; Dighe et al., 2020).

5.3 CURRENT CRISIS

Nutraceutical dietary components created from herbal/natural raw materials (Sharma et al., 2020; Rane et al., 2020a–c) that aid in the treatment and prevention of diseases. This is a fast-growing industry which is up to 7–12% per year, with more people in the world using these natural products. The world's nutraceuticals market reaches up to $ 450 billion by 2015. The consumers of India have an awareness of standard nutraceutical ingredients is severely less, and the manufacturers have a need to take up the cause and advertise their products to the Indian masses (Ahire et al., 2021a, Surana et al., 2021). Maximum growth of the world's nutraceuticals market has been seen in the last year. In India, quenchers and functional foods are more likely to be used to witness much higher growth rates when it is compared to dietary supplements for more than five years (Ajit et al., 2012; Rajasekaran et al., 2008).

5.4 WHAT ARE VIRUSES?

Viruses are micro-particles of genetic material may be DNA or RNA that are enclosed by a protein (Jarouliya & Keservani, 2019b) coat. They have fatty envelope covering. Viruses also have a fatty "envelope" covering. They cannot reproduce on their own. They are dependent on organisms for their survival that they infect (host). Viruses get a drop, but they perform various essential functions for humans, animals, and the environment. Some viruses are helpful in protecting the host from the many other infections. They even participate in the process of evolution by transferring genes among different species.

After hearing the word "virus," people think of disease-causing viruses like the common cold, influenza, chickenpox, HIV, SARS-CoV-2 (Ahire & Kshirsagar, 2021; Gunjal et al., 2020), and many others. Viruses are responsible for affecting many regions of the body that includes systems including reproduction, respiratory, and gastrointestinal systems. They even affect the liver, brain, and skin. Viruses are also there in many cancers (Charles et al., 2020).

5.5 WHAT IS A VIRAL INFECTION?

A viral infection is a multiplication of a harmful virus within the body. They are not able to multiply themself without the assistance of a host. Viruses contaminate a host by inserting their dietary matter into the cells. A virus multiplies itself and kills the host cell to form a new virus particle free of an active viral infection (Talele et al., 2022). In some of the cases, virus particles "bud" off the host cell over a period of time before killing the host cell. New virus particles are then free to infect other cells. Symptoms of the viral illness occur as a result of cell damage, tissue destruction, and the associated immune response (Charles et al., 2020). Figure 5.2 represents respiratory viral infections.

5.5.1 TYPES OF VIRAL INFECTIONS (DANIEL ET AL., 2019)

i. Respiratory viral infections;
ii. Rhinovirus;
iii. Seasonal influenza;
iv. Respiratory syncytial virus;
v. Viral skin infections.

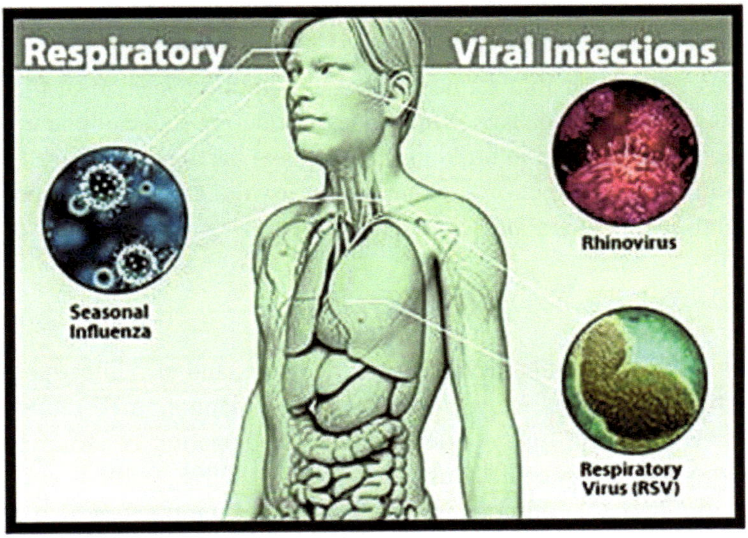

FIGURE 5.2 Respiratory viral infections.

5.6 POTENTIAL NUTRIENTS FOR PREVENTION OF VIRAL INFECTIONS

Various natural compounds available shows the antiviral property in treating viral infection or for healing applications. A with nutrients can help in preventing the chances of causing chronic diseases and reduces viral infections. Nutrients consist of vitamins (vitamins A, D, C, E, B6, and B12), minerals (calcium and magnesium), trace elements (zinc, copper, selenium, etc.), carbohydrates, proteins, fats, and water. The multinutrient provide a large amount of nutritional value for the whole body (Cardiovascular, skin, liver, and immune support). So, a balanced diet rich in multi-nutrients definitely helps in the improvement of immunity by maintaining respiratory and pulmonary health (Daniel et al., 2019).

Examples of respiratory diseases include (Daniel et al., 2019):

- Flu;
- Common cold;
- Respiratory syncytial virus infection;
- Adenovirus infection;
- Para influenza virus infection;
- SARS.

5.7 ROLE OF VITAMINS IN ANTIVIRAL IMMUNITY

Vitamins are responsible for supporting the immune system of the body at 3 levels, i.e., physical barrier antibody production and cellular immunity. Vitamins C and E help in building the physical barriers. Vitamins C, D, and E help in immune functions. Vitamin C is involved in antibody production (Carvajal-Millan et al., 2021).

5.7.1 ROLE OF VITAMIN A (RETINOL)

Vitamin A belongs to the family of retinyl-esters and also known as retinoic acid. Different studies show how natural and manufactured retinoids have protective effect on many viruses, including hepatitis B virus, influenza, norovirus, and cytomegalovirus (Angulo et al., 1998; Trottier et al., 2008; Lee et al., 2016). Food containing vitamin A. Vitamin A is also called an anti-inflammatory vitamin because of its important role in stimulating the feedback to the immune system. Vitamin A has importance in the therapy of several infectious diseases, such as pneumonia (Mahapatra et al., 2020). It has been found that children who are suffering from a deficiency of vitamin A they lead to be at a larger risk of death and illness because of respiratory tract infections which are more common in children (Angulo et al., 1998). Studies have shown that the infection has been worsened in children with already present Vitamin A deficiency, and its supplementation has been shown to lower the risk of death. Vitamin A is obtained from orange/yellow fruits and vegetables (Lee et al., 2018; Shakoor et al., 2021).

5.7.2 ROLE OF VITAMIN D (ERGOCALCIFEROL)

Vitamin D is called "sunlight hormone" or "sunshine vitamin" because it is mainly obtained from sunlight. Vitamin D synthesis is affected by lack of sun exposure to human, season change, use of excessive sunscreen, indoor lifestyle, clothing style, air pollution, less calcium intake, malabsorption, lack of maternal Vitamin D, and obesity (Jarouliya & Keservani, 2019a) (Vitamin D is present in adipose tissue) (Finklea et al., 2011; Hari et al., 2009; Aranow et al., 2011). Vitamin D is a steroid hormone, and it is an immune system modulator too. Vitamin D acts by suppressing and opposing infection by increasing anti-pathogen peptides. Current reviews suggest that vitamin D regulates the natural responses of the immune system to respiratory viral infections. Another study found that the use of vitamin D in improving the response to antiviral treatments in patients suffering from HIV and hepatitis C. Deaths in aged people are most common because of infections like bronchitis, pneumonia, and influenza, as they have weak immunity. According to research, vitamin D is more helpful in supporting the first line of defense with age. Thus, it prevents chronic respiratory infections (Abu et al., 2011). Figure 5.3 shows sources of vitamin D.

The Vitamin D that is important for humans are Vitamin D2 or Ergocalciferol, which is synthesized from Ergo sterol in plants, and Vitamin D3 or Cholecalciferol, which is synthesized naturally from cholesterol in animals. To the body, they can be supplied from the diet and Vitamin D from fortified products (Herrmann et al., 2017; Dusso et al., 2005). Hence, for the human body, the main source of Vitamin D is its synthesis in the skin. Vitamin D is involved in host defense through an autocrine pathway in monocytes and macrophages in humans, which is followed by stimulation of toll-like receptors (Kroner et al., 2015; Adams et al., 2009).

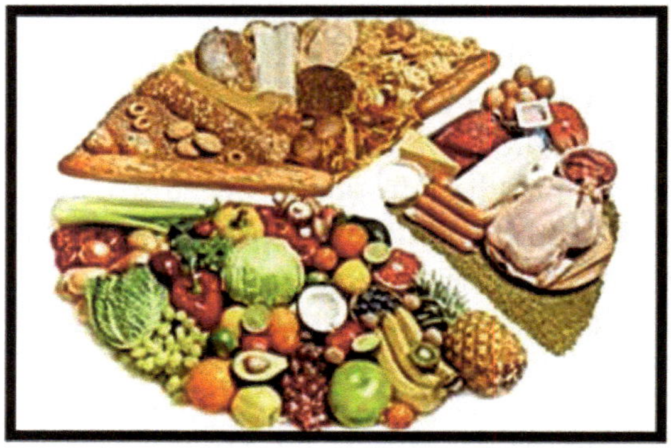

FIGURE 5.3 Sources of vitamin D (sources of vitamin D: natural sunlight, organ meats (liver), fatty fish (salmon, sardines, herring, pilchards, and tuna), egg yolks, fish oils and dairy products like milk and yogurt).

5.7.3 ROLE OF VITAMIN B

Vitamin B is found naturally and is involved in RBC production process. All the vitamins that are of B complex type are very important for normal physiological cell function (Zhang et al., 2018). Vitamin B helps the body to utilize nutrients (carbohydrates, fat, and protein) for the skin health and cells of brain and other tissues (Puneet et al., 2021). Figure 5.4 represents vitamin B-rich foods.

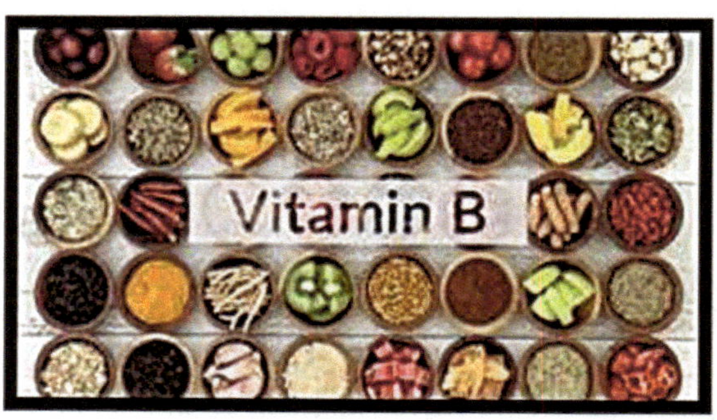

FIGURE 5.4 Vitamin B-rich food (sources of vitamin B: fish, cheese, cashew, milk, salmon, cereal, chicken, and spinach).

5.7.4 ROLE OF VITAMIN C

Vitamin C has antiviral properties; many studies have shown that vitamin C help in reducing the risk associated with respiratory tract infections (Carr et al., 2017). Vitamin C is required for biochemical reactions, which are catalyzed by monooxygenases, dioxygenases (Skylar et al., 2018; Subramani et al., 2014).

5.7.5 ROLE OF VITAMIN E

Vitamin E, which is fat-soluble, is a good antioxidant, and it improves host immune functions. Vitamin E deficiency boosts both humoral and cellular immunity (Moriguchi et al., 2000; Jayawardena et al., 2020).

5.8 ROLE OF VITAMINS IN VIRAL PNEUMONIA

Pneumonia is high in developing and developed countries in the world (Hui et al., 2021). With the increasing many virus infections, COVID-19 has resulted in severe pneumonia; there is a need for more efficient designs to test different therapeutics individually as well as in combination for treating pneumonia. Vitamin C is used in the prevention and also treating of pneumonia . Been introduced in the 1930s based on clinical observations of a favorable effect of vitamin C on patients suffering from pneumonia in countries like Germany. Vitamin C is given in large doses through oral or either intravenous route was claimed to be beneficial in patients with viral pneumonia and they appear to be safe (Arabi et al., 2020; Bohnholtzer et al., 1937; Gander et al., 1936; Klenner et al., 1951; Cathcart et al., 1981).

5.8.1 SYMPTOMS OF VIRAL PNEUMONIA IN ADULTS AND CHILDREN

The symptoms of pneumonia occur when the lungs are inflamed as they try to protect from viruses. As a result, this inflammation starts blocking the oxygen flow and exchange of gas in the lungs, as shown in Figure 5.6. The primary symptoms of pneumonia are flu symptoms. They include fever, chills, dehydration, fatigue, loss of appetite, malaise, clammy skin or sweating, fast breathing, shallow breathing, shortness of breath, wheezing, coughing, or fast heart rate (Stacy et al., 2019).

Advantages of nutraceuticals (Navya et al., 2021):

- It improves the health of an individual;
- It boosts the immune system;
- It helps in the prevention of chronic diseases;
- Helps in improving sleeping pattern;

- Relieves anxiety.

5.9 CONCLUSION

This chapter helps us to understand in detail about vitamins, nutraceuticals, viral infection, as well as the role of vitamins in vital infection prevention. Vitamins are lot beneficial in the treatment of viral infections. Different vitamins have different roles in the treatment or prevention of diseases. Nutraceuticals are very much important for preventing and treating diseases.

ACKNOWLEDGMENTS

We thank the Mahatma Gandhi Vidyamandir's Pharmacy College, Panchavati, Nashik, Maharashtra, India, for their constant support and providing all facilities to complete this work. Also, many thanks to all the known and unknowns who helped us right from the writing till the publishing of this chapter.

KEYWORDS

- **chronic diseases**
- **immune system**
- **nutraceuticals**
- **pneumonia**
- **viral infection and immunity**
- **virus**
- **vitamins**

REFERENCES

Abu-Mouch, S., Fireman, Z., Jarchovsky, J., Zeina, A. R., & Assy, N., (2011). Vitamin D supplementation improves sustained virologic response in chronic hepatitis C (genotype 1)-naïve patients. *World J. Gastroenterol., 17*, 5184–5190.

Adams, J. S., Ren, S., Liu, P. T., Chun, R. F., Lagishetty, V., & Gombart, A. F., (2009). Vitamin D-directed rheostatic regulation of monocyte antibacterial responses. *J. Immunol., 182*(7), 4289–4295.

Ahire, E. D., & Kshirsagar, S. J. (2021). Immune responses induced by different vaccine platforms against coronavirus disease-19. *Journal: Exploration of Immunology*, 243–257.

Ahire, E. D., Sonawane, V. N., Surana, K. R., & Talele, G. S., (2021). Drug discovery, drug-likeness screening, and bioavailability: Development of drug-likeness rule for natural products. In: *Applied Pharmaceutical Practice and Nutraceuticals* (pp. 191–208). Apple Academic Press.

Ahire, E. D., Surana K. R., Sonawane V.N., Pagar K. R., Gunjal S. S., & Talele S. G., (2020). Influence of allopathy, homeopathy, ayurveda and Unani systems of medicine in the management of COVID-19. *COVID-19 Pandemic: Questions, Answers and Hypotheses, 1.*

Ajit, S., (2012). *Nutraceuticals – Critical Supplement for Building a Healthy India, Ernst and Young, FICCI Task Force on Nutraceuticals*, pp. 1–80.

Alamgir, N. M., (2018). Vitamins, nutraceuticals, food additives, enzymes, anesthetic aids and cosmetics. *Progress in Research Book Series*, 407–534.

Angulo, A., Chandraratna, R. A., LeBlanc, J. F., & Ghazal, P., (1998). Ligand induction of retinoic acid receptors alters an acute infection by murine cytomegalovirus. *J. Virol., 72*(6), 4589–4600.

Anup, K. C., Snehal, S. M., & Sushma, M. R., (2021). *Current Trends in Social and Preventive Pharmacy, 1,* 25–28.

Arabi, Y. M., Fowler, R., & Hayden, F. G. (2020). Critical care management of adults with community-acquired severe respiratory viral infection. *Intensive Care Med., 46*, 315–328.

Aranow, C., (2011). Vitamin D and the immune system. *J. Investig. Med., 59*, 881–886.

Avrelija, C., & Walter, C., (2010). The role of functional foods, Nutraceuticals, and food supplements in intestinal health. *Nutrients, 2*, 611–625.

Bohnholtzer, E., (1937). Contribution to the question of pneumonia treatment with vitamin C. *Dtsch Med. Wochenschr, 63*, 1001–1003.

Carr, A. C., & Maggini, S., (2017). Vitamin C and immune function. *Nutrients, 9*(11), 1211.

Carvajal-Millan, E., Yaser, A. Z., & Haghi, A. K., (2021). *Natural Food Products and Waste Recovery: Healthy Foods, Nutrition Design, and Extraction of Valuable Compounds*. CRC Press.

Cathcart, R. F., (1981). Vitamin C, titrating to bowel tolerance, anascorbemia, and acute induced scurvy. *Med. Hypotheses, 7*, 1359–1376.

Charles, P. D., (2020). *What's a Virus? Viral Infection Types, Symptoms, Treatment*. On health.

Chauhan, B., Kumar, G., Kalam, N., & Ansari, S. H., (2013). Current concepts and prospects of herbal nutraceutical: A review. *J. Adv. Pharm. Technol. Research, 4*(1), 4–8.

Daniel, M., & Jill, S. S., (2019). *Viral Diseases 101*, Healthline.

Defelice, S. L., (1995). The nutraceutical evolution: Its impact on food industry R and D. *Trends Food Sci Techno, 6,* 59–61.

Dickinson, A., & Mackay, D., (2014). Health habits and other characteristics of dietary supplement users: A review. *Journal of Nutrition, 13*, 14.

Dighe, S. A., Nalkar, R. S., & Kakad, S. B., (2020). *A Review on Nutraceuticals and its Role in Treatment of Disease, 9*(12), 1285–1297.

Dusso, A. S., Brown, A. J., & Slatopolsky, E., (2005). Vitamin D. *Am. J. Physiol. Renal. Physiol., 289*(1), F8–28.

Eknath, B. K., Bhaskar, A. M., Rahul, D. K., & Kailash, R. B., (2020). *Concise Course in Social Pharmacy, 1,* 37–48.

Foods, H., & Design, N. (2021). *Natural Food Products and Waste Recovery, 1,* 1–334.

Gander, J. N., (1936). Vitamin C in the treatment of pneumonia. *Münch Med Wochenschr, 83,* 2074–2077.

Hamid, N., Azar, B., & Mahmoud, R. K., (2014). A new concept in nutraceuticals as an alternative to pharmaceuticals. *International Journal of Preventive Medicine, 5*(12), 1487–1499.

Herrmann, M., Farrell, C. L., Pusceddu, I., Fabregat-C, N., & Cavalier, E., (2017). Assessment of vitamin D status – a changing landscape. *Clin. Chem. Lab Med., 55*(1), 3–26.

Hui, L. L., Nelson, A. S. E., Lin, S. L., & Zhao, J. V. (2021). The role of vitamin C in pneumonia and COVID-19 infection in adults with European ancestry: A Mendelian randomization study. *European Journal of Clinical Nutrition.*

Jarouliya, U., & Keservani, R. K., (2019a). Pathways leading to child obesity; Chapter 12. In: Debasis, B., (ed.), *Global Perspectives on Childhood Obesity: Current Status, Consequences and Prevention* (2nd edn., pp. 137–146). Academic Press, Elsevier. ISBN: 9780128128404.

Jarouliya, U., & Keservani, R. K., (2019b). Protein function as cell surface and nuclear receptor in human diseases; Chapter 1. In: Sanjay, B., & Debarshi, K. M., (eds.), *Medicinal Chemistry with Pharmaceutical Product Development* (pp. 1–32). Apple Academic Press, CRC Press, Taylor & Francis Group. ISBN: 9781771887106.

Jayawardena, R., Sooriyaarachchi, P., Chourdakis, M., Jeewandara, C., & Ranasinghe, P. (2020). Enhancing immunity in viral infections, with special emphasis on COVID-19: A review. *Diabetes Metabolite Syndrome Clinical Research, 14*(4), 367–382.

Jian, W., Sanjay, G., Mattheos, A. G. K., & Yajun, Y. (2016). *Microbial Production of Value-added Nutraceuticals, 37,* 97–104.

Keservani, R. K., Kesharwani, R. K., Sharma, A. K., Vyas, N., & Chadoker, A., (2010b). Nutritional supplements: An overview. *International Journal of Current Pharmaceutical Review and Research, 1*(1), 59–75.

Keservani, R. K., Kesharwani, R. K., Vyas, N., Jain, S., Raghuvanshi, R., & Sharma, A. K., (2010a). Nutraceutical and functional food as future food: A review. *Der Pharmacia Lettre, 2*(1), 106–116.

Keservani, R. K., Sharma, A. K., & Jarouliya, U. (2015). Protein and peptide in drug targeting and its therapeutic approach. *Ars Pharmaceutica (Internet), 56*(3), 165–177.

Keservani, R. K., Sharma, A. K., & Kesharwani, R. K. (2017). An overview and therapeutic applications of nutraceutical and functional foods. *Recent Advances in Drug Delivery Technology*, 160–201. ISBN:9781522507543.

Keservani, R. K., Sharma, A. K., & Kesharwani, R. K. (2020). *Nutraceuticals and Dietary Supplements: Applications in Health Improvement and Disease Management.* CRC Press. ISBN: 9781771888738.

Kharb, S., & Singh, V., (2004). Nutraceuticals in health and disease prevention. *Indian Journal of Clinical Biochemistry, 19*(1), 50–53.

Klenner, F. R., (1951). Massive doses of vitamin C and the virus diseases. *South Med. Surg., 113,* 101–107.

Kögl, F., & Tönnis, B., (1936). Über das bios-problem. *Darstellung Von Krystallisiertem Biotin aus Eigelb.* 20. Mitteilung über pflanzliche Wachstumsstoffe.

Kroner, J. C., Sommer, A., & Fabri, M., (2015). Vitamin D every day to keep the infection away? *Nutrients, 7*(6), 4170–4188.

Lee, G. Y., & Han, S. N., (2018). The role of vitamin E in immunity. *Nutrients.*

Mahapatra, D. K., Talele, S. G., & Haghi, A. K., (2020). *Applied Pharmaceutical Science and Microbiology: Novel Green Chemistry Methods and Natural Products.* CRC Press.

Maria, G. C., Thomas, G. W., & Guglielmo, C., (2020). The role of vitamins in oral health. A systematic review and meta-analysis. *International Journal of Environmental Research and Public HEALTH, 17*(3), 938.

Moriguchi, S., & Muraga, M., (2000). Vitamin E and immunity. *Vitamins and Hormones, 59,* 305–336.

Namdeo, S., Bhaskar, B., Sunil, D., & Pratik, K., (2014). Nutraceuticals: A review on current status. *Research Journal of Pharma and Tech, 7*(1), 110–113.

Navya, K. (2021). *Nutraceuticals Benefits*, Onlymyhealth.

Nitu, S., Sumeet, D., Rageeb, M. D. U., & Pralhad, K. K., (2019). Health and disease. *Textbook of Social and Preventive Pharmacy, 1,* 8–21.

Olaiya, C. O., Soetan, K. O., & Esan, A., (2016). Role of nutraceuticals, functional foods, and value-added products in prevention and treatment of chronic diseases. *African Journal of Food Science, 10*(10), 185–193.

Parveen, S. S., & Srinivas, P., (2017). The role of vitamins and trace elements in oral health: A systematic review. *International Journal of Medical Reviews, 4*(1), 22–31.

Puneet, K., Mandeep, K., & Sumit, J., (2021). *Role of Vitamins and Minerals as Immunity Boosters in COVID-19, 29,* 1001–1016.

Rajasekavan, A., (2017). *General Perspective- The Future of Drug Discovery,* 108.

Rane, B. R., Bharath, M. S., Patil, R. R., Keservani, R. K., & Jain, A. S. (2020b). Novel approaches in nutraceuticals; Chapter 11. In: Rajesh, K. K., Raj, K. K., & Anil, K. S., (eds.), *Enhancing the Therapeutic Efficacy of Herbal Formulations Through Novel Drug Delivery Systems* (pp. 241–266). IGI Global International Publisher, Pennsylvania, USA. ISBN13: 9781799844532.

Rane, B. R., Patil, A. S., Keservani, R. K., & Jain, A. S., (2020a). Novel approaches in herbal formulation; Chapter 2. In: Rajesh, K. K., Raj, K. K., & Anil, K. S., (eds.), *Enhancing the Therapeutic Efficacy of Herbal Formulations Through Novel Drug Delivery Systems* (pp. 43–68). IGI Global International Publisher, Pennsylvania, USA. ISBN13: 9781799844532.

Rane, B. R., Tadavi, S, A., & Keservani, R. K., (2020c). Naturopathy; Chapter 12. In: Anil, K. S., Raj, K. K., & Surya, P. G., (eds.), *Herbal Product Development* (pp. 321–347). Apple Academic Press, CRC Press, Taylor & Francis Group. ISBN: 9781771888776.

Sascha, S., & Annabell, P., (2016). Health-beneficial nutraceuticals—Myth or reality? *European Journal of Applied Microbiology and Biotechnology, 101*(3), 951–961.

Shakoor, H., Feehan, J., Mikkelsen, K., Al Dhaheri., A. S., Ali, H. I., & Platat, C., (2021). Be well: A potential role for vitamin B in COVID-19. *Maturitas, 144,* 108–111.

Sharma, A. K., Keservani, R. K., & Gautam, S. P., (2020). *Herbal Product Development.* Apple Academic Press, CRC Press, Taylor & Francis Group. ISBN: 9781771888776.

Shilpa, P. C., Priyatam, V. P., & Mahesh, N. P. (2017). Nutraceuticals: Review. *World Journal of Pharmacy and Pharmaceutical Sciences, 6*(8), 681–739.

Singh, P., Kesharwani, R. K., & Keservani, R. K., (2017a). Antioxidants and vitamins: Roles in cellular function and metabolism. In: *Sustained Energy for Enhanced Human Functions and Activity* (pp. 385–407). Academic Press. ISBN:9780128054130.

Singh, P., Kesharwani, R. K., & Keservani, R. K., (2017b). Protein, carbohydrates, and fats: Energy metabolism. In: *Sustained Energy for Enhanced Human Functions and Activity* (pp. 103–115). Academic Press. ISBN:9780128054130.

Skylar, A. S., Katharive, P. S., & Marp, P. L., (2018). Nutraceuticals A review. *Dermatol. Ther., 8*, 5–16.

Stacy, S., & Shannon, J. (2019). *Viral Pneumonia: Symptoms, Risk Factors, and More.* Healthline.

Subrrramni, T., Yeap, S. K., Omar, A. R., Aziz, S. A., & Rahman, N. M., (2014). Vitamin suppresses cell death in MCF -7 human breast cancer cells induced by Jall MoL. *International Journal of Environmental Research and Public Health, 18*, 305–313.

Surana, K. R., Ahire, E. D., Sonawane, V. N., & Talele, S. G., (2021). Biomolecular and molecular docking: A modern tool in drug discovery and virtual screening of natural products. In: *Applied Pharmaceutical Practice and Nutraceuticals* (pp. 209–223). Apple Academic Press.

Surana, K. R., Ahire, E. D., Sonawane, V. N., Talele, S. G., & Talele, G. S., (2021). Informatics and methods in nutrition design and development. *Natural Food Products and Waste Recovery: Healthy Foods, Nutrition Design, and Extraction of Valuable Compounds*, 33.

Talele, S. G., Ahire, E. D., Surana, K. R., Sonawane, V. N., & Talele, G. S., (2022). Coronavirus disease (COVID-19): A past and present perspective. *Asian Journal of Pharmaceutical Research, 12*(1), 45–53.

Tomisiav, M., & Benedette, C., (2021). What are nutraceuticals? *1,* 1–7.

Tomislav, M., & Benedette, C. (2021). *What are Nutraceuticals.* Medical and Life Science.

Trottier, C., Chabot, S., Mann, K. K., Colombo, M., Chatterjee, A., & Miller, W. H. Jr., (2008). Retinoids inhibit measles virus *in vitro* via nuclear retinoid receptor signaling pathways. *Antiviral Res., 80*(1), 45–53.

Zhang, Y., Zhou, W., Yan, J., Liu, M., Zhou, Y., & Shen, X. (2018). A review of the extraction and determination methods of thirteen essential vitamins to the human body: An update from *Molecules, 23*(6), 1484.

CHAPTER 6

Vitamins as Nutraceuticals for Microbial Infections

ASHWINI V. SHELKE,[1] KHEMCHAND R. SURANA,[2] VAISHALI N. PARDESHI,[1] TUSHAR N. LOKHANDE,[3] and SUNIL K. MAHAJAN[4]

[1]*Department of Pharmaceutical Chemistry, Mahatma Gandhi Vidyamandir's Pharmacy College, Panchavati, Nashik, Maharashtra, India*

[2]*Department of Pharmaceutical Chemistry, Shreeshakti Shaikshanik Sanstha, Divine College of Pharmacy, Satana, Nashik, Maharashtra, India*

[3]*Maharashtra Educational Society's H. K. College of Pharmacy, Oshiwara, Jogeshwari (W), Maharashtra, India*

[4]*Department of Pharmaceutical Chemistry, M.G.V's Samajshri Prashant Dada Hiray, College of Pharmacy, Malegaon, Nashik, Maharashtra, India*

ABSTRACT

Nutrition and immunity, as well as the likelihood and severity of infection, have long been linked. For health and function, all cells, especially immune cells, necessitate nutrients as a component of a good diet. Each component of the body's immune response necessitates many micronutrients, such as vitamins. While chronic or severe infections cause nutritional problems or worsen the nutritional condition of those who are infected. Therefore, it is essential for all of us to focus on our diet and nutritional status. We must get the correct nutrients in our diet for our immune system to function at its best to fight against various microbial infections. Our immunological system is

Preventive and Therapeutic Role of Vitamins as Nutraceuticals. Khemchand R. Surana, Eknath D. Ahire, Raj K. Keservani, & Rajesh K. Kesharwani (Eds.)

a complicated network of immune cells that fight germs and viruses that cause disease. Some vitamins can also help to recover healthy again faster by killing harmful germs. Furthermore, the output of the advent of selective, multidrug-resistant bacteria is the rise of antimicrobial resistance as a critical worldwide health issue. Finding innovative strategies to treat bacterial infections, particularly those caused by Gram-negative organisms, is critical. Vitamins could be useful to treat some microbial diseases, and they could be administered as nutraceuticals. A vitamin is an important micronutrient that an organism needs in small amounts for proper metabolic activity. It is an organic molecule (or chemically connected set of molecules, i.e., vitamins).

6.1 VITAMINS IN MICROBIAL INFECTION

On a day-to-day basis, we are exposed to a variety of potentially hazardous germs. Our immunity, which is composed of a complicated network of stages and pathways throughout the body, protects us from microorganisms and diseases. It recognizes foreign invaders like bacteria, viruses, and parasites and takes immediate action (Chandra, 1997; Surana et al., 2020). The term 'nutraceutical' refers to natural foods or supplements that have therapeutic properties. It is a substance that can be regarded as food or the component of a food that has medical or health advantages, including illness prevention and treatment. Dr. Stephen DeFelice invented the term Nutraceutical in 1989, combining the phrases "nutrition" and "pharmaceutical" (Kalra, 2003; Keservani et al., 2010a, b). Nutraceuticals, which are described as substances such as isolated nutrients, dietary supplements, diets, and herbal items (Sharma et al., 2020; Rane et al., 2020a–c), may help to avoid the inflammatory cascade and hypercoagulation by exerting anti-inflammatory and antioxidant properties. Essential vitamins such as Vitamin C and zinc, for example, can aid in the production of immune cells, such as white blood cells and antibodies, which are necessary for a healthy immune system. Essential nutrients like vitamins are unable to be produced in the body, either entirely or in adequate amounts, and must therefore be received through the diet. Natural substance's pharmacological capabilities have gotten a lot of interest in the area of complementary and alternative therapies for a number of disorders. As a result, the food industry is focusing on nutraceuticals (Keservani et al., 2017, 2020), which are bioactive compounds found in foods or natural products that can provide health advantages along with their intrinsic nutritional value, particularly for the therapeutic treatment of chronic diseases. As a result, the aim of this chapter is to discuss in detail the significance of various vitamins as nutraceuticals in the treatment and prevention of microbial illness (Surana et al., 2021).

Vitamins are organic bio-molecules that must be absorbed by diet, with the exception of vitamin D. Vitamins have a crucial part in vital activities, such as anti-oxidant, pro-oxidant, anti-inflammatory, and metabolic activities. Most vitamins are made up of vitamins, which are groups of linked molecules. Vitamin E, for example, has eight vitamers: four tocotrienols and four tocopherols. Vitamins are compounds that your body requires for appropriate growth and development. A single dietary deficiency can change the immunological response of the organism. Deficits in folic acid, as well as vitamins A, B6, C, D, and E, have been shown in animal experiments to modify immunological responses (Beisel, 1982; Talele et al., 2022). These nutrients aid the immunity system in a variety of ways, including acting like antioxidants (Singh et al., 2017) to guide healthy cells, promoting immune cell growth and activity, and creating antibodies (Semba, 2012; Surana et al., 2018). According to epidemiological studies, persons who are malnourished are more susceptible to viral, bacterial, and many other diseases. There has been numerous research examining nutritional intakes in relation to various infections (Ahire et al., 2020).

Our body necessitates 13 vitamins. Some publications include choline in their list of 14 vitamins; however, major health organizations only list 13.

Carotenoids (vitamin A), thiamine (vitamin B_1), riboflavin (vitamin B_2), niacin (vitamin B_3), pantothenic acid (vitamin B_5), pyridoxine (vitamin B_6), biotin (vitamin B_7), folic acid or folate (vitamin B_9), cobalamins (vitamin B_{12}), ascorbic acid (vitamin C), calciferols (vitamin D), tocopherols and tocotrienols and phylloquinone and menaquinones (vitamin K) (Oyarzun et al., 2001; Bender, 2003). All these vitamins can be obtained from various natural sources, as shown in Table 6.1.

6.1.1 VITAMIN A (RETINOL)

Vitamin A is found to have anti-inflammatory action because of its critical role in supporting the immune system's response; through T helper cell regulation, surface IgA and the production of cytokines, it regulates humoral and cell-mediated immunity. Vitamin A also has proved to be beneficial in the therapy of a variety of viral disorders, including measles-associated pneumonia. Vitamin A supplementation has been researched extensively as a possible adjunct to therapy for preventing the incidence of ALRTIs, i.e., Acute Lower Respiratory Tract Infections, as well as lowering the severity

TABLE 6.1 Sources for Vitamins as Nutraceutical

Sl. No.	Name of Vitamin	Synonym	Food Sources	Role in Body
1.	B1	Thiamine	Beans, fortified, enriched, or whole-grain products such as pasta and cereals.	It helps the body to process some carbohydrates and protein.
2.	B2	Riboflavin	Fortified cereals, dark meat chicken, milk asparagus, almonds, breads, and cooked beef.	It supports many body processes, such as converting food into energy. It also assists your body makes red blood cells.
3.	B3	Niacin	Fortified cereals, meat, fish, whole grains and poultry.	Changing food into energy; helps with digestion and the production of cholesterol.
4.	B6	Pyridoxine	Spinach, bananas, fortified cereals, peas, soy-based meat substitutes, baked potatoes, eggs, meat, and chicken.	Helps the body for metabolism of proteins and stored sugar. It also Supports the nervous system.
5.	B12	Cobalamins	Fortified foods, poultry, crabs, beef, and salmon.	Helps in the production of red blood cells and cell division.
6.	C	Ascorbic acid	Green and red bell peppers, tomatoes, cauliflower, broccoli, berries, potatoes, brussels sprouts, cabbage, spinach, and citrus fruits.	It is needed for the synthesis of certain chemical messengers in the brain. Also, boost the immune system and helps to prepare collagen.
7.	D	Ergocalciferol	Cod liver oil, egg yolks, cereals, fortified milk and cheese.	Maintains the health of bones and helps the process of calcium in the body, important for immune system function; may act as an anticancer agent.
8.	E	Tocopherols and tocotrienols	Leafy green vegetables, soybean, canola, sunflower, vegetable oils, hazelnuts, and almonds.	It protects cells from damage and acts as an antioxidant.
9.	B9	Folic acid	Fortified cereals, dark leafy vegetables, garbanzo beans, lentils, and grain products.	It prevents birth defects, promotes cell development, helps red blood cell formation, and promotes heart health.
10.	K	Phylloquinone and menaquinones	Fruits such as grapes, kiwi, fruits, avocado, cabbage, broccoli, Brussels sprouts, leafy green vegetables like parsley, chard, and kale.	Maintains bone health and helps in blood clotting.

and speeding recovery. It has been discovered that children with vitamin A deficiency have a greater risk of death and illness in case of respiratory tract infections (Wiseman et al., 2017). Vitamin A is found in animal goods such as fish, liver, and dairy products as all-trans-Retinol or Vitamin A and in plant foods such as oranges, leafy vegetables, ripe yellow fruits, pumpkin, carrots, squash, and spinach as all-trans-beta-carotene or provitamin A.

6.1.2 VITAMIN B_1 (THIAMINE)

Humans require vitamin B1 (thiamine) as nutrition. Viral, bacterial, and fungal infections were resistant in vegetable crop plants, thiamine-treated rice, and Arabidopsis (Arabidopsis thaliana). In rice and other plants, thiamine administration causes the transitory expression of pathogenesis-related (PR) genes. Furthermore, thiamine therapy increases the strength and speed of PR gene expression along with the activity of protein kinase C. In Arabidopsis mutants, thiamine inhibited bacterial infection (Pyung et al., 2005). Nutraceuticals to obtain Vitamin B1 are Pork, whole meal grains, brown rice, vegetables, potatoes, liver, eggs.

6.1.3 VITAMIN B_2 (RIBOFLAVIN)

Vitamin B2, often known as Riboflavin, is the vital component of the vitamin B complex. Flavin adenine dinucleotide (FAD) and Flavin mononucleotide (FMN) are two essential cofactors involved in many oxidative-reduction reactions and energy metabolism that make up riboflavin. Riboflavin is an antioxidant that also has photosensitizing effects. Riboflavin has the ability to generate ROS, i.e., Reactive Oxygen Species and alter immunological responses. When administered alone or in combination with other anti-infectives, riboflavin has a strong antibacterial effect. Antimicrobial medications should focus on the riboflavin production pathway. UVA, in conjunction with riboflavin, has antibacterial properties (Nuratiqah et al., 2022). Nutraceutical sources for Vitamin B2 are dairy products, bananas, green beans, and asparagus.

6.1.4 VITAMIN B_3 (NIACIN)

It is suggested in The Journal of Clinical Investigation that nicotinamide (NAM), additionally called nutrition B3 boosts the neutrophil-related killing of Staphylococcus aureus. Antibiotic-resistant bacteria, inclusive of methicillin-resistant *S. aureus* (MRSA), have emerged and spread, making the improvement of recent antimicrobial strategies a top priority. Professor Adrian Gompart stated, "This could provide us a new technique to treat Staph infections, which can be lethal, and it could be beneficial to use in combination with current medications" (Andrew, 2012). Nutraceutical sources for niacin Meat, fish, eggs, many vegetables, mushrooms, tree nuts.

6.1.5 VITAMIN B_5 (PANTOTHENIC ACID)

Pantothenic acid, often known as vitamin B5, is light yellowish viscous oil that is water and ethanol soluble. Vitamin B5, also known as pantothenic acid or pantothenate, comes under the category of water-soluble vitamin, which is generated by microbes and plants, but not by animals (Smith & Song, 1996). Coenzyme A (CoA), an important cofactor for the TCA cycle, is a precursor to vitamin B5. In the clinical therapy of tuberculosis, vitamin B5 supplementation may provide an extra therapeutic advantage. Vitamin B5 suppressed the *in vivo* germination of Mycobacterium TB through regulating innate and adaptive immunity (Wenting et al., 2018). Vitamin B5 was found to cure the mycobacterial infection in mice by enhancing macrophage maturation and increasing separation of Th1 and Th17 cells. In animal-sourced meals, it is present in high proportions as phosphopantetheine or coenzyme A (Nuraly et al., 2022). Nutraceutical sources for vitamin B5 are Meat, broccoli, and avocados.

6.1.6 VITAMIN B_6 (PYRIDOXINE)

Vitamin B6 is needed for the production of important immune system cells that aid in the fight against dangerous bacteria. B6 specifically helps your body generate T-cells, which are immune cells that assist your body eliminate contaminated cells and trigger your immune system response. B6 deficiency is uncommon, according to experts, and most people should be able to receive enough vitamin B6 through their diet. Meat, vegetables, tree nuts, and bananas are good sources of vitamin B6 (Parra et al., 2018).

6.1.7 VITAMIN B7 (BIOTIN)

B7 it is the B-complex vitamin (Biotin). Because it is required for appropriate cellular metabolism and function, biotin is an important vitamin for optimal human health. The vitamin functions as a cofactor of five carboxylases that is essential for fatty acid, glucose, and amino acid metabolism (McMahon, 2002). Resources from food Leafy green veggies, raw egg yolk, liver, and peanuts.

6.1.8 VITAMIN B_9 (FOLIC ACID OR FOLATE)

Vitamin B9 (folic acid) is a water-soluble important vitamin that the body converts to tetrahydrofolic acid. This conversion is required for proper erythropoiesis, purine and thymidylate production, amino acid metabolism (glycine and methionine), and histidine metabolism (Hillman, 1995). Folic acid is used to suppress and treat folic acid deficiency in nutritional anemias and megaloblastic anemias, also in pregnancy, infancy, and childhood. To lower the prospect of exoderm abnormalities and different birth complications, B vitamin is given to ladies who are progressing to get pregnant also as within the early months of physiological state (Jennifer, 2007). Nutraceutical sources for vitamin B9 leafy vegetables, pasta, bread, cereal, and liver.

6.1.9 VITAMIN B_{12} (COBALAMINS)

Cobalamin, often known as vitamin B12, is a corrinoid molecule with a corrin ring and a core cobalt molecule. In both bacteria and mammals, cobalamin is a precursor for the enzymes methyl malonyl-CoA mutase (MCM) and methionine synthase (MetH), which are involved in the synthesis of amino acids and degradation of fatty- and amino acid, respectively (Roth et al., 1996). As a result, cobalamin is important for homeostatic functioning. Because there are numerous forms of cobalamin, researchers looked forward to the impact of various forms of cobalamin on gut flora in several studies. The rate of *Acinetobacter* spp. increased after methyl cobalamin administration, while the rate of *Enterobacteriaceae* spp., *Bacteroides* spp., and Ruminococcaceae spp. decreased. Methylcobalamin was found to have a positive connection with Pseudomonas bacteria in this investigation (Yuanyuan et al., 2018).

6.1.10 VITAMIN C (ASCORBIC ACID)

On a cellular level, vitamin C aids various actions of the adaptive and innate immune systems. It assembles in the immune system's phagocytic cells, such as neutrophils, and promotes microbe death via chemotaxis, phagocytosis, the production of ROS, i.e., Reactive oxygen species and eventually microbial destruction (Jing, 2018). Vitamin C is a water-soluble vitamin which acts as an antioxidant and a cofactor for regulatory enzymes while also providing electrons. It aids the production of cortisol, vasopressin, and catecholamines, in particular. Vitamin C is necessary for both the adaptive and innate immune system to function properly. Vitamin C aids in epithelial and endothelial barrier function, as well as maintaining vasodilation and lowering proinflammatory mediators (May et al., 2013). Vitamin C improves phagocytosis, chemotaxis, and the production of ROS, i.e., reactive oxygen species, reducing necrosis and tissue damage (Carr et al., 2017). Vitamin C supplementation boosts the immunity system in humans by keeping the oxidation ability of cells and protecting the system from reactive oxygen species (ROS). Vitamin C helps to lessen the risk, severity, and duration of various infectious diseases (Shaik-Dasthagirisaheb et al., 2013; Gombart et al., 2020). Furthermore, vitamin C levels might drop during illness; consequently, in extreme situations, substantial doses of intravenous Vitamin C are required to compensate for the fast turnover of the vitamin (Rosengrave et al., 2017). Many enzymes require it as a cofactor. By retaining ions of metals in the reduced state, it improves the operation of several enzymes throughout the body. It also works as an antioxidant, reducing inflammation and tissue damage caused by immunological reactions (Chien et al., 2004). In the US, the Soviet Union, the United Kingdom, and Japan, RCTs examining the effectiveness of vitamin C were done among soldiers, young boys, and the elderly. Vitamin C supplementation was found to dramatically lower the incidence of infections of the respiratory tract in several investigations (Hemila et al., 2013). Vitamin C's usefulness has also been investigated in hospitalized patients in the United States, Egypt, and Iran who were admitted for a variety of reasons, including severe sepsis, surgical complications, burns, lung contusions, and heart disorders (Wang et al., 2019). In these patients, vitamin C has been demonstrated to minimize the duration of stay in the critical care unit and the need for mechanical breathing (Hemila et al., 2019). During flu season or other times of illness, people often seek out certain meals or vitamin supplements that are said to boost immunity. Vitamin C is abundant in chicken soup, citrus fruits, and honey-infused tea.

6.1.11 VITAMIN D (ERGOCALCIFEROL)

It is a steroid hormone and immunity system modulator which increases macrophage activity while lowering the expression of inflammatory cytokines. It also boosts the production of AMPs, i.e., antimicrobial peptides, which are found in neutrophils, monocytes, natural killer cells, and respiratory epithelial cells (Mawson, 2013). Vitamin D suppresses infection while also boosting anti-pathogen peptides to defend against it (Charan et al., 2012). Vitamin D supplementation decreases the risk of acute respiratory tract infections (most of which are thought to be caused by viruses) by 12% to 75%, according to evidence from various clinical trials and pooled studies (Urashima et al., 2010). Both the seasonal and pandemic flu caused by the H1N1 virus in 2009 were studied (Gysin et al., 2016; Martineau et al., 2017). Supplementation had a positive effect on patients of all ages, including those with pre-existing chronic conditions (Arihiro et al., 2019). If people who were infected received dosages of vitamin D more than 1000 IU, flu symptoms were reduced and recovery was faster (Zhou et al., 2018). Individuals with vitamin D insufficiency show higher benefits than those who have the appropriate amount of vitamin D. Maintaining proper vitamin D levels is very crucial. Vitamin D is created in our skin when we are exposed to sunshine, and blood concentration of vitamin D tends to be low in the late winter and early spring due to limited solar exposure (Borel et al., 2015). Vitamin D's biosignaling role in the metabolism is widely recognized, but this metabolite has also been related to the risk of generating disorders like cancer, infectious diseases, and depression over time. The active metabolite of vitamin D [1,25$(OH)_2$D3 or calcitriol] regulates gene transcription after attaching to its nuclear receptor, as well as having many impacts on the immunological and inflammatory response. Vitamin D might work against respiratory infections in a variety of ways, according to Grant et al. recent analysis (Grant et al., 2020). Because vitamin D insufficiency has been linked to a high risk of respiratory infections, it is reasonable to give vitamin D to healthy people and COVID-19 patients (Fabio et al., 2020).

6.1.12 VITAMIN E (TOCOPHEROLS AND TOCOTRIENOLS)

Vitamin E is a group of critical micronutrients that includes lipid-soluble tocopherols and tocotrienols that have potent antioxidant and immunomodulatory properties. Vitamin E supplementation has been related to enhanced resistance to a variety of infections, particularly in the elderly, who are at higher risk of vitamin E deficiency due to a lack of vitamin E in their diet (Angel et al., 2006; Kang et al., 2004). *Burkholderia cenocepacia* is a Gram-negative bacterium that causes significant respiratory infections in cystic fibrosis sufferers. Vitamin E can be utilized to boost bactericidal antibiotic killing by interfering with lipocalin binding, according to a study.

Vitamin E, when taken with bactericidal antibiotics, increases bacterial death *in vivo-in vitro*, according to a study (Marwa et al., 2018). According to studies published between 2010 and 2020, vitamin E is a promising adjunct antibiotic therapy option for infectious disorders caused by MDR (multi-drug-resistant) bacteria such as *Burkholderia cenocepacia*, Pseudomonas aeruginosa and methicillin-resistant Staphylococcus aureus (MRSA) (Minnja et al., 2020). Another study found that vitamin E has antibacterial properties against MRSA when taken alone or in conjunction with daptomycin. Significant bacterial suppression was related to elevated markers of tissue healing and immunological alterations in mice treated with either vitamin E alone or vitamin E in combination with daptomycin (Elisa et al., 2011). Nutraceutical sources for vitamin E are many fruits, nuts, vegetables, and seed oils.

6.1.13 VITAMIN K (PHYLLOQUINONE AND MENAQUINONES)

Vitamin K is a biologically active chemical found in functional foods that is necessary in the coagulation process, where it is required for the production of prothrombin, along with the production of proteins found in plasma, kidneys, and possibly other organs (Klack et al., 2006). The pharma industry has shown increased interest in substances isolated from natural products like vitamins that have antimicrobial properties in recent years in light of the development of bacterial resistance to antibiotics, which is responsible for the lack of efficacy in the treatment of many existing infections. Menadione's antibiotic-modifying action in multiresistant strains of Staphylococcus aureus, Pseudomonas aeruginosa, and Escherichia coli was investigated *in vitro*. Vitamin K3 also known as Menadione, is a lipid-soluble vitamin and a lipophilic chemical that causes disruptions in the bacterial membrane, resulting in damage to the membrane's essential constituents, allowing higher permeability. Menadione (vitamin K) increases the antibacterial action of medicines by permeabilizing the cell membrane. Menadione was particularly efficient against *S. aureus* 358 and, in particular, *E. coli* 27, pathogens with various morphologies (Jacqueline et al., 2017). Water-soluble and fat-soluble vitamins are the two types of vitamins. There are 13 vitamins in humans: four fat-soluble vitamins (A, D, E, and K) and nine water-soluble vitamins (8-B vitamins and vitamin C). Vitamins soluble in water dissolve rapidly in water and are expelled from the body in large quantities to the point where urine output is a good analyzer of vitamin consumption (Fukuwatari et al., 2008). Because they are not as easily stored, it is necessary to consume them on a more regular basis (Bellows et al., 2015). Nutraceutical sources for vitamin K are Leafy green vegetables. Examples, Spinach, egg yolks, liver.

6.2 CONCLUSION

Because of the rise and spread of antibiotic-resistant bacteria, finding new antimicrobial techniques is a top concern. Vitamins could provide a novel strategy to treat potentially fatal diseases, and they could be administered in conjunction with conventional antibiotics. Vitamins protect the body's immune system on three levels: physical barrier (such as skin and mucous membranes), cellular immunity, and antibody synthesis. Vitamins E and C aid in the reinforcement of physical barriers. On a cellular level, vitamins C, D, and E support the immunological function. Vitamin C is also involved in the formation of antibodies. Vitamin A acts as a growth and differentiation regulator for cells and tissues, among other biochemical functions. The B complex vitamins function as cofactors (coenzymes) or precursors for enzymes, and Vitamin D regulates mineral metabolism in bones and other organs in a hormone-like manner. Vitamin D would possibly work towards respiratory infections in numerous ways. Vitamin E can be carried out to enhance bactericidal antibiotic killing; vitamin C, curcumin, and glycyrrhizic acid, in combination, enhance interferon production and regulate the inflammatory response, suggesting that the combination of these molecules may be useful in regulating the immune response to cope with SARS-CoV-2 infections; Antioxidants encompass vitamins C and E. Among nutraceuticals, Vitamin E, vitamin C, carotenoids, and sure minerals (Zn, Mn, Cu, and Se), in addition to polyphenols (flavonoids, phenolic acids, stilbenes, lignans), have a synergistic impact in maintaining redox equilibrium, and so provide medicinal or health benefits. Furthermore, our system is advanced and has an impact with the aid of using perfect stability of the various elements, now no longer simply a diet, and now no longer in particular with the aid of using any single food or nutrition. A well-balanced, vitamin-and mineral-rich diet, combined with healthy lifestyle variables similar to acceptable sleep, exercise, and low stress, permits the body to best fight infection and disease.

ACKNOWLEDGMENTS

We thank the Mahatma Gandhi Vidyamandir's Pharmacy College, Panchavati, Nashik, Maharashtra, India, for their constant support and providing all facilities to complete this work. Also, many thanks to all the known and unknowns who helped us right from the writing till the publishing of this chapter.

KEYWORDS

- **ascorbic acid**
- **immunological**
- **microbial infection**
- **nutraceuticals**
- **riboflavin**
- **thiamine**
- **vitamers**
- **vitamins**

REFERENCES

Ahire, E. D., Sonawane, V. N., & Surana, K. R., (2020). Role of drug repurposing in current treatment strategies against COVID-19; systemic review. *Pharm. Reson.*, 24–29.

Ahire, E. D., Sonawane, V. N., Surana, K. R., Jadhav, K. R., Sonawane, D. D., & Shah, A. A., (2020). Convalescent plasma therapy: A promising approach in the treatment of COVID-19. *Int J Pharm. Sci. Res.*, *11*, 4078–4086.

Andrew, J., (2012). Antibacterial vitamin. *Nature Reviews-Microbiology, 10*(10).

Angel, D. M., Ramon, H. J., & Martınez-Martınez, L., (2006). Extended-spectrum b-lactamase-producing *Escherichia coli* and *Klebsiella pneumoniae* in Spanish hospitals: 2nd multicenter study. *Enferm. Infecc. Microbiol. Clin.*, *27*, 503–510.

Arihiro, S., Nakashima, A., Matsuoka, M., Suto, S., Uchiyama, K., Kato, T., Mitobe, J., et al., (2019). Randomized trial of vitamin D supplementation to prevent seasonal influenza and upper respiratory infection in patients with inflammatory bowel disease. *Inflammatory Bowel Diseases, 25*(6), 1088–1095.

Bellows, L., & Moore, R., (2015). *Water-Soluble Vitamins*. Colorado State University.

Bender, D. A., (2003). *Nutritional Biochemistry of the Vitamins*. Cambridge, U.K.: Cambridge University Press.

Borel, P., Caillaud, D., & Cano, N. J., (2015). Vitamin D bioavailability: State of the art. *Critical Reviews in Food Science and Nutrition, 55*(9), 1193–1205.

Carr, A. C., & Maggini, S., (2017). Vitamin C and immune function. *Nutrients*, *9*, 1211.

Carr, A. C., Rosengrave, P. C., Bayer, S., Chambers, S., Mehrtens, J., & Shaw, G. M., (2017). Hypovitaminosis C and vitamin C deficiency in critically ill patients despite recommended enteral and parenteral intakes. *Crit. Care, 21*, 300.

Chandra, R. K., (1997). Nutrition and the immune system: An introduction. *Am. J. Clin. Nutr., 66*(2), 460S–463S.

Chandra, R. K., (1997). Nutrition and the immune system: An introduction. *The American Journal of Clinical Nutrition, 66*(2), 460S–463S.

Charan, J., Goyal, J. P., Saxena, D., & Yadav, P., (2012). Vitamin D for prevention of respiratory tract infections: A systematic review and meta-analysis. *Journal Of Pharmacology & Pharmacotherapeutics, 3*(4), 300.

Chen, L., Hu, C., Hood, M., Zhang, X., Zhang, L., Kan, J., & Du, J. (2020). A novel combination of vitamin C, curcumin, and glycyrrhizic acid potentially regulates immune and inflammatory response associated with coronavirus infections: A perspective from system biology analysis. *Nutrients, 12*, 1193.

Chien, C. T., Chang, W. T., Chen, H. W., Wang, T. D., Liou, S. Y., Chen, T. J., Chang, Y. L., et al., (2004). Ascorbate supplement reduces oxidative stress in dyslipidemic patients undergoing apheresis. *Arteriosclerosis, Thrombosis, and Vascular Biology, 24*(6), 1111–1117.

Elisa, P., Oscar, C., Alessandra, B., Fiorenza, O., Carmela, S., Andrea, G., & Mauro, P., (2011). Vitamin E supplementation in old mice induces antimicrobial activity and improves the efficacy of daptomycin in an animal model of wounds infected with methicillin-resistant *Staphylococcus aureus*. *Journal of Antimicrobial Chemotherapy, 66*(9), 2184–2185.

Fabio, I., Massimiliano, M., Massimo, M., Francesco, F., Claudio, M. M., Paolo, S., Giancarlo, C., & Letizia, S., (2020). Diet supplementation, probiotics, and nutraceuticals in SARS-CoV-2 infection: A scoping review. *Nutrients, 12*, 1718.

Fukuwatari, T., & Shibata, K., (2008). Urinary water-soluble vitamins and their metabolite contents as nutritional markers for evaluating vitamin intakes in young Japanese women. *Journal of Nutritional Science and Vitaminology, 54*(3), 223–229.

Gombart, A. F., Pierre, A., & Maggini, S., (2020). A review of micronutrients and the immune system–working in harmony to reduce the risk of infection. *Nutrients, 12*, 236.

Grant, W. B., Lahore, H., McDonnell, S. L., Baggerly, C. A., French, C. B., Aliano, J. L., & Bhattoa, H. P., (2020). Evidence that vitamin D supplementation could reduce the risk of influenza and COVID-19 infections and deaths. *Nutrients, 12*, 988.

Guillin, O. M., Vindry, C., Ohlmann, T., & Chavatte, L., (2019). Selenium, selenoproteins, and viral infection. *Nutrients, 11*(9), 2101.

Gysin, D. V., Dao, D., Gysin, C. M., Lytvyn, L., & Loeb, M., (2016). Effect of vitamin D3 supplementation on respiratory tract infections in healthy individuals: A systematic review and meta-analysis of randomized controlled trials. *Plos One, 11*(9), 1–17.

Hemila, H., & Chalker, E., (2019). Vitamin C can shorten the length of stay in the ICU: A meta-analysis. *Nutrients, 11*(4), 708.

Hemila, H., & Louhiala, P., (2013). Vitamin C for preventing and treating pneumonia. *Cochrane Database of Systematic Reviews*, (8), Article no. CD005532.

Hillman, R. S., (1995). Hematopoietic agents: Growth factors, minerals, and vitamins. *Goodman and Gilman's The Pharmacological Basis of Therapeutics*, 1311–1340.

Jacqueline, C. A., Maria, F. B., Morais, B., Gla′ucia, M. M. G., Saulo, R. T., Maria, A. F., Lucindo, J. Q., et al., (2017). Menadione (vitamin K) enhances the antibiotic activity of drugs by cell membrane permeabilization mechanism. *Saudi Journal of Biological Sciences, 24*(1), 59–64.

Jennifer, M., (2007). *Folic Acid.* Medical Communication Consultants.

Jing, L. (2018). Evidence is stronger than you think: A meta-analysis of vitamin C use in patients with sepsis. *Li. Critical Care, 22*, 258.

Kalra, E. K., (2003). Nutraceutical definition and introduction. *AAPS PharmSci., 5*(3), 27–28.

Kang, C. I., Kim, S. H., & Kim, D. M., (2004). Risk factors for ciprofloxacin resistance in bloodstream infections due to extended-spectrum b-lactamase-producing *Escherichia coli* and *Klebsiella pneumoniae. Microb. Drug Resist., 10*, 71–76.

Keservani, R. K., Kesharwani, R. K., Sharma, A. K., Vyas, N., & Chadoker, A., (2010b). Nutritional supplements: An overview. *International Journal of Current Pharmaceutical Review and Research, 1*(1), 59–75.

Keservani, R. K., Kesharwani, R. K., Vyas, N., Jain, S., Raghuvanshi, R., & Sharma, A. K., (2010a). Nutraceutical and functional food as future food: A review. *Der Pharmacia Lettre, 2*(1), 106–116.

Keservani, R. K., Sharma, A. K., & Kesharwani, R. K. (2017). An overview and therapeutic applications of nutraceutical and functional foods. *Recent Advances in Drug Delivery Technology*, 160–201. ISBN:9781522507543.

Keservani, R. K., Sharma, A. K., & Kesharwani, R. K. (2020). *Nutraceuticals and Dietary Supplements: Applications in Health Improvement and Disease Management.* CRC Press. ISBN: 9781771888738.

Klack, K., & Carvalho, J. F., (2006). Vitamina K: Metabolismo, fontes e interac¸a˜o com o anticoagulante varfarina. *Rev. Bras. Reumatol., 46*, 398–406.

Kohler, T., Pechere, J. C., & Plesiat, P., (1999). Bacterial antibiotic efflux systems are of medical importance. *Cell. Mol. Life Sci., 56*, 771–778.

Maqbool, A., & Stallings, V. A., (2008). Update on fat-soluble vitamins in cystic fibrosis. *Current Opinion in Pulmonary Medicine, 14*(6), 574–581.

Martineau, A. R., Jolliffe, D. A., Hooper, R. L., Greenberg, L., Aloia, J. F., Bergman, P., Dubnov-Raz, G., et al., (2017). Vitamin D supplementation to prevent acute respiratory tract infections: Systematic review and meta-analysis of individual participant data. *BMJ, 2*(15), 356–i6583.

Marwa, M. N., & Miguel, A. V., (2018). Vitamin E increases antimicrobial sensitivity by inhibiting bacterial lipocalin antibiotic binding. *mSphere- American Society for Microbiology, 3*(6), Article no. e00564–18.

Maton, A., Hopkins, J., McLaughlin, C. W., Johnson, S., Warner, M., Lahart, D., & Wright, J. D., (1993). *Human Biology and Health.* Article No. 32308337.

Mawson, A. R., (2013). Role of fat-soluble vitamins A and D in the pathogenesis of influenza: A new perspective. *Infectious Dis.* Article no. 246737.

May, J. M., & Harrison, F. E., (2013). Role of vitamin C in the function of the vascular endothelium. *Antioxid. Redox Signal, 19*, 2068–2083.

Mc Mahon, R. J., (2002). Biotin in metabolism and molecular biology. *Annu. Rev. Nutr., 22*, 221–239.

Minnja, S., Hartmann, S. M., Stefan, B., & Markus, M. H., (2020). Vitamin E as promising adjunct treatment option in the combat of infectious diseases caused by bacteria including multi-drug resistant pathogens – Results from a comprehensive literature survey. *European Journal of Microbiology and Immunology, 10*(4), 193–201.

Nuraly, S. A., Ilya, D., & Mohammed, S. R. (2022). Role of vitamins in maintaining structure and function of intestinal microbiome. *Comprehensive Gut Microbiota,* 320–334.

Nuratiqah, F., Voon, K. C., Pei, P. C., Wai, F. L., Chee, W. L., Rusliza, B., Sui, K. C., & Tze, Y. L., (2022). Riboflavin as a promising antimicrobial agent? A multi-perspective review. *Current Research in Microbial Sciences, 3*, 100111.

Parra, M., Stahl, S., & Hellmann, H., (2018). Vitamin b_6 and its role in cell metabolism and physiology. *Cells*, 7 (7), 84.

Pyung, A., Soonok, K., & Yong-Hwan, L., (2005). Vitamin B1 functions as an activator of plant disease resistance. *Plant Physiology*, *7*(138), 1505–1515.

Rane, B. R., Bharath, M. S., Patil, R. R., Keservani, R. K., & Jain, A. S. (2020b). Novel approaches in nutraceuticals; Chapter 11. In: Rajesh, K. K., Raj, K. K., & Anil, K. S., (eds.), *Enhancing the Therapeutic Efficacy of Herbal Formulations Through Novel Drug Delivery* (pp. 241–266). IGI Global International Publisher, Pennsylvania, USA. ISBN13: 9781799844532.

Rane, B. R., Patil, A. S., Keservani, R. K., & Jain, A. S., (2020a). Novel approaches in herbal formulation; Chapter 2. In: Rajesh, K. K., Raj, K. K., & Anil, K. S., (eds.), *Enhancing the Therapeutic Efficacy of Herbal Formulations Through Novel Drug Delivery Systems* (pp. 43–68). IGI Global International Publisher, Pennsylvania, USA. ISBN13: 9781799844532.

Rane, B. R., Tadavi, S. A., & Keservani, R. K., (2020c). Naturopathy; Chapter 12. In: Anil, K. S., Raj, K. K., & Surya, P. G., (eds.), *Herbal Product Development* (321–347). Apple Academic Press, CRC Press, Taylor & Francis Group. ISBN: 9781771888776.

Roth, J., Lawrence, J., & Bobik, T., (1996). Cobalamin (Coenzyme B12): Synthesis and biological significance. *Annual Review of Microbiology*, *50*, 137–181.

Semba, R. D., (2012). The discovery of the vitamins. *Int. J. Vitam. Nutr. Res.*, *82*(5), 310–315.

Shaik-Dasthagirisaheb, Y. B., Varvara, G., Murmura, G., Saggini, A., Caraffa, A., Antinolfi, P., Tetè, S., et al., (2013). Role of vitamins D, E, and C in immunity and inflammation. *J. Biol. Regul. Homeost. Agents*, *27*, 291–295.

Sharma, A. K., Keservani, R. K., & Gautam, S. P., (2020). *Herbal Product Development*. Apple Academic Press, CRC Press, Taylor & Francis Group. ISBN: 9781771888776.

Singh, P., Kesharwani, R. K., & Keservani, R. K. (2017). Antioxidants and vitamins: Roles in cellular function and metabolism. In: *Sustained Energy for Enhanced Human Functions and Activity* (pp. 385–407). Academic Press. ISBN:9780128054130.

Surana, K. R., Ahire, E. D., Sonawane, V. N., Talele, S. G., & Talele, G. S., (2021). Informatics and methods in nutrition design and development. *Natural Food Products and Waste Recovery: Healthy Foods, Nutrition Design, and Extraction of Valuable Compounds*, 33.

Surana, K., Chaudhary, B., Diwaker, M., & Sharma, S. (2018). Benzophenone: A ubiquitous scaffold in medicinal chemistry. *MedChemComm*, *9*(11), 1803–1817.

Talele, S. G., Ahire, E. D., Surana, K. R., Sonawane, V. N., & Talele, G. S., (2022). Coronavirus disease (COVID-19): A past and present perspective. *Asian Journal of Pharmaceutical Research*, *12*(1), 45–53.

Tang, A. M., Graham, N. M., & Saah, A. J., (1996). Effects of micronutrient intake on survival in human immunodeficiency virus type 1 infection. *American Journal of Epidemiology*, *143*(12), 1244–1256.

Urashima, M., Segawa, T., Okazaki, M., Kurihara, M., Wada, Y., & Ida, H., (2010). Randomized trial of vitamin D supplementation to prevent seasonal influenza A in schoolchildren. *The American Journal of Clinical Nutrition*, *91*(5), 1255–1260.

Vincenti, A., Bertuzzo, L., Limitone, A., D'Antona, G., & Cena, H., (2021). Perspective: Practical approach to preventing subclinical B12 Deficiency in elderly population. *Nutrients, 13(6), 1913.*

Vitamin and Mineral Requirements in Human Nutrition, (2004). pp. 340–341. World Health Organization and Food and Agriculture Organization of the United Nations.

Wang, Y., Lin, H., Lin, B. W., & Lin, J. D., (2019). Effects of different ascorbic acid doses on the mortality of critically ill patients: A meta-analysis. *Annals of Intensive Care*, *9*(1), 58.

Wenting, H., Shengfeng, H., & Xialin, D. (2018). Vitamin B5 reduces bacterial growth by regulating innate immunity and adaptive immunity in mice infected with *Mycobacterium tuberculosis*. *Front. Immunol.*, *9*, 365.

Wessels, I., Maywald, M., & Rink, L., (2017). Zinc is a gatekeeper of immune function. *Nutrients, 9*(12), 1286.

Yuanyuan, X., Shasha, X., & Kun, Y., (2018). Cobalamin (vitamin B12) induced a shift in microbial composition and metabolic activity in an *in vitro* colon simulation. *Front. Microbiol.*, *11*(16), 2780.

Zhou, J., Du, J., Huang, L., Wang, Y., Shi, Y., & Lin, H., (2018). Preventive effects of vitamin D on seasonal influenza A in infants: A multicenter, randomized, open, controlled clinical trial. *The Pediatric Infectious Disease Journal*, *37*(8), 749–754.

CHAPTER 7

Vitamins as Nutraceuticals for COVID-19

PANKAJ R. AHER,[1] KHEMCHAND R. SURANA,[2] EKNATH D. AHIRE,[3] SUNIL K. MAHAJAN,[4] and SANJAY J. KSHIRSAGAR[3]

[1]*Department of Pharmaceutical Chemistry, Loknete Dr. J. D. Pawar College of Pharmacy, Manur, Kalwan, Nashik, Maharashtra, India*

[2]*Department of Pharmaceutical Chemistry, Shreeshakti Shaikshanik Sanstha, Divine College of Pharmacy, Satana, Nashik, Maharashtra, India*

[3]*Department of Pharmaceutics, MET's Institute of Pharmacy, Bhujbal Knowledge City, Adgaon, Nashik, Maharashtra, India*

[4]*Department of Pharmaceutical Chemistry, M.G.V's Samajshri Prashant Dada Hiray, College of Pharmacy, Malegaon, Nashik, Maharashtra, India*

ABSTRACT

The coronavirus of 2019 (COVID-19) has caused international outbreaks and main loss of life. The disruption to public health and financial well-being has exceeded the direct results of COVID-19. The clinical outcomes of COVID-19 range from person to person. Some humans may also haven't any signs, even as others may also have signs inclusive of fever, headache, nasal congestion, chronic dry cough, and/or stomach signs and symptoms. People with this circumstance may also have acute respiration distress syndrome (ARDS), leading to problem respiration and reducing blood oxygen levels that require oxygen assistance, even mechanical ventilation. Other severe problems can consist of abnormal blood contact, emotional problems, damage to the cardiovascular system, and multiple organ failure, which may lead to death. Unfortunately, SARS-CoV-2 appears to have a massive effect on those maximums at risk in society, which includes those who are

Preventive and Therapeutic Role of Vitamins as Nutraceuticals. Khemchand R. Surana, Eknath D. Ahire, Raj K. Keservani, & Rajesh K. Kesharwani (Eds.)

physically weak, consisting of the elderly and people with comorbidities. Existing reusable treatment options, such as prophylactic and therapeutic agents, can reduce the devastation of the epidemic. Emerging evidence of capability applications in different medical conditions has caused the investigation of vitamins as a treatment for COVID-19. This consists of a variety of vitamins, likely Vitamin D, C, Folate, and Vitamin B, all of which might be presently under clinical research. In this study, we thoroughly understood the proof surrounding vitamins, including the prophylaxis dietary supplements and COVID-19 treatment.

7.1 INTRODUCTION

The epidemic has caused severe public health disruption globally and has gone beyond the direct effects of COVID-19. People need more safety through the use of plenty of nutritious foods and nutritional dietary supplements. Nutraceuticals are described as health advantages in addition to their fundamental dietary value through prophylaxis and/or treatment of a disease or illness (Keservani et al., 2010a, b, 2017, 2020; Lordan et al., 2021). Dietary supplements are supposed to increase the dietary value someone may need because of dietary deficiencies or malnutrition, which has led to a spike in the sale of dietary supplements, nutraceuticals, and various products with the effect of "strengthening the immune system." According to available clinical information, the European Food Safety Authority (EFSA) competent clinical panel has decided that the following six vitamins are vital for the healthful maintenance of the immune system: D, C, A (and ß-carotene), and B-group vitamins (especially B6, Folate, and B12) (Lordan, 2021). The patient's nutritional status plays a vital position in the immune system function and in the patient's general health outcomes following various diseases that have additionally been highlighted in relation to COVID-19 (Costagliola et al., 2021). The diverse dietary effects of vitamins have been previously investigated *in vitro*, *in vivo*, and clinically against several pathogenic viruses, including polio, influenza, and different respiratory viruses. Indeed, vitamin D supplements have been bonded to possible safety again respiratory infections, and vitamin D deficiency or lacking may increase people's chance of seasonal flu. Vitamin D deficiency is likewise a major risk issue for HIV-positive patients, as deficiency may have an adverse effect at the time of HIV (Shakoor et al., 2021). However, support may play a shielding role, and despite the fact that similar studies are needed as a result, researchers have targeted their interest at the ability to find a route to prevent COVID-19 with nutraceuticals such as vitamin D (Bae & Kim, 2020).

Coronavirus (COVID-19) is a global public health problem resulting from the novel coronavirus SARS-CoV-2 and represents a prime risk to health care worldwide. It was first diagnosed in a set of patients with symptoms of pneumonia in the city of Chinas, Wuhan, in late 2019 (Alexander et al., 2020). Originally, it was named 2019 nCoV but was renamed COVID-19 by the World Health Organization. It is taken into consideration to be much more likely or similar to the Middle East Respiratory Syndrome (MERS) and the Serious Respiratory Syndrome (SARS) virus (Galmés et al., 2020). The virus may be transmitted from individual to individual through respiration drops, contact, and formulas. SARS-CoV-2 has main types: 'Type L' (70%) and 'S' (30%), and the type L is very large, aggressive, and contagious. Symptoms of COVID-19 vary from blurred vision to severe and encompass fever, dry cough, pneumonia, malaise, and acute respiratory distress syndrome (Corrao et al., 2021). Currently, there are different permitted COVID-19 treatments, but prevention strategies include social isolation, public hygiene, and wearing a face mask (Subedi et al., 2021). Current best practices for decreasing COVID-19 (Ahire et al., 2021). Recent evidence has suggested that dietary help can also additionally play a supportive role in COVID-19 patients. Administration of better doses than recommended nutritional dietary supplements, including vitamins D, C, and E, may have useful consequences, probably decreasing SARS-CoV-2 viral infections and duration of hospital stay (Tahir et al., 2020). These nutrients are fine known for his or her antioxidant (Singh et al., 2017) properties and immunomodulatory (Keservani et al., 2015) consequences. Deficiency of those nutrients can reason immune system dysfunction and increase the chances of pathological infection. In fact, vitamin deficiencies were diagnosed in high-risk groups of COVID-19 sufferers, including the elderly, which increases morbidity and mortality (Lammi & Arnoldi, 2021). Overall, in addition, studies are needed before compelling evidence-based design. However, nutritional status plays an important role in outpatient outcomes, and those products can assist in delaying deficits. For example, evidence suggests that vitamin D lacking can be associated with a better incidence of infection and importance of COVID-19, suggesting that vitamin D supplementation may keep prophylactic or therapeutic value. A huge number of clinical organizations are actually recommending vitamin D supplementation for those at high risk of COVID-19. The reason why vitamin D and different vitamins may be treated as nutritious foods and dietary supplements is simply the beginning; here, we're looking for out how effective those nutraceutical vitamins and nutritional dietary supplements are in the COVID-19 disaster. It is well-known that older ones are much more likely to be malnourished and to compromise their immune system through immunosenescence, which greatly increases their risk of adverse effects from COVID-19 and makes adequate nutrients doubly important. The position of nutrients A, C, and D in immunization is discussed, and its status in a patient infected with SARS-CoV-2 and its potential therapeutic role (Wong et al., 2021).

7.2 NUTRACEUTICALS AND SUPPLEMENTS AMID THE PANDEMIC

The term Nutraceutical is an integrated time period for foods and drugs that, in particular, displays food or a part of it that has medicinal or health benefits. Known examples of nutritious foods are milk, diverse vegetables, fruit juice, etc., as those foods additionally play an important role in health benefits (Grant & Lordan, 2021). Along with conventional therapies, the usage of adjunctive of these nutraceuticals can be useful in the treatment and/or prevention of COVID-19. Here, we have summarized some nutraceuticals examined to be used in COVID-19. Globally, vitamin D, C and nutritional dietary supplements are a few of the most important interventions under investigation (Singh et al., 2021). Vitamin C is the only supplement this is being investigated for its long-term association with increasing immune function, lesser time period of the intensive care unit (ICU) or hospitalization, and decreasing mechanical ventilation time for those who are critically ill (Tramontana et al., 2020). However, it remains to be visible whether vitamin C can affect the clinical course of sufferers with COVID-19; that's the situation of a few clinical trials (Barrea et al., 2022). Both healthful and vulnerable people need to consider dietary supplementation or vitamin C supplementation if they suspect that they lack vitamins (A, B, E, and K), trace elements (selenium, copper, etc.), and natural products (elderberry), echinacea, rosemary, curcumin, bee propolis, etc.), melatonin, phosphatidylserine, collagen, and various different components in sand and nutrients are all taken into consideration to enhance prophylactic and potential therapies in opposition to COVID-19 (Infusino et al., 2020). Nutraceuticals and supplements also are taken into consideration in the treatment of COVID-19 cardiovascular symptoms (van Kempen & Deixler, 2021).

7.2.1 VITAMINS

Vitamin micronutrients play a crucial role in the proper formation and proper functioning of proteins in addition to in a number of physiological approaches and signaling pathways in the human body (Brenner et al., 2020). Vitamin C (ascorbic acid) is a water-soluble vitamin this is proposed to have antioxidant, anti-inflammatory, and immunomodulatory properties. In addition, also it acts as an enzyme cofactor for many biosynthetic pathways and might increase the endogenous synthesis of catecholamines (Samad et al., 2021). Vitamin C has been studied traditionally to be used in many viral and non-viral infections, which include herpes zoster infection, flu infection, and the common cold (Ashok et al., 2020). However, because of conflicting results and limited quality studies, using vitamin C in these indicators is not constantly recommended. There are numerous ongoing research inspecting using vitamin C in the treatment of COVID-19. Although now no longer directly related to COVID-19, vitamin C has additionally been examined to be used in septic shock and ARDS, each of which can be traces of COVID-19 infection; however, studies have found conflicting results for these indicators. Serious patients will also be deficient in vitamin C (Rodriguez-Leyva & Pierce, 2021). Several research have located that maximum septic patients have hypovitaminosis C. Since vitamin C cannot be produced externally, critically ill patients can also additionally need vitamin C supplementation. Dose-dependent IV management is preferred when used in critically ill patients (Pisoschi et al., 2022). Although aspect effects are uncommon in over-the-counter (OTC) doses, in high doses which have been studied for septic shock and ARDS, potential aspect effects consist of nausea, abdominal pain, and calcium oxalate nephropathy, and glucose-6-phosphate dehydrogenase, lack of hemolysis (Tiwari et al., 2022). Blood sugar levels in the care place might not be as bad as vitamin C and glucose are structurally similar. Vitamins D and E also are examined as those fat-soluble vitamins can also additionally have anti-inflammatory and anti-inflammatory properties (Žmitek et al., 2021). In each case, vitamin D supplementation is of interest as low vitamin D stages can be related to an accelerated risk of ARDS and infectious diseases, inclusive of upper respiratory infections (Bianconi et al., 2021). Vitamin D may additionally alter the immune response, facilitate the production of antibiotic peptides in the lungs to assist in preventing respiratory infections, and promote the expression of ACE2 genes. Since the ACE2 gene is less in the regulation of COVID-19, using vitamin D can also additionally help maintain the regulation of the renin-angiotensin-aldosterone system. Vitamin D may additionally lessen cytokine depletion (Ahvanooei et al., 2021). Although side effects are uncommon, vitamin D-associated toxicity can also additionally consist of nausea, confusion, hypercalcemia, belly pain, polyuria, and dehydration. Due to factors such as heterogeneity within the studies and absence of excessive-quality evidence, it is tough to provide specific recommendations for using vitamins C, D, and E in this patient population; therefore, patients need to obtain as a minimum a number of their recommended daily vitamins (Di Renzo et al., 2020).

7.2.2 VITAMIN D

Vitamin D is a fat-soluble steroid hormone mostly found in types of cholesterol, ergocalciferol (vitamin D2) and cholecalciferol (vitamin D3), each of which might be produced constantly in the dermis found in 7-dehydrocholesterol in response to mild-ultraviolet (UVB) in the sun (Figure 7.1). Vitamin D is also observed in meal sources together with fish, milk, eggs, and supplements. It is thought that 200–800 IU of vitamin D is needed daily, which is often difficult to attain with the aid of using diet alone, but exposure to UVB mild is a main contributor to the preservation of vitamin D levels (Horowitz & Freeman, 2020). 1,25-(OH)2D]; however, this molecule has a half-life of some hours and is most commonly found in less concentration. Thus, vitamin D status is measured with the aid of using a measurement of serum 25-hydroxyvitamin D, a small biologically active precursor moiety with a half-life of up to 15 days found in high concentrations 1,000 times in serum (Mattioli et al., 2020). Modern house style, clothing, and seasonal lighting significantly have an effect on the amount of sun exposure. Although the concentration of vitamin D in the blood may also last for several weeks, the vitamin D stored in fatty tissue can last as long as three months (Mehrotra & Jadhav, 2021). There also are significant differences in 25-hydroxyvitamin D levels amongst people because of physical and environmental factors. Factors such as impurities, dark skin tone, age, and pre-current situations, together with obesity (Jarouliya & Keservani, 2019a), can growth a person's threat of vitamin D deficiency. But this is nevertheless debated (Galanakis, 2020).

7.2.2.1 VITAMIN D AND THE PANDEMIC

At the beginning of the epidemic, it turned into thought that the onset of SARS-CoV-2 and the severity of COVID-19 could be related to the patient's vitamin D levels. Previously, observational studies have reported institutions among low serum levels of 25-hydroxyvitamin D and the risk of serious respiratory infections. Indeed, modification in vitamin D supplements may also reduce the threat of developing respiratory infections (Souza et al.,

2020). The first instances of COVID-19 have been reported in Chinas Wuhan in late November 2019 before the onset of winter and unfolded unexpectedly in most of the northern hemisphere. Outbreaks seem exacerbated during the winter, with decreased levels of vitamin D in the south; at periods of time, the southern hemisphere infection rates remain lower, with vitamin D levels higher. This has led researchers to impeach whether or not there is a seasonal complication of SARS-CoV-2 infection and whether or not vitamin D levels may play a role (Chirumbolo, 2021). Figure 7.1 represents a schematic representation of vitamin D sources and synthesis in humans.

7.2.2.2 IMMUNOMODULATORY ROLE OF VITAMIN D

Vitamin D is a fat-soluble steroid hormone precursor derived from the ultraviolet B (UVB) rays of 7-dehydrocholesterol (7-DHC) in the skin epidermis, where its miles converted right into a circulating precursor of cholecalciferol. In the liver, cholecalciferol is hydroxylated to form 25-hydroxyvitamin D, which is converted to the active hormone 1,25-hydroxyvitamin D (1, 25 (OH)2D) in the nephron (Rezaei et al., 2021; Ali et al., 2021). Vitamin D has different roles in the body's systems, including both innate and mutant immune responses, as shown in Figure 7.2.

Vitamin D improves innate cellular immunity by promoting the expression of antimicrobial peptides, consisting of catholicizing and defensins. Defensins keep strong adhesion to the gap, adhere, and enhance anti-oxidative gene expression. Influenza-like infections are regarded to most severely damage the integrity of epithelial tight junctions, which will increase the risk of infection and pulmonary edema (Handu et al., 2021). Vitamin D is known for retaining the integrity of such compounds, with low levels of vitamin D receptor expression leading to increased expression of claudin-2 and inflammation (Jayawardena & Misra, 2020). Vitamin D additionally promotes the secretion of monocytes to macrophages while growing superoxide production, phagocytosis, and viral destruction. In addition, vitamin D is capable of regulating the immune response by suppressing T-helper-type 1 (Th1) cell activity and lowering the production of anti-inflammatory cytokines by Th2 cells, and indirectly suppressing Th1 cell divides pro-inflammatory (Ashok, Ravivarman, & Kayalvizhi, 2020).

Lacking Vitamin D has been recommended to increase the incidence and severity of COVID-19 infections. Patients with COVID-19 have been time and again proven to have low amounts of vitamin D, meaning that plasma concentrations are a part of the control. Therefore, supplementation

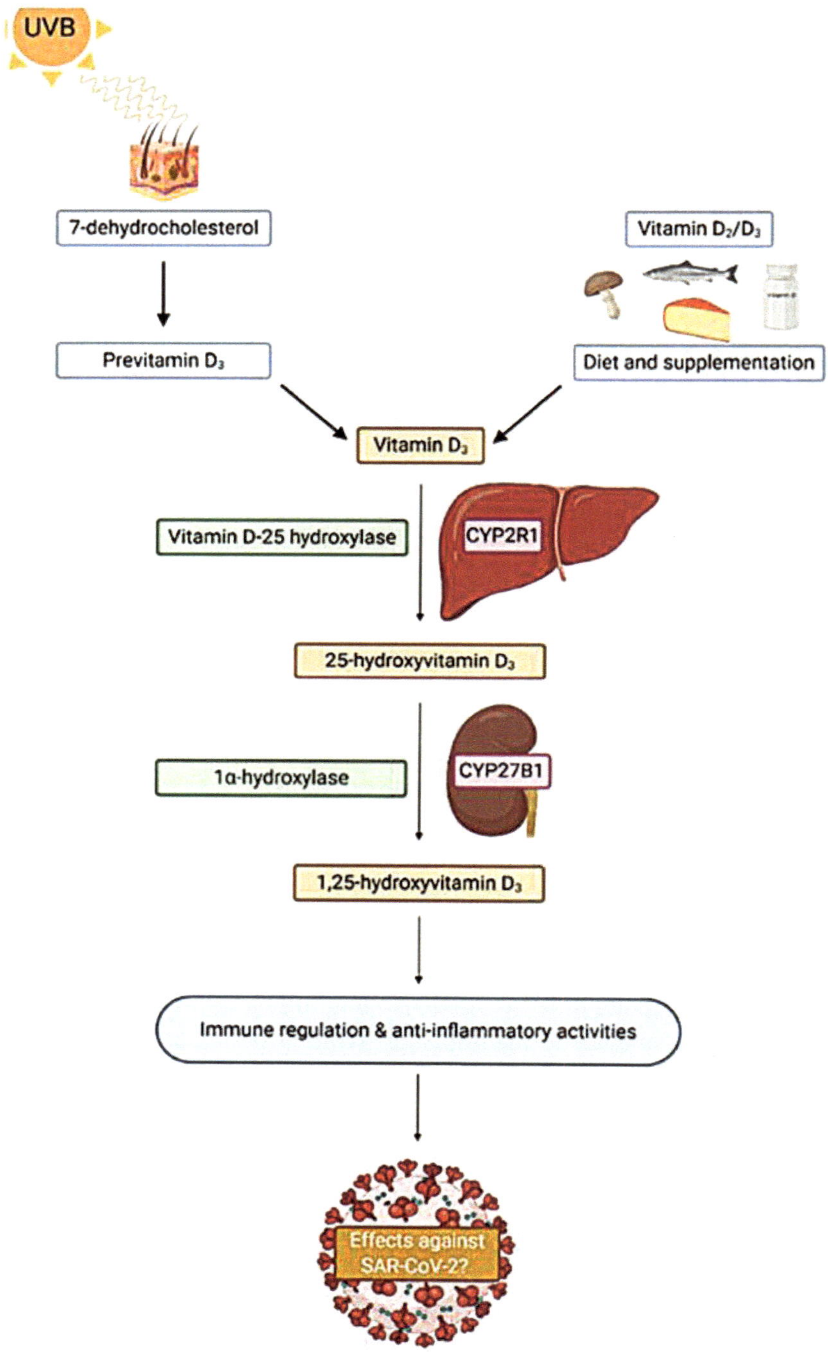

FIGURE 7.1 Schematic representation of vitamin D sources and synthesis in humans.

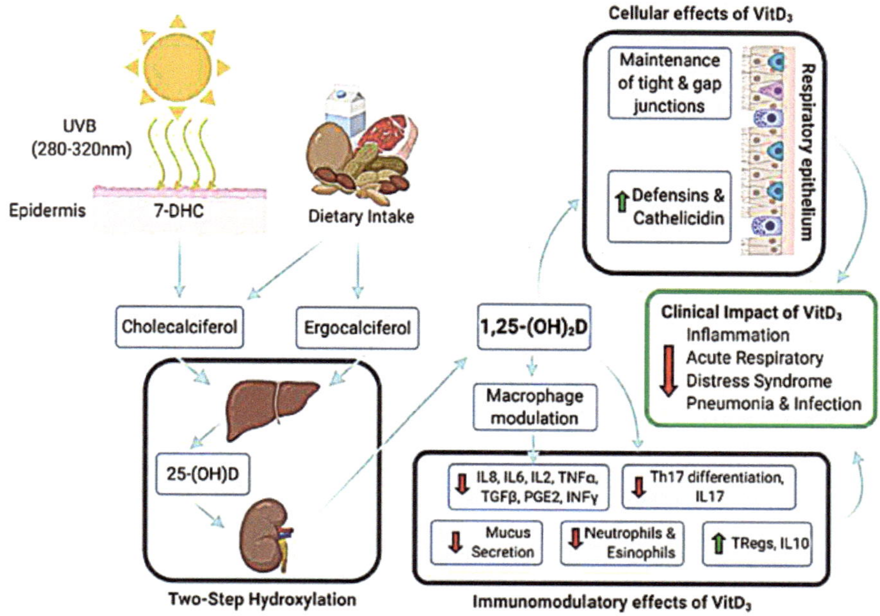

FIGURE 7.2 Immunomodulatory actions of vitamin D [IL: Interleukin; TNF: Tumor necrosis factor; IFN: Interferon; Th: T-Helper; 7-DHC: 7-Dehydrocholesterol; and PGE2: Prostaglandin E2].

of vitamin D is recommended to increase immunity against COVID-19 and reduce mortality; however, this theory is useful to be tested in human trials. It has been advised that adequate vitamin D levels might also additionally help protect the respiratory epithelium from pathogenic attacks, decreasing the threat of infection (Singh et al., 2021). Pre-print studies in Israel also found that vitamin D is related to morbidity, even after corrective sociodemographic variability and comorbidity (Borges et al., 2021). These findings are primarily based totally on additional studies; however, for now, these results need to be confirmed. However, large bio-bank studies conclude that vitamin D lacking becomes not adhere to the incidence of COVID-19, nor did it explain the difference in demographic differences in infection rates (Hunter et al., 2020). It seems that the association between vitamin D and COVID-19 is highly dependent on statistical evaluation and does not continue to be constant after the correction of important, complicated variables, including comorbidity and sociodemographic characteristics. Although it isn't always clear whether or not vitamin D status influences infection levels, there may be evidence that it does play a role in reducing the severity of the disease

(Nimer et al., 2022). COVID-19-associated mortality rates vary from country to country, and the southern hemisphere is lower than the Northern Hemisphere. Another theory that explains this pattern is that people in the northern hemisphere are at greater risk of vitamin deficiencies because of a loss of sun exposure in winter as compared to the summer solstice during the monsoon months (January–May) (Borkhade & Sawal, 2021). It has additionally been shown that countries with high stages of vitamin D deficiency often have a better burden of COVID-19 morbidity and mortality. Evidence has clearly shown that mortality rates are high in COVID-19 patients deficient in vitamin D, possibly because of vitamin D deficiency due to increased use of supplements. In addition, C-reactive protein (CRP), an anti-inflammatory and surrogate marker for cytokine storm, was significantly exposed to sufferers with extreme signs and symptoms of COVID-19 and became related to vitamin D deficiency showed an association between vitamin D deficiency and severe COVID-19 (Quiles et al., 2020). Participants with vitamin D deficiency have been much more likely to have coagulopathy and suppress immune function. Mechanical understanding of the role of the virus has diagnosed the number of proteins (Jarouliya & Keservani, 2019b) that it could regulate, yet no definite evidence has been discovered. However, with to be evidence now, many groups are starting to review whether or not support should be commended more widely (Pouramini et al., 2021).

7.2.2.3 PROTECTIVE ROLE OF VITAMIN D IN VIRAL INFECTION

Vitamin D supplements are recognized to assist in reducing the occurrence and severity of viral infections, and there is a negative correlation between upper respiratory tract infections and serum levels of 25-hydroxyvitamin D (Ooi & Pak, 2021). While the impact of vitamin D on SARS-CoV-2 infection has now no longer been demonstrated, supplementation may reduce inflammatory cytokines and later reduce the severe respiration depression related to COVID-19 mortality. A number of human clinical trials have been registered to determine the impact of vitamin D supplementation in COVID-19 patients (Costagliola et al., 2021).

7.2.3 IMMUNOMODULATORY ROLE OF VITAMIN C

Vitamin C, or ascorbic acid, is a water-soluble component which can interact with humans. Vitamin C acts as an anti-oxidant this is capable of eradicating reactive oxygen species (ROS), as a result protecting biomolecules, inclusive of proteins, lipids, and nucleotides, from oxidative damage and dysfunction (Uddin et al., 2021). Vitamin C is gathered in leukocytes at a concentration of 50,100 instances higher than plasma. During infection, the vitamin C found in leukocytes is used up immediately. Disruption of the balance among antioxidant defenses and oxidant production can modify many signaling pathways that encompass inflammatory signals, such as nuclear factor κB (NF-κB) (Michienzi & Badowski, 2020). Increased oxidative levels result in the activation of NF-κB, which causes the emergence of cascade by nuclear aspect κB (NF-κB). The quit result of the continuous production of oxidative species and inflammatory mediators. NF-κB is concerned with the inflammatory response, pathogenesis of certain diseases, and viral infections. NF-κB inhibition can be a treatment modality against viral infections. Vitamin C is well-known for providing protection against infectious diseases. Indeed, support is known to support breathing mechanisms, preventing bacterial infections and reducing their duration and intensity, in addition to having antihistamine compounds that can improve flu-like symptoms (Papadopoulou et al., 2020). Interestingly, patients with intense breathing infections such as pneumonia or tuberculosis have reduced vitamin C plasma concentrations, and, in addition, vitamin C administration reduces the severity and duration of pneumonia in elderly patients. This is the key to the protective motion against respiratory infections, making it an exciting target for COVID-19 for use as Nutraceuticals (Hamid et al., 2021).

7.2.3.1 VITAMIN C AND IMMUNE RESPONSES IN COVID-19

Cytokine storm at some point of COVID-19 infection will increase because the disease progresses, and vitamin C has been suggested as an antidote to this. For example, pro-inflammatory cytokines IL-1β and TNF-α increase rapidly after infection, and the potent response resulting from this stimulates the continuous preservation of IL-6 and IL-8, promoting an additional inflammatory state. TNF-α is presently being investigated to assist the access of SARS-CoV-2 into host cells (Lehberger et al., 2021). Vitamin C is understood to reduce levels of pro-inflammatory cytokines, which include TNF-α, and increase anti-inflammatory cytokines (IL-10). Clinical studies have proven that taking 1 g/day of vitamin C will increase the release of IL-10 by mononuclear blood cells. IL-10 acts as an antagonistic response to IL-6 and regulates inflammation, which is important for COVID-19. Older people are more susceptible to infections because of immune system characteristics and immunosenescence (Hacışevki & Baba, 2020). Data show that COVID-19 patients are at high risk for pneumonia. In any other development, a small study on inflammatory biomarkers and specific respiratory restrictions turned into noted following intravenous administration of vitamin C. Therefore, vitamin C supplementation is a sensible choice for people lacking micronutrient risk of COVID-19 infection to help with prevention and support (Hernández et al., 2021).

7.2.4 VITAMIN A

Vitamin A may be achieved from an animal source in a pre-existing way or from non-animal sources in the previous way (pro-vitamin A carotenoids). Most carotenoids have immune functions in humans and animals: these compounds are associated with the right production and cytotoxic activity of subset lymphocytes, promote the release of certain cytokines, or have the potential for neutrophil/macrophage phagocytosis (Giovane et al., 2021). Deficiency of vitamin-A is leads to multiple immunosuppression disorders and degenerative reactions. In addition, side effects can increase in the event of obesity. Thus, malnutrition of this vitamin-A is associated with an increased risk of measles and diarrhea, while its increase is associated with decreased morbidity and mortality caused by infectious diseases (pneumonia-related pneumonia, HIV infection, and malaria) (Alzaben, 2020). In addition, vitamin A and different retinoids also exhibit important immune responses, including the ability to increase the effectiveness of type 1 interferons (IFN-I), an important antibacterial cytokine released by the innate immune system towards viral infections (Ooi, 2022). However, coronaviruses such as SARS-CoV-2 may suppress IFN-I-based antiviral response as part of their infection path. Therefore, retinoids have recently been identified as adjuvants that enhance IFN-I-mediated antiviral responses, the impact of which may also be examined in mixture with antibiotics currently studied in pre-SARS-CoV-2, particularly the ones primarily based totally on IFN-I mediated. At the same time, less Vitamin A levels are associated (though not significantly) with COVID-19 disease and death (Pedrosa et al., 2021). The GWA study revealed a number of genes associated with one-of-a-kind levels of carotenoids as well retinoids in the human plasma. Circulating carotenoid levels are associated with the chance of various complications, such as metabolic syndrome, while there is controversy about this effect and circulatory levels of retinol (Peng et al., 2021). In this context, the most important and significant genetic variant related to carotenoid plasma attention is rs6564851, with

BCO1 SNP as its biological mechanism being broadly described and related to different plasma carotenoid levels. This SNP is found in near proximity to genes including 15,150-monooxygenase 1 (BCO1), an enzyme expressed in the small intestine, liver, and other tissues such as adipocyte, which mediates the isometric separation of carotene and different pro-vitamin A carotenoids. Rs6564851 can be the most obvious genetic biomarker to evaluate the genetic risk of Vitamin A deficiency (Medoro et al., 2022).

7.3 FOLATE

Folate (or Vitamin B9) performs a crucial function in the metabolism of single carbon-mediated amino acids and Nucleic acid metabolism, in addition to DNA methylation. In addition, Folate is also crucial for the immune-mediated response of Th-1 and the proper production of antibodies (Lavie & Holick, 2011). Therefore, low levels of Folate consumption may also purpose an imbalance in the T and NK cell-mediated immune response and reduced antibody production. Although scientific evidence is still deficient, Folate may also play a prominent role in regulating COVID-19: it may play a role in the inhibition of furan (a modification involved in SARS-CoV-2 spike protein cleavage) and therefore prevent this step needed for the virus to reach the host cells (Mullin et al., 2021). In addition, disruption of the homocysteine metabolic pathway because of COVID-19 infection has recently been suggested as one of the leading causes of death of infected cells. Therefore, Folate, together with Vitamins B6 and B12, must be taken into consideration in the treatment of SARS-CoV-2 infections to suppress those problems. Regarding the relationship between the Folate diet and COVID-19 instances and mortality, the suboptimal situation is positively, however now no longer strongly related to those epidemiological parameters, even though it is much less effective than vitamins D, A, and C (Farzana et al., 2022). In addition, the prevalence of MTHFR 677TT genotype varies according to population, and it's been referred to that folic acid administration can smooth out genotype-caused differences. These data, brought to the reality that unused folic acid in plasma is associated with a lower in the cytotoxicity of natural killer cells, make this SNP a marker to consider complying with nutritional guidelines for proper immune function. Therefore, taking the C677T SNP as a marker to assess genetic predisposition to low Folate status, as well as dietary/healing strategies, should be considered to cover this issue (Ahire et al., 2020).

7.4 VITAMIN B6

It has been defined as a very good dietary supplement for Vitamin B6 (additionally referred to as Pyridoxine). Essential for maintaining the cytotoxic activity of NK cells, the improvement of proper lymphocytes, and the production of B-cell antibodies. Otherwise, unwanted use of this vitamin is related to low concentrations of circulating lymphocytes, impaired lymphocyte maturation, and decreased antibody-based responses. In an equal way as folate, the proper supply of Vitamin B6 (and B12) to patients affected by COVID-19 has been suggested as a part of a treatment regimen, even with formula supplements, with the intention to control metabolic metabolism disorders. Homocysteine pathway as a result of SARS-CoV-2 infection (Ahire et al., 2021). The recommended Vitamin B6 requirements are 1.6 mg/day for women and 1.7 mg/day for men and 25 mg/day for both sexes. Following the pattern of the vitamins analyzed above, the specified amounts increase in pregnancy or breastfeeding (1.8 and 1.7 mg/day, respectively) and PRI and UL decrease in infants and toddlers. There is some equality concerning Vitamin B6 consumption levels among the reviewed countries. In addition, no clear association with epidemiologic COVID-19 signs is determined in this micronutrient (Ahire et al., 2020).

7.5 VITAMIN B12

Adequate Vitamin B12 consumption is also crucial for immune production and clonal proliferation. Thus, its deficiency adheres with a low amount of circulating lymphocytes and adjusted antibody-based responses. Vitamin B12 has recently been suggested as a capacity treatment against COVID-19 (Ahire et al., 2021). This evidence changed into collected by *silico* methods geared toward detecting malignant cell fashions against SARS-CoV-2 by combining genetic series with information associated with preceding remedies towards SARS-CoV and the MERS virus. In summary, this visual experiment changed primarily based totally on the identity of antimicrobial compounds, vitamins, antimicrobials, and different systemic drugs which could resist the two proteases that had to process and extract synthetic non-structural proteins from corona bacteria, so as to speak, protease type 3-C (M-pro) and papain-like protease (Plpro) (Talele et al., 2022). In addition, based on the fact that SARS-CoV-2 infection is related to the proliferation of cellular metabolism and the homocysteine pathway causing major complications from COVID-19, the right supply of Vitamin B12 and Folate mentioned above, and Vitamin B6 should be important for COVID-19 patients. Therefore, this evidence supports the significance of this diet plan or supplements in the immune system and the fight against COVID-19 (Adams et al., 2020).

7.6 THE ROLE OF NUTRITIONAL SUPPLEMENTATION IN COVID-19

Adequate levels of vitamins C, D, and E are crucial during COVID-19 to reduce symptoms and decrease the duration of respiratory infections. Research additionally helps the function of zinc-like minerals as they have antiviral results and can enhance immune response and suppress viral replication (Mentella et al., 2021). Therefore, the usage of adequate quantities of vitamins and minerals in meals is crucial to make certain the proper response of the immune system. Fruits (Keservani et al., 2016b), vegetables, meat, fish, poultry, and dairy products are proper sources of those vitamins and minerals. Supporting the immune system during COVID-19 diet high in amount of vitamins D, C, and E, zinc, and omega-3 fatty acids may be more beneficial (Hamulka et al., 2020). It is noteworthy, however, that a lot of the proof surrounding the usage of those compounds in patients with COVID-19 is; the use of doses that are too high for food. The addition of excessive doses of those compounds during COVID-19 infection has shown good results and, given their low-chance profile, is a reasonable addition to affected person care. However, similar studies need to be completed to decide the effective dose of vitamins C, E, D, omega-3 fatty acids, and zinc to protect people or reduce the signs and symptoms of COVID-19 (Lordan et al., 2021).

7.7 CONCLUSION

The effects of vitamins C, D, and E on an immune system and the potential benefits for those suffering from COVID-19 are presented. These are especially important for vulnerable older people, who represent an unbalanced burden of sickness and death in these times. All the mentioned elements play a possible role in supporting COVID-19 patients. The addition of adequate doses of vitamin D, C may have a positive effect on COVID-19 infection. However, clinical trials based on dietary supplementation with COVID-19 are lacking. Other clinical studies are effectively registered and currently underway to determine the efficacy of certain nutrients in patients with COVID-19. Hopefully, the results of this study will determine the important use of micronutrients during SARS-CoV-2 infection. It is also important to investigate other important micronutrients that shield the body, such as vitamin B in COVID-19, in order to further evaluate the role of nutrition in the effects of disease. According to the balance, in view of the unpredictable risk profile of the nutritional supplement, measured against known and potential benefits, it seems appropriate to ensure adequate, if not high, intake of these essential vitamins and minerals as a treatment for both vulnerable and disadvantaged people from COVID-19.

Nutritional therapy should be part of patient care in order to survive this life-threatening disease (COVID-19), as well as better and shorter recovery. Most importantly, nutritional testing and the provision of nutritional supplements are important steps for the proper functioning of the immune system in the human body. Malnourished patients are more likely to come from lower socioeconomic groups; therefore, nutritional support is important in the risk group as well as older adults with weakened immune systems.

ACKNOWLEDGMENTS

We thank you to the Dr. J. D. Pawar College of Pharmacy, Manur, METs, Institute of Pharmacy, Adgaon, Nashik, and Mahatma Gandhi Vidyamandir's Pharmacy College, Panchavati, Nashik, Maharashtra, India, for their constant support and providing all facilities to complete this work. Also, many thanks to all the known and unknowns who helped us right from the writing till the publishing of this chapter.

KEYWORDS

- **COVID-19**
- **immune systems**
- **minerals**
- **nutraceuticals**
- **nutritional therapy**
- **viral infection**
- **vitamin C**
- **vitamin D**

REFERENCES

Acosta-Ampudia, Y., Monsalve, D. M., Rojas, M., Rodríguez, Y., Gallo, J. E., Salazar-Uribe, J. C., Santander, M. J., Cala, M. P., Zapata, W., Zapata, M. I., & Manrique, R., (2021). COVID-19 convalescent plasma composition and immunological effects in severe patients. *Journal of Autoimmunity*, *118*, 102598.

Adams, K. K., Baker, W. L., & Sobieraj, D. M., (2020). COVID-19? Myth busters: Dietary supplements and COVID-19. *Annals of Pharmacotherapy*, *54*(8), 820–826.

Ahire, E. D., & Kshirsagar, S. J. (2021). Immune responses induced by different vaccine platforms against coronavirus disease-19. *Journal: Exploration of Immunology*, 243–257.

Ahire, E. D., Sonawane, V. N., & Surana, K. R., (2020). Role of drug repurposing in current treatment strategies against COVID-19; systemic review. *Pharm. Reson.*, 24–29.

Ahire, E. D., Sonawane, V. N., Surana, K. R., & Talele, G. S., (2021). Drug discovery, drug-likeness screening, and bioavailability: Development of drug-likeness rule for natural products. In: *Applied Pharmaceutical Practice and Nutraceuticals* (pp. 191–208). Apple Academic Press.

Ahire, E. D., Sonawane, V. N., Surana, K. R., Jadhav, K. R., Sonawane, D. D., & Shah, A. A., (2020). Convalescent plasma therapy: A promising approach in the treatment of COVID-19. *Int. J. Pharm. Sci. Res.*, *11*, 4078–4086.

Ahire, E. D., Surana K. R., Sonawane V.N., Pagar K. R., Gunjal S. S., & Talele S. G., (2020). Influence of allopathy, homeopathy, ayurveda and Unani systems of medicine in the management of COVID-19. *COVID-19 Pandemic: Questions, Answers and Hypotheses, 1.*

Ahvanooei, M. R., Norouzian, M. A., & Vahmani, P., (2021). Beneficial effects of vitamins, minerals, and bioactive peptides on strengthening the immune system against COVID-19 and the role of cow's milk in the supply of these nutrients. *Biological Trace Element Research*, 1–14.

Alexander, J., Tinkov, A., Strand, T. A., Alehagen, U., Skalny, A., & Aaseth, J., (2020). Early nutritional interventions with zinc, selenium, and vitamin D for raising anti-viral resistance against progressive COVID-19. *Nutrients*, *12*(8), 2358.

Ali, A. M., Kunugi, H., Abdelmageed, H. A., Mandour, A. S., Ahmed, M. E., Ahmad, S., & Hendawy, A. O., (2021). Vitamin K in COVID-19—Potential anti-COVID-19 properties of fermented milk fortified with bee honey as a natural source of vitamin K and probiotics. *Fermentation*, *7*(4), 202.

Alzaben, A. S., (2020). The potential influence of vitamin A, C, and D and zinc supplements on the severity of COVID-19 symptoms and clinical outcomes: An updated review of the literature. *Current Research in Nutrition and Food Science Journal*, *8*(3), 703–714.

Ashok, A. D., Ravivarman, J., & Kayalvizhi, K., (2020). Nutraceutical properties of recommended horticultural crops to develop the human immune system against COVID-19. *Int. J. Chem. Stud.*, *8*(4), 105–112.

Ashok, A., Ravivarman, J., & Kayalvizhi, K., (2020). Nutraceutical value of salad vegetables to combat COVID-19. *J. Pharmacol. Phytochem.*, *9*(3), 2144–2148.

Bae, M., & Kim, H., (2020). The role of vitamin C, vitamin D, and selenium in the immune system against COVID-19. *Molecules*, *25*(22), 5346.

Barrea, L., Grant, W. B., Frias-Toral, E., Vetrani, C., Verde, L., De Alteriis, G., Docimo, A., et al., (2022). Dietary recommendations for post-COVID-19 Syndrome. *Nutrients*, *14*(6), 1305.

Bianconi, V., Mannarino, M. R., Figorilli, F., Cosentini, E., Batori, G., Marini, E., Lombardini, R., et al., (2021). Prevalence of vitamin D deficiency and its prognostic impact on patients hospitalized with COVID-19. *Nutrition, 91*, 111408.

Borges, L., Gennari-Felipe, M., Dias, B. B., & Hatanaka, E., (2021). Melatonin, zinc, and vitamin C: Potential adjuvant treatment for COVID-19 patients. *Frontiers in Nutrition, 8.*

Borkhade, A., & Sawal, A. (2021). *Assessing the Role of Vitamins for COVID-19 Treatment, 33*(60A), 710–717.

Brenner, H., Holleczek, B., & Schöttker, B., (2020). Vitamin D insufficiency and deficiency and mortality from respiratory diseases in a cohort of older adults: Potential for limiting the death toll during and beyond the COVID-19 pandemic. *Nutrients, 12*(8), 2488.

Chandra, R. K., (1997). Nutrition and the immune system: An introduction. *Am. J. Clin Nutr., 66*(2), 460S–463S.

Chirumbolo, S., (2021). Nutraceuticals and dietary supplements should not be used to treat COVID-19 as pharmaceuticals. *Nutrition.* Burbank, Los Angeles County, Calif.

Corrao, S., Mallaci, B. R., Lo Monaco, M., Natoli, G., Cavezzi, A., Troiani, E., & Argano, C., (2021). Does evidence exist to blunt inflammatory response by nutraceutical supplementation during the COVID-19 pandemic? An overview of systematic reviews of vitamin D, vitamin C, melatonin, and zinc. *Nutrients, 13*(4), 1261.

Costagliola, G., Nuzzi, G., Spada, E., Comberiati, P., Verduci, E., & Peroni, D. G., (2021). Nutraceuticals in viral infections: An overview of the immunomodulating properties. *Nutrients, 13*(7), 2410.

Costagliola, G., Spada, E., Comberiati, P., & Peroni, D. G., (2021). Could nutritional supplements act as therapeutic adjuvants in COVID-19? *Italian Journal of Pediatrics, 47*(1), 1–5.

Di Renzo, L., Gualtieri, P., Pivari, F., Soldati, L., Attinà, A., Cinelli, G., Leggeri, C., et al., (2020). Eating habits and lifestyle changes during COVID-19 lockdown: An Italian survey. *Journal of Translational Medicine, 18*(1), 1–15.

Farzana, M., Shahriar, S., Jeba, F. R., Tabassum, T., Araf, Y., Ullah, M., Tasnim, J., et al., (2022). Functional food: Complementary to fight against COVID-19. *Beni-Suef University Journal of Basic and Applied Sciences, 11*(1), 1–18.

Galanakis, C. M., (2020). The food systems in the era of the coronavirus (COVID-19) pandemic crisis. *Foods, 9*(4), 523.

Galmés, S., Serra, F., & Palou, A., (2020). Current state of evidence: Influence of nutritional and nutrigenetic factors on immunity in the COVID-19 pandemic framework. *Nutrients, 12*(9), 2738.

Giovane, R. A., Di Giovanni-Kinsley, S., & Keeton, E. (2021). Micronutrients for potential therapeutic use against COVID-19; a review. *Clinical Nutrition ESPEN, 46*, 9–13.

Grant, W. B., & Lordan, R. (2021). Vitamin D for COVID-19 on trial: An update on prevention and therapeutic application. *Endocrine Practice.*

Hacışevki, A., & Baba, B., (2020). An overview of vitamins and minerals in the prevention of COVID-19 infection. *Gazi Medical Journal*, 523–527.

Hamid, H., Thakur, A., & Thakur, N. S., (2021). Role of functional food components in COVID-19 pandemic: A review. *Ann. Phytomed. Int. J, 10.*

Hamulka, J., Jeruszka-Bielak, M., Górnicka, M., Drywień, M. E., & Zielinska-Pukos, M. A., (2020). Dietary supplements during the COVID-19 outbreak. results of Google trends analysis supported by PLifeCOVID-19 online studies. *Nutrients, 13*(1), 54.

Handu, S., Jan, S., Chauhan, K., & Saxena, D. C., (2021). Vitamin D fortification: A perspective to improve immunity for COVID-19 infection. *Functional Food Science, 1*(10), 50–66.

Horowitz, R. I., & Freeman, P. R., (2020). Three novel prevention, diagnostic, and treatment options for COVID-19 urgently necessitate controlled randomized trials. *Medical Hypotheses, 143*, 109851.

Hunter, J., Arentz, S., Goldenberg, J., Yang, G., Beardsley, J., Mertz, D., & Leeder, S., (2020). Rapid review protocol: Zinc for the prevention or treatment of COVID-19 and other coronavirus-related respiratory tract infections. *Integrative Medicine Research, 9*(3), 100457.

Infusino, F., Marazzato, M., Mancone, M., Fedele, F., Mastroianni, C. M., Severino, P., Ceccarelli, G., et al., (2020). Diet supplementation, probiotics, and nutraceuticals in SARS-CoV-2 infection: A scoping review. *Nutrients, 12*(6), 1718.

Jarouliya, U., & Keservani, R. K., (2019a). Pathways leading to child obesity; Chapter 12. In: Debasis, B., (ed.), *Global Perspectives on Childhood Obesity: Current Status, Consequences and Prevention* (2nd edn., pp. 137–146). Academic Press, Elsevier. ISBN: 9780128128404.

Jarouliya, U., & Keservani, R. K., (2019b). Protein function as cell surface and nuclear receptor in human diseases; Chapter 1. In: Sanjay, B., & Debarshi, K. M., (eds.), *Medicinal Chemistry with Pharmaceutical Product Development* (pp. 1–32). Apple Academic Press, CRC Press, Taylor & Francis Group. ISBN: 9781771887106.

Jayawardena, R., & Misra, A., (2020). A balanced diet is a major casualty of COVID-19. *Diabetes & Metabolic Syndrome, 14*(5), 1085.

Keservani, R. K., Kesharwani, R. K., Sharma, A. K., & Jarouliya, U., (2015). Dietary supplements, nutraceutical and functional foods in immune response (immunomodulators); Chapter 20. In: Debasis, B., Harry, G. P., & Anand, S., (eds.), *Nutraceutical and Functional Foods in Human Life and Disease Prevention* (pp. 343–358). Boca Raton, Fl. CRC Press, Taylor and Francis. ISBN: 9781482237214.

Keservani, R. K., Kesharwani, R. K., Sharma, A. K., Vyas, N., & Chadoker, A., (2010b). Nutritional supplements: An overview. *International Journal of Current Pharmaceutical Review and Research, 1*(1), 59–75.

Keservani, R. K., Kesharwani, R. K., Vyas, N., Jain, S., Raghuvanshi, R., & Sharma, A. K., (2010a). Nutraceutical and functional food as future food: A review. *Der Pharmacia Lettre, 2*(1), 106–116.

Keservani, R. K., Sharma, A. K., & Kesharwani, R. K. (2016). Medicinal effect of nutraceutical fruits for the cognition and brain health. *Scientifica*, 10. Article ID 3109254. doi: 10.1155/2016/3109254.

Keservani, R. K., Sharma, A. K., & Kesharwani, R. K. (2017). An overview and therapeutic applications of nutraceutical and functional foods. *Recent Advances in Drug Delivery Technology*, 160–201. ISBN:9781522507543.

Keservani, R. K., Sharma, A. K., & Kesharwani, R. K. (2020). *Nutraceuticals and Dietary Supplements: Applications in Health Improvement and Disease Management*. CRC Press. ISBN: 9781771888738.

Lammi, C., & Arnoldi, A. (2021). Food-derived antioxidants and COVID-19. *Journal of Food Biochemistry, 45*(1), e13557.

Lavie, C. J., & Holick, M. F., (2011). Vitamin D supplementation for cardiovascular disease prevention. *JAMA, 306*(14), 1546–1548.

Lehberger, M., Kleih, A. K., & Sparke, K., (2021). Panic buying in times of coronavirus (COVID-19): Extending the theory of planned behavior to understand the stockpiling of non-perishable food in Germany. *Appetite, 161*, 105118.

Lordan, R. (2021). Notable developments for vitamin D amid the COVID-19 pandemic, but caution warranted overall: A narrative review. *Nutrients, 13*(3), 740.

Lordan, R., Rando, H. M., & Greene, C. S. (2021). Dietary supplements and nutraceuticals under investigation for COVID-19 prevention and treatment. *Msystems, 6*(3), e00122–21.

Mattioli, A. V., Sciomer, S., Cocchi, C., Maffei, S., & Gallina, S., (2020). Quarantine during COVID-19 outbreak: Changes in diet and physical activity increase the risk of cardiovascular disease. *Nutrition, Metabolism and Cardiovascular Diseases, 30*(9), 1409–1417.

Medoro, C., Cianciabella, M., Magli, M., Daniele, G. M., Lippi, N., Gatti, E., Volpe, R., et al., (2022). Food involvement, food choices, and bioactive compounds consumption correlation during COVID-19 PANDEMIC: How food engagement influences consumers' food habits. *Nutrients, 14*(7), 1490.

Mehrotra, N., & Jadhav, K., (2021). Nutraceuticals: Potential prospect for COVID-19 management. *Annals of Phytomedicine-an International Journal*, S85–S102.

Mentella, M. C., Scaldaferri, F., Gasbarrini, A., & Miggiano, G. A. D., (2021). The role of nutrition in the COVID-19 pandemic. *Nutrients, 13*(4), 1093.

Michienzi, S. M., & Badowski, M. E., (2020). Can vitamins and/or supplements provide hope against coronavirus? *Drugs in Context, 9*.

Mullin, G. E., Limektkai, B., Wang, L., Hanaway, P., Marks, L., & Giovannucci, E. (2021). Dietary supplements for COVID-19. *Coronavirus Disease-COVID-19*, 499–515.

Nimer, R. M., Khabour, O. F., Swedan, S. F., & Kofahi, H. M., (2022). The impact of vitamin and mineral supplements usage prior to COVID-19 infection on disease severity and hospitalization. *Bosnian Journal of Basic Medical Sciences*.

Ooi, R. S. E., (2022). *Disinfectants, Face Masks and Nutraceutical Supplementation Against COVID-19*. Doctoral dissertation, Tunku Abdul Rahman University College.

Ooi, S. L., & Pak, S. C., (2021). Nutraceuticals in immune function. *Molecules, 26*(17), 5310.

Papadopoulou, S. K., Mantzorou, M., Koutridou, D., Tassoulas, E., Sakellaropoulou, S., Biskanaki, F., Xatziapostolou, E., & Papandreou, D., (2020). COVID-19 disease, obesity, and micronutrients: An updated narrative review of the literature. *Nutrition & Food Science*.

Pedrosa, L. F., Barros, A. N., & Leite-Lais, L., (2021). Nutritional risk of vitamin D, vitamin C, zinc, and selenium deficiency on risk and clinical outcomes of COVID-19: A narrative review. *Clinical Nutrition ESPEN*.

Peng, M. Y., Liu, W. C., Zheng, J. Q., Lu, C. L., Hou, Y. C., Zheng, C. M., Song, J. Y., et al., (2021). Immunological aspects of SARS-CoV-2 infection and the putative beneficial role of vitamin D. *International Journal of Molecular Sciences, 22*(10), 5251.

Pisoschi, A. M., Pop, A., Iordache, F., Stanca, L., Geicu, O. I., Bilteanu, L., & Serban, A. I., (2022). Antioxidant, anti-inflammatory and immunomodulatory roles of vitamins in COVID-19 therapy. *European Journal of Medicinal Chemistry*, 114175.

Pouramini, A., Kafi, F., & Hassanzadeh, S., (2021). Vitamin D and COVID-19 infection; recent findings. *J. Ren. Endocrinol., 7*, e19.

Quiles, J. L., Rivas-García, L., Varela-López, A., Llopis, J., Battino, M., & Sánchez-González, C., (2020). Do nutrients and other bioactive molecules from foods have anything to say in the treatment against COVID-19? *Environmental Research, 191*, 110053.

Rezaei, H., Khiali, S., Rezaei, H., Rezaee, H., Baghi, H. B., Pourghasem, M., & Entezari-Maleki, T., (2021). Potential roles of vitamins in the management of COVID-19: A comprehensive review. *Pharmaceutical Sciences*, *27*(COVID-19), S29–S49.

Rodriguez-Leyva, D., & Pierce, G. N., (2021). The impact of nutrition on the COVID-19 pandemic and the impact of the COVID-19 pandemic on nutrition. *Nutrients*, *13*(6), 1752.

Samad, N., et al., (2021). Fat-soluble vitamins and the current global pandemic of COVID-19: Evidence-based efficacy from literature review. *Journal of Inflammation Research*, *14*, 2091.

Shakoor, H., Feehan, J., Al Dhaheri, A. S., Ali, H. I., Platat, C., Ismail, L. C., Apostolopoulos, V., & Stojanovska, L., (2021). Immune-boosting role of vitamins D, C, E, zinc, selenium, and omega-3 fatty acids: Could they help against COVID-19? *Maturitas*, *143*, 1–9.

Singh, P., Kesharwani, R. K., & Keservani, R. K. (2017). Antioxidants and vitamins: Roles in cellular function and metabolism. In: *Sustained Energy for Enhanced Human Functions and Activity* (pp. 385–407). Academic Press. ISBN:9780128054130.

Singh, S., Singh, C. M., Ranjan, A., Kumar, S., & Singh, D. K., (2021). Evidence suggesting a possible role of vitamin D in COVID-19: The missing link. *Indian Journal of Pharmacology*, *53*(5), 394.

Souza, A. C. R., Vasconcelos, A. R., Prado, P. S., & Pereira, C. P. M., (2020). Zinc, vitamin D and vitamin C: Perspectives for COVID-19 with a focus on physical tissue barrier integrity. *Frontiers in Nutrition*, 295.

Subedi, L., Tchen, S., Gaire, B. P., Hu, B., & Hu, K., (2021). Adjunctive nutraceutical therapies for COVID-19. *International Journal of Molecular Sciences*, *22*(4), 1963.

Tahir, A. H., Javed, M. M., & Hussain, Z. (2020). Nutraceuticals and herbal extracts: A ray of hope for COVID-19 and related infections. *International Journal of Functional Nutrition*, *1*(2), 1.

Talele, S. G., Ahire, E. D., Surana, K. R., Sonawane, V. N., & Talele, G. S., (2022). Coronavirus disease (COVID-19): A past and present perspective. *Asian Journal of Pharmaceutical Research*, *12*(1), 45–53.

Tiwari, A., Singh, G., Singh, U., Sapra, L., Rana, V., Sharma, V., Srivastava, R. K., & Sharma, S., (2022). Edible mushrooms: The potential game changer in alleviating vitamin D deficiency and improving human health. *International Journal of Food Science & Technology*, *57*(3), 1367–1377.

Tramontana, F., Napoli, N., El-Hajj, F. G., & Strollo, R., (2020). The D-side of COVID-19: Musculoskeletal benefits of vitamin D and beyond. *Endocrine*, *69*(2), 237–240.

Uddin, M. S., Millat, M., Baral, P. K., Ferdous, M., Uddin, M., Sarwar, M., & Islam, M. S., (2021). The protective role of vitamin C in the management of COVID-19: A review. *Journal of the Egyptian Public Health Association*, *96*(1), 1–8.

Van, K. T. A., & Deixler, E., (2021). SARS-CoV-2: Influence of phosphate and magnesium, moderated by vitamin D, on energy (ATP) metabolism and on severity of COVID-19. *American Journal of Physiology-Endocrinology and Metabolism*, *320*(1), E2–E6.

Wong, Y., Chan, C. H., Venkatakrishnan, K., Chiu, H. F., Shen, Y. C., Glovinskaia, O., Han, Y. C., & Wang, C. K., (2021). Impact of dietary nutrients (functional foods/nutraceuticals) and micronutrients on COVID-19: A review. *Journal of Food Bioactives*, *15*.

Wong, Y., Chan, C. H., Venkatakrishnan, K., Chiu, H. F., Shen, Y. C., Glovinskaia, O., Han, Y. C., & Wang, C. K., (2021). Impact of dietary nutrients (functional foods/nutraceuticals) and micronutrients on COVID-19: A review. *Journal of Food Bioactives*, *15*.

Žmitek, K., Hribar, M., Lavriša, Ž., Hristov, H., Kušar, A., & Pravst, I., (2021). Socio-demographic and knowledge-related determinants of vitamin D supplementation in the context of the COVID-19 pandemic: ASSESSMENT of an educational intervention. *Frontiers in Nutrition, 8*, 290.

PART III

Functional Activity of Vitamins in Brain Health and Obesity Management

CHAPTER 8

Vitamins as Nutraceuticals for Hypertension

KSHITIJ S. VARMA,[1] TUSHAR N. LOKHANDE,[2] RAMESH A. HEROLE,[3] KHEMCHAND R. SURANA,[4] and SUNIL K. MAHAJAN[5]

[1]*Department of Pharmaceutical Chemistry, Mahatma Gandhi Vidyamandir's Pharmacy College, Panchavati, Nashik, Maharashtra, India*

[2]*Department of Pharmaceutical Chemistry, Maharashtra Educational Society's H. K. College of Pharmacy, Oshiwara, Jogeshwari (W), Maharashtra, India*

[3]*Department of Pharmaceutical Chemistry, K. K. Wagh Institute of Pharmacy, Chandori, Niphad, Nashik, Maharashtra, India*

[4]*Department of Pharmaceutical Chemistry, Shreeshakti Shaikshanik Sanstha, Divine College of Pharmacy, Satana, Nashik, Maharashtra, India*

[5]*Department of Pharmaceutical Chemistry, M.G.V's Samajshri Prashant Dada Hiray, College of Pharmacy, Malegaon, Nashik, Maharashtra, India*

ABSTRACT

Hypertension is a significant risk factor for a variety of disorders, including cardiovascular disease, vascular diseases, and kidney failure. Many studies are concentrating their attention on various diet formulas (dietary approaches), with a particular emphasis on micro- and macronutrients, as well as a transformed lifestyle and conventional antihypertensive medicines. Micronutrients (vitamins) play an important role in blood pressure regulation because they help macronutrient function and boost the antihypertensive effects of some

Preventive and Therapeutic Role of Vitamins as Nutraceuticals. Khemchand R. Surana, Eknath D. Ahire, Raj K. Keservani, & Rajesh K. Kesharwani (Eds.)

antihypertensive drugs. Even though multiple studies have shown the favorable benefits of micronutrients on blood pressure control, nutritionists and clinicians are still divided as to which combinations or unique nutrients (nutritional approach) correlate to improved Hypertension regulation. Oxidative stress, hyperactivity of the renin-angiotensin system, irritation, hypercholesterolemia, and vascular resistance are all risk factors that can be modulated to achieve goals and lower cardiovascular risks. We look at recent medical studies that looked at characteristics of biological and pharmaceuticals of various nutraceuticals, including ascorbic acid, vitamin E, vitamin B complex, and vitamin D, in terms of preventing and treating hypertension. As a result, the essential function of vitamins in the management, prevention, or delay of hypertension and its related problems, as well as its method of blood pressure regulation, has received substantial support from clinical trials.

8.1 INTRODUCTION

A chronic, consistent rise in blood (arterial) pressure above 140/90 (Systolic/Diastolic BP) mmHg (obtained from The National Department of Health Excellence recommendations) is referred to as hypertension (Giles et al., 2009). Hypertension is defined as "office systolic (SBP) levels 140 mmHg, perhaps diastolic (DBP) levels 90 mmHg," according to the 2017–2018 European Society for Cardiology and European Society for Hypertension recommendations. The 2018 European Society for Cardiology and European Society for High blood pressure guidelines for the therapy of arterial hypertension presented uncontroversial research based on improved boiling point control rates by encouraging simple and effective options for treatment (Williams et al., 2018). Table 8.1 shows categorizing blood pressure in adults as per the definition of hypertension. Primary hypertension (90–95%) and secondary hypertension (5–10%) are the two kinds of hypertension, both of which are produced primarily by genetic, epigenetic, and lifestyle variables (particularly dietary patterns) (Venkatakrishnan, Chiu, & Wang, 2020).

TABLE 8.1 Categorizing Blood Pressure in Adults as per the Definition of Hypertension.

Frequency	Ideal	Average	High	Light Hypertension	Careful Hypertension	Scathing Hypertension	Abnormal Systolic Hypertension
Systolic (mmHg)	<120	120–129	130–139	140–159	160–179	≥180	>140
Diastolic (mmHg)	<80	80–84	85–89	90–99	100–109	≥110	<90

Source: Adapted from Katsanos et al. (2017)

8.1.1 EPIDEMIOLOGY

Vascular disease is the result of a delicate balancing act involving vascular injury and healing. The endothelium, which lies between blood and the vascular smooth muscle, secretes a variety of chemicals that help maintain vascular homeostasis and health. Endothelial dysfunction is caused by a variety of insults to the endothelium, which can lead to hypertension and many other cardiovascular disorders. Endothelial dysfunction, venous and cardiac muscle fibers dysfunction, loss of arterial flexibility with reduced arterial compliance, and enhanced systemic vascular resistance may be hemodynamic markers of wounded endothelium and smooth muscle linked to finite reactions of inflammation, oxidative stress or immune dysfunction of arteries resulting to endothelial dysfunction, venous, and cardiac muscle fibers dysfunction, loss of arterial flexibility with reduced arterial compliance, and increased vascular resistance. The combination between genetics and environment leads to hypertension. Because of heredity, environmental factors, and prescription drug use, macronutrients, as well as micronutrients, are critical in the control of blood pressure. As a result, they are more likely to be consumed by those with increased blood pressure and coronary heart disease. These flaws will have a significant impact on current as well as long-term cardiac function outcomes such as high blood pressure, myocardial infarction, stroke, and renal disease. Diagnosing and treating these dietary deficiencies will lower blood pressure while also improving venous health, endothelial dysfunction, venous biology, and cardiovascular event.

According to epidemiology, diet and related nutrient intake play an etiologic effect on hypertension. The transition from the Paleolithic to the modern diet has resulted in a nutritional illness epidemic. Some of these disorders include high blood pressure, atherosclerosis, heart disease, myocardial infarction, heart failure, cerebrovascular accident, kidney diseases, type 2 diabetes, metabolic syndrome, and obesity (Houston, 2007; Eaton, Eaton, & Konner, 1997).

Although we share 99.9% of our genetic composition with our Paleolithic predecessors, our dietary, vitamin, and element intakes are dramatically different (Houston & Harper, 2008). Through complicated nutrient-gene interactions, neurobiological, and nutrient-caveolae interactions, and nutrient-caveolae interactions, macronutrient as well as micronutrient varieties, production of reactive oxygen species from reactive oxidative species and reactionary nitrogen species, and inflammatory processes including cell adhesion molecules, chemokines, signal transduction & immune deficiency vascular dysfunction of T and B Cells, an increased incidence of high blood pressure (Layne et al., 2011; Dandona et al., 2010; Houston, 2014; Talmud & Waterworth, 2000; Lundberg & Yan, 2011; Zhao, Lee, & Hwang, 2011). Vascular and myocardial dysfunction and hypertension are triggered by decreased nitric oxide absorption, increased angiotensin II and endothelin, and endothelial activation. Nutritionally-related diseases have increased exponentially as a result of poor nutrition combined with fatness and a sedentary lifestyle. The comparatively small intake of omega 3 polyunsaturated fatty acids, rise in omega 3 polyunsaturated fatty acids, fat content, and trans-fatty acids, in addition to current diets' relatively high Na+/K+ proportion, have all contributed to high blood pressure, heart disease, infarction, heart failure, cerebrovascular disease, and renal disease (Houston & Harper, 2008; Houston, 2011; Broadhurst, 1997).

8.1.2 PATHOPHYSIOLOGY

Essential hypertension is an unknown origin; however, it often starts in the 5th or 6th decade of life, is frequently related to increasing salt intake and obesity, and has a strong association with family history, suggesting a hereditary susceptibility (Weber et al., 2014). Secondary hypertension is accompanied by specific factors such as renal impairment, chronic renal failure, sleep apnea, and adrenal illnesses (Weber et al., 2014). Possible mechanisms involved in the maintenance of regular blood pressure are disrupted in both scenarios, and as a result, the nervous system, angiotensinogen system, endothelial function, sodium, and fluid retention have all been extensively studied to determine mechanisms in the disease's development (Carretero & Oparil, 2000; Delacroix, Chokka, & Worthley, 2014).

8.1.2.1 HEART RATE AND VASCULAR RESISTANCE

Heart rate and vascular resistance are important factors in maintaining normal blood pressure. It has been proposed that elevated cardiac output caused by sympathetic impairment is the trigger for the improvement of Hypertension and that increases in Vascular resistance are essentially the physiologic reaction to facilitate pressure changes and restore health (Carretero & Oparil, 2000; Delacroix, Chokka, & Worthley, 2014; Mayet & Hughes, 2003).

8.1.2.2 SYMPATHETIC NERVOUS SYSTEM

The significance of the nervous system in the establishment and improvement of heart rate has been extensively studied over the last decade, and it has been determined that the sympathetic nervous system of the heart, peripheral vascular system, and kidneys leads to increased heart rate, increased arterial pressure, and fluid retention, is significant in the formation and maintenance of such a disease (Mark, 1996). Sympathetic overdrive is frequently accompanied by reduced parasympathetic tone, which exacerbates the disease (Kim, 1999), as indicated by the Coronary Artery Risks Developing among Young Adults study. Furthermore, multiple investigations have shown evidence of sympathetic overactivity in individuals with hypertension by showing elevations in norepinephrine spillover, confirming that sympathetic overactivity is a key component in the disease's etiology. The hepatic sympathetic nervous system, which affects blood pressure via two routes, the efferent and afferent, is a key part of the development and management of hypertension. The efferent pathway transmits messages from the nervous system to the kidney, increasing renin release and thus activating the renin-angiotensin-aldosterone system, increasing sodium and water retention, all of which result in increased circulating volumes and thus higher blood pressures. In addition to the aforementioned mechanisms, the efferent pathway reduces renal blood flow, and the kidney responds by activating the afferent pathway, which sends signals to the sympathetic nerves, aggravating sympathetic overactivity and maintaining high blood pressure (Cain & Khalil, 2002).

8.1.2.3 RENIN-ANGIOTENSIN-ALDOSTERONE SYSTEM

The Renin-angiotensin-aldosterone system facilitates the management of normal blood pressure and is triggered by two mechanisms: Sympathetic nervous system stimulation and glomerular under perfusion (Cain & Khalil, 2002; Cody, 1997; Sarzani, 2008). These stimuli cause renin to be released from the juxtaglomerular apparatus, which reduces angiotensinogen into inactive angiotensin I, which is then converted into angiotensin II by endothelium-bound angiotensin-converting enzyme, which is a strong vasoconstrictor (Ferrario, 2006; Piepho & Beal, 2000; Simoes, Silva, & Flynn, 2012).

8.1.2.4 ENDOTHELIAL DYSFUNCTION

It is unclear whether endothelial dysfunction is just a factor or an outcome of hypertension; there is strong evidence relating endothelial dysfunction to hypertension (Cardillo et al., 1998). There is a correlation between the severity of hypertension and the extent of endothelial dysfunction (Panza et al., 1993). The main cause of endothelial dysfunction in hypertension is a decrease in nitric oxide availability, which occurs as a result of oxidative stress within those people (Panza et al., 1995). Although effective antihypertensive medication restores reduced nitric oxide generation, endothelium-dependent vasorelaxation remains changed, implying that once hypertension is developed, it is irreversible (Panza, Quyyumi, Brush, & Epstein, 1990). This evidence, together with research showing that inhibiting endothelium-derived production of nitric oxide causes hypertension in people, suggests that endothelial dysfunction plays a possible etiological role in the onset of hypertension (Benjamin et al., 2004; Sander, Chavoshan, & Victor, 1999).

8.1.2.5 VASOACTIVE SUBSTANCES

One of the principal molecules involved in managing vascular tone is endothelin, a powerful vasoconstrictor. Hickey et al. discovered it in 1985. It is produced by epithelial cells and has a paracrine or autocrine action on vascular endothelial cells, counteracting the calming effects of nitrous oxide (Hickey et al., 1985; Wagner et al., 1992). Infusion of endothelin-1 causes an elevation in blood pressure in both animals and humans (Vierhapper et al., 1990), and inhibiting the system utilizing antagonists reverses the phenomena. Interestingly, the plasma concentration of endothelin-1 is typical in those with essential hypertension, suggesting that the activation of this system may be important only in certain forms of hypertension, including salt-sensitive hypertension as well as renal hypertension (Krum et al., 1998).

8.2 NUTRACEUTICAL TREATMENT FOR HYPERTENSION

Dr. Stephen L. De Felice, MD, the founder and chief executive of the Foundation for Innovation In Medicines, invented the term "nutraceutical" as a combination of "nutrition" and "pharmaceutical" (Das et al., 2012). Over time, the phrase "nutraceuticals" has changed, and nomenclature differs by country." A food (or a part of food) that delivers medicinal or health advantages, including the prevention of and treatment of disease," according to the definition (Keservani et al., 2010a, b, 2017, 2020; Dillard & German, 2000; Olas, 2018; Surana et al., 2021a).

Nutraceuticals, also known as natural functional ingredients or bioactive phytochemicals (Keservani & Sharma, 2014; Keservani et al., 2016a, b), are compounds obtained from foods that are utilized in the form of tablets, capsules, potions, as well as liquids to deliver physiological benefits or prevent serious illness (Kailasapathy, 2009). Functional foods are "products which have been shown to possess pharmacological advantages and/or contribute to chronic disease when consumed as part of a routine diet" (Chumphukam et al., 2019). According to a current cross-sectional study, nutraceuticals were taken by 82.5% of cardiovascular patients as health-promoting activities (Aykan & Aykan, 2018; Surana et al., 2021). Figure 8.1 represents a diagrammatic Description of the Concept of Nutraceuticals.

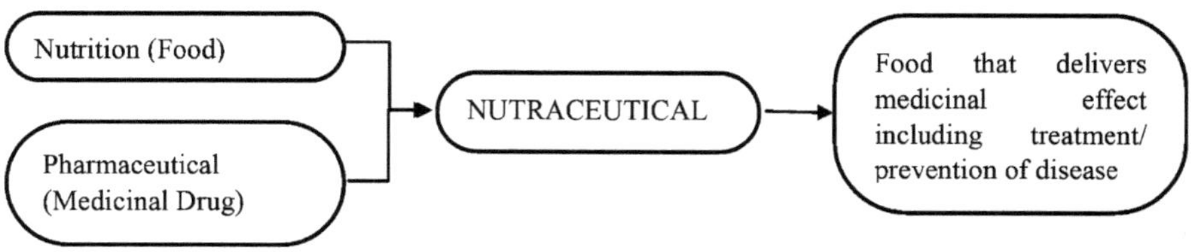

FIGURE 8.1 Diagrammatic description of the concept of nutraceuticals.
Source: Modified from Das et al. (2012)

Blood pressure-reducing nutraceuticals can be divided based on their mode of action and chemical composition:

i. Foods:
   Example: Tea and Cocoa.
ii. Nutrients:
   Examples: Magnesium, Calcium, Vitamin C, Soluble fibers, Omega 3 poly-unsaturated fatty acids.
iii. Non-nutrient nutraceuticals:
   Example: Coenzyme Q10, lycopene, prebiotics (Cicero et al., 2019; Kokate, Purohit, & Gokhale, 2002; Olas, 2018; Sirtori, Arnoldi, & Cicero, 2015).

8.3 ROLE OF NUTRACEUTICALS IN HYPERTENSION

The proceeding is a few parameters to reflect about:

- As a protective impact through multiple methods such as vascular tone modulation, blood pressure regulation, vascular smooth muscle activities, and endothelium maintenance (Keservani et al., 2015; Parker et al., 2010; Somjen et al., 2005; Margolis et al., 2008).

- It affects calcium-phosphate homeostasis and appears to have anti-inflammatory and immunoregulatory properties (Keservani et al., 2015; Dozio et al., 2015).
- Acting as a nutrition as well as a therapeutic agent (Lawson, 1998).
- Enhancing angiogenesis is linked to inflammatory indicators. These findings indicate the health advantage of consuming lycopene daily (Kim et al., 2011).
- It is essential for cell function in mammalian tissues and protects the cell from death, inflammatory processes, and necrosis is necessary for cell function (Donnarumma, Trivedi, & Lefer, 2017).

8.4 VITAMINS

Vitamins are micronutrients that have several roles in human development and growth. Vitamins that are both water and lipid-soluble are important for the absorption and stimulation of macronutrients such as carbs, proteins, and lipids. As a result, vitamins are critical for overall health management since they have a variety of biological functions, such as antioxidant (Singh et al., 2017), anti-inflammatory, and immunomodulatory properties (Maqbool et al., 2018). Vitamins are effective in lowering blood pressure whether used alone or in conjunction with other nutrients or functional meals in several studies (Venkatakrishnan, Chiu, & Wang, 2020; Czernichow et al., 2004; Chen et al., 2002; Surana et al., 2021c). Table 8.2 shows chemical name, year of discovery, discovered by scientists, country, and source of vitamins used in hypertension.

8.4.1 VITAMINS USED FOR HYPERTENSION

We will concentrate on important vitamins such as:

- Vitamin D/calciferol;
- Vitamin E/tocopherol;
- Vitamin B6/pyridoxine;
- Vitamin B12/cobalamin/cyanocobalamin;
- Vitamin C/ascorbic acid.

Above vitamins are shown to have better blood pressure-regulating effects than other vitamins.

TABLE 8.2 Chemical Name, Year of Discovery, Discovered by Scientists, Country, and Source of Vitamins Used in Hypertension.

Vitamins	Vitamin D	Vitamin E	Vitamin B6	Vitamin V12	Vitamin C
Chemical Name	Calciferol	Tocopherol	Pyridoxine	Cobalamin	Ascorbic acid
Discovered by	Elmer McCollum	Herbert M Evans	Paul Gyorgy	George H. Whipple, etc.	Albert Szent-Gyorgyi
Discovered in Year	1922	1922	1934	1926	1928
Sources	Sunlight, fish, etc.	Vegetable oil, dairy products, etc.	Bananas, chicken, etc.	Meat, dairy products, etc.	Liver, leafy vegetables, etc.

Source: Modified from Christian (2015)

8.5 ROLE OF IMPORTANT VITAMINS IN HYPERTENSION

8.5.1 VITAMIN D/CALCIFEROL

Vitamin D, also known as cholecalciferol, a vitamin that is fat-soluble, helps to maintain calcium homeostasis and hence the appropriate functioning of the musculoskeletal, circulatory, and neurological systems. Oily fish, such as salmon, herring, egg yolk, and red meat, are dietary sources of vitamin D, which will then be converted to activated vitamin D3 (1,25-dihydroxycholecalciferol) by sunshine exposure (Slominski et al., 2020). Several observational (survey), cross-sectional, and experimental investigations have found a link between Vitamin D (its activated form D3) and blood pressure, as well as its consequences such as cardiovascular disease. However, certain clinical studies and epidemiological investigations have found that vitamin D or its active metabolites, such as 1,25-dihydroxycholecalciferol or vitamin D3, had little or only a minor hypotensive impact (Kunutsor, Apekey, & Steur, 2013; Judd et al., 2008).

8.5.1.1 BLOOD PRESSURE REGULATING MECHANISM

Vitamin D affects calcium homeostasis (particularly calcium intake and metabolism) through interacting with voltage-dependent Ca^{++} channels and by regulating the Renin-angiotensin-aldosterone system by directly modulating renin synthesis, which in turn modulates parathyroid hormone release (Morvaridzadeh et al., 2020; Lee et al., 2010). As a result, co-supplementing vitamin D with calcium resulted in improved blood pressure-controlling function. Furthermore, vitamin D has been demonstrated to promote endothelial function by suppressing vascular resistance (by increasing nitric oxide generation) and calcification (by preserving vascular tone) while also lowering inflammatory responses. As a result, vitamin D is beneficial in preventing cardiovascular disease-related problems (Sugden et al., 2008; Yuan et al., 2007).

8.5.1.2 CLINICAL EVIDENCE

Vitamin D revealed a substantial drop in diastolic (3.1 mm Hg) in patients with hypertension, but still no major changes in systolic blood pressure, according to a comprehensive study and meta-analysis study. Overall, the author found that people who took Calciferol supplements had mild hypotensive activity in hypertension patients but no changes in normotensive people (Witham, Nadir, & Struthers, 2009). Burgaz (Burgaz, Orsini, Larsson, & Wolk, 2011) found that blood Calciferol content is oppositely related to hypertension in a meta-analysis that included numerous cross-section tests. A meta-analysis of eight prospective studies found that vitamin D (25-hydroxyvitamin D) levels are inversely proportional to the frequency of HT (Kunutsor, Apekey, & Steur, 2013). However, Beveridge and colleagues (Beveridge et al., 2015) conducted a meta-analysis that included data from 46 clinical studies and found that vitamin D supplementation did not affect blood pressure. Nonetheless, Golzarand and colleagues demonstrated in meta-analysis research (Golzarand et al., 2016) that daily Vit D3 (dosage > 800 IU per day) for even more than 6 months might significantly lower Systolic and Diastolic in normal and hypertensive participants. In people experiencing Calciferol deficiency and hypertension, recent retrospective studies and meta-analysis reports have documented that oral Vit D3 ingestion can considerably lower systole and diastole (He & Hao, 2019).

Overall, oral supplementation increases Vitamin D3 levels, which has an inverse relationship with blood pressure and can be coupled with other elements or macronutrients (adjuvant treatment) for a better hypotensive impact in patients with hypertension with vitamin insufficiency.

8.5.2 VITAMIN E/TOCOPHEROL

Vitamin E is an essential lipid-soluble antioxidant vitamin with a huge range of functions. Nuts (almonds, peanuts, cashews), soy products (sunflower, soybean), raisins, leafy greens, and red bell pepper are high in vitamin E

(Rizvi et al., 2014). Although existing evidence suggests that supplementing with tocopherol can help to reduce blood pressure (Boshtam et al., 2002; Emami et al., 2019), a few studies have found that Vitamin E had little or no effect on blood (Palumbo et al., 2000; Mottram et al., 1999). To improve vascular function, adding 10–15 milligrams (RDA) of Vitamin E by ingesting Vitamin E-rich foods as described above helps to maintain normal Vitamin E levels.

8.5.2.1 BLOOD PRESSURE REGULATING MECHANISM

Vitamin E has been proven to have mild hypotensive characteristics by increasing Nitrous oxide (vasodilation) and prostaglandins I/E production, decreasing arterial stiffness, and maintaining vascular smooth muscle function (Plantinga et al., 2007; Dakshinamurti & Dakshinamurti, 2001). Vitamin E and also its metabolites have a natriuretic (diuretic) effect by blocking the 70 prostaglandins K+ and Ca++ channels in the upper limbs of the Henle loops and therefore regulating blood pressure (Hensley et al., 2004). Furthermore, vitamin E contains potent antioxidant as well as anti-inflammatory capabilities (which improve vascular function) and so reduces blood pressure (Dakshinamurti & Dakshinamurti, 2001).

8.5.2.2 CLINICAL EVIDENCE

The increase in serum Tocopherol was significantly lower in severe gestational hypertension individuals (pre-eclampsia) compared to normotensive pregnant women, according to a study conducted by Gratacos and colleagues (Gratacos et al., 1998). Another clinical investigation found that supplementing using 200 IU/day over 27 weeks resulted in a significant reduction in systolic (24%) and diastolic (12.5%) in moderate hypertension participants when compared to placebo (Boshtam et al., 2002). Emami and colleagues (Emami et al., 2019) recently published a systematic review and meta-analysis that included 18 studies with 839 participants and found that vitamin E supplementation resulted in a substantial reduction in systolic (3.4 mm Hg) when matched to a placebo, although no changes in diastolic. Vitamin E supplementation may improve overall vascular health (by increasing nitric oxide bioavailability), but it is more beneficial in elderly hypertension and severe pregnant hypertensive patients. However, further research is needed before Vitamin E may be recommended for the treatment of hypertension patients.

8.5.3 VITAMIN B COMPLEX

8.5.3.1 VITAMIN B6/PYRIDOXINE AND VITAMIN B12/ COBALAMIN/CYANOCOBALAMIN

Vitamin B complex is a variety of water-soluble vitamins that includes pyridoxine and cyanocobalamin, two of which have been indicated to have blood pressure-lowering characteristics. Milk, yolk, fatty meat, and pistachio are good sources of vitamin B6, whereas liver, yolks, salmon, and red meat are good sources of vitamin B12. Pyridoxine and cyanocobalamin require several values are 1.3–1.8 milligrams and 1.5–2.4 grams, respectively, which can be met by eating pyridoxine and cyanocobalamin-rich foods as previously described. Few investigations have been undertaken on animals to show that pyridoxine and cyanocobalamin may play a function in blood circulation (Dakshinamurti et al., 2014; Lal, Dakshinamurti, & Thliveris, 1996). Low levels of serum of pyridoxine and cyanocobalamin are related to higher blood pressure in humans, according to a human study (Dakshinamurti & Dakshinamurti, 2001; Aybak et al., 1995).

8.5.3.2 BLOOD PRESSURE REGULATING MECHANISM

Vitamin B6 deficiency causes a decrease in serotonin as well as gamma-aminobutyric acid generation (neurotransmitters), which results in a significant reduction in phospholipid content in the brain, which changes Ca++ transfer and metabolism (by acting as a Ca++ channel blocker), resulting in positive blood pressure regulation (Dakshinamurti & Dakshinamurti, 2001; Dakshinamurti, Lal, & Ganguly, 1998). Vitamin B6 has also been proclaimed to increase diuretic activity by modulating the sympathetic nervous system and improving glutathione production, as well as reduce inflammation by suppressing homocysteine levels, lowering cardiovascular disease risk and blood pressure indirectly (Houston, 2018; Aybak et al., 1995). Furthermore, vitamin B12 supplementation has been associated with a depletion in homocysteine levels and, consequently a reduction in blood pressure (Dakshinamurti & Dakshinamurti, 2001).

8.5.3.3 CLINICAL EVIDENCE

Only a few clinical studies have been managed to investigate the link between Vitamin B6 or B12 and hypertension, but the evidence is insufficient to establish its blood pressure-lowering properties (Dakshinamurti

& Dakshinamurti, 2001; Aybak et al., 1995). As a result, supplementing or consuming Pyridoxine or cyanocobalamin is not immediately suggested in the treatment of hypertension and its complications. For a more hypotensive response, vitamin B6 or B12 might collaborate with other hypotensive nutrition and traditional antihypertensive medications.

8.5.4 VITAMIN C/ASCORBIC ACID

Vitamin C, or ascorbic acid, is a water-soluble antioxidant that promotes the development and growth of bodily tissues, particularly collagen synthesis and wound healing. Citrus (orange, lemons, and grapefruits), kiwi fruit, and berries are all good sources (Walingo, 2005). Existing research demonstrated that a low vitamin C serum level in people was linked to increased blood pressure (hypertension), implying an inverse relationship between vitamin C and BP. As a result, maintaining a normal vitamin C level is critical for maintaining good cardiovascular health (by supplying 70–90 milligrams) as well as enhancing the effectiveness of some conventional antihypertensive drugs like amlodipine and so positively modulating blood pressure (Mahajan et al., 2007; Ness, Chee, & Elliott, 1997).

8.5.4.1 BLOOD PRESSURE REGULATING MECHANISM

Vitamin C, or ascorbate, has been indicated to have hypotensive characteristics by increasing the generation of nitrous oxide (an anti-oxidant and vasodilation) and prostaglandin, hence maintaining endothelial function and functioning as an angiotensin receptor blocker, decreasing blood pressure (Plantinga et al., 2007). Vitamin C also increases erythrocyte $Na+/K+$ ATPases, diuretics activities ($Na+$ excretion), and is implicated in cytosolic $Ca++$ reductions (Ca channels blocker), all of which inhibit vascular constriction by regulating SNS and therefore positively controlling blood pressure (Houston, 2018; Cicero et al., 2019). Furthermore, vitamin C has been shown to have potent antioxidant as well as anti-inflammatory properties, suggesting that it may improve endothelial function by increasing NO levels (Duffy et al., 1999).

8.5.4.2 CLINICAL EVIDENCE

According to McRae (2006), hypertensive participants who were supplied with ascorbic acid at 500 milligrams/day for 6 weeks had a substantial reduction in their systolic through 3.9 mm Hg and diastolic to 2.1 mm

Hg, demonstrating a negative link among vitamin C and blood pressure. Juraschek et al. (2012) conducted a meta-analysis of control trials and found that ascorbic acid supplementation (500 mg/day) during 8 weeks in hypertensive participants resulted in a substantial reduction in systolic (4.8 mm Hg) without affecting diastolic levels. Another systematic review and meta-analysis involving 44 clinical trials found that vitamin C supplement reduces the risk of cardiovascular disease by enhancing endothelial function and vascular tone (Ashor et al., 2014).

In a meta-analysis study, Guan and colleagues found that adjunct with Vitamin C (500 mg/day) resulted in a substantial reduction in both systolic (4.09) and diastolic (2.30) in basic or primary hypertension individuals. As a result, the foregoing studies emphasize the role of vitamin C in regulating blood pressure and suggest that it be used in conjunction with certain common antihypertensive medications (Guan, Dai, & Wang, 2020). Figure 8.2 represents a diagrammatic description of major micronutrient potential blood pressure-regulating mechanisms.

8.6 MECHANISM OF ACTION

8.6.1 VITAMIN D/CALCIFEROL

Vitamin D may play an individual and direct effect on blood pressure and insulin metabolic activity control. Dietary modification for Calciferol has indeed been manifested to lower blood pressure without affecting calcium levels, implying that it has a direct influence on blood pressure regulation. Both Ca-regulating hormones have a transmitter or receptors in vascular tissue. Under long-term care of patients experiencing intermittent hypercalcemia, vitamin D was found to reduce blood pressure. Short-term supplementation with vitamin D3 plus calcium is more potent than Ca^{++} alone in lowering systolic pressure (Dakshinamurti & Lal, 1996; Hanni et al., 1995; Boucher, 1998; Kurtz & Morris, 1986; Bukoski & McCarron, 1986).

8.6.2 VITAMIN E/TOCOPHEROL

In vitro, a-tocopherol suppresses thrombin-induced endothelin secretion, at least in part, by inhibiting Protein kinase C. Insulin sensitivity is getting better. Antioxidant status has improved. Nitrous oxide and nitric oxide levels have increased. Increased Mg^{++} levels in the membrane and intracellularly. Serum glutathione levels have increased. It lowers oxygenated low-density lipoprotein (Wen et al., 1996; Pezeshk & Derick, 2000; Iino et al., 1977).

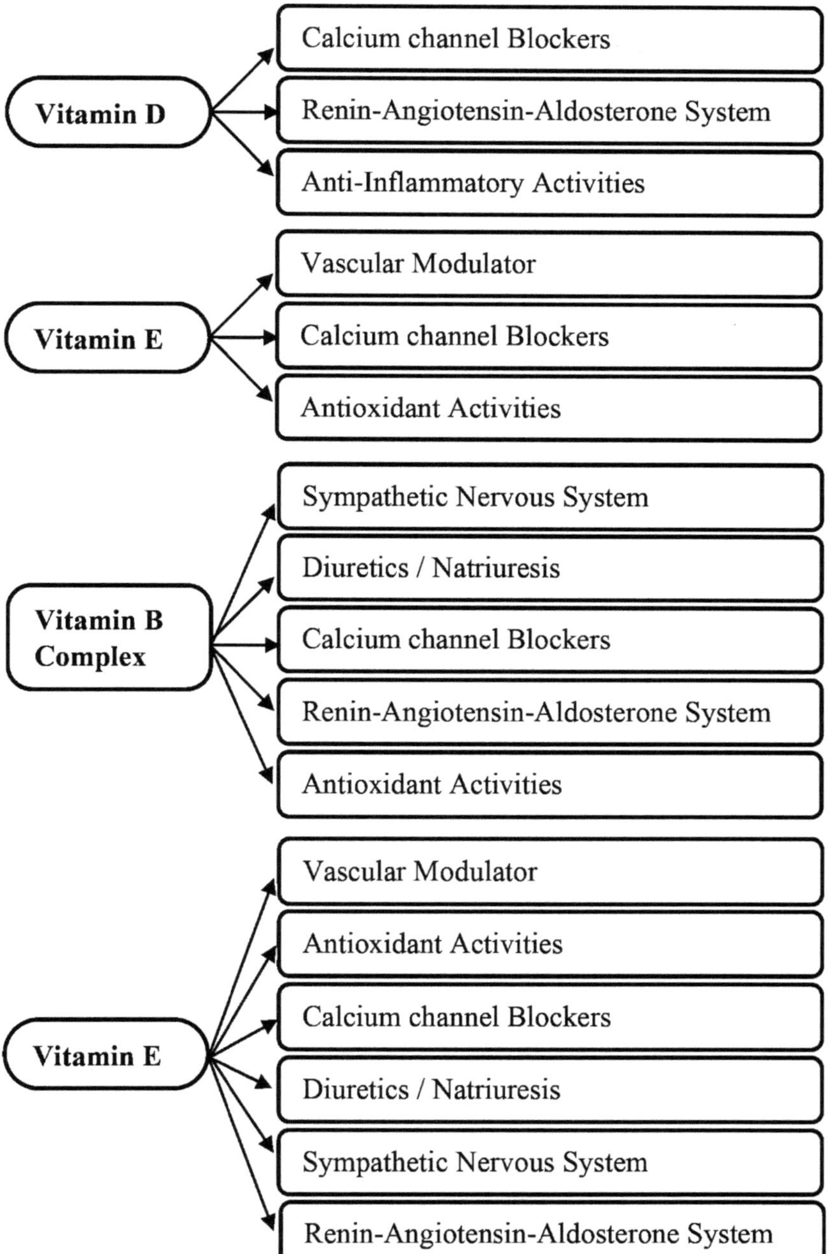

FIGURE 8.2 Diagrammatic description of major micronutrient potential blood pressure-regulating mechanisms.

Source: Modified from Fang et al. (2021)

8.6.3 VITAMIN B COMPLEX (VITAMIN B6/PYRIDOXINE)

The following are suggested pathways of high arterial pressure in vitamin B complex-deficient living creatures:

- Destruction of neurons, including serotonin and benzodiazepines, in the nervous system and brain stem, leading to a rise in sympathetic stimulation.
- Increased sympathetic nervous system activity in the periphery.
- Increased Ca++ uptake and intracellular Ca++ release in smooth muscles.
- Increased glucocorticoid and mineralocorticoid end-organ responsiveness (aldosterone).
- Aldehyde level has increased.
- Develops insulin resistance (Bender, 1999; Weber, 2014).

8.6.4 VITAMIN C

1. In hypertension, hyperlipidemia, heart disease, and smokers reduce erectile dysfunction and increase endothelial vasodilation while also lowering blood pressure and vascular resistance.
2. Urination problems.
3. Prostacyclin I2 and nitric oxide levels should be increased.
4. Reduce steroid synthesis in the adrenal glands.
5. Achieve a more balanced sympathovagal system.
6. Lower Ca++ in the cytosol.
7. Vitamin E, glutathione, and uric acid are all recycled by this antioxidant.
8. Neutralizes neuroendocrine peptides (neuroendocrine peptides) in the body.
9. It lowers thromboxane A2 and lowers thrombosis.
10. Lowers lipids (lowering total cholesterol, low-density lipoproteins, triglycerides, and increasing high-density lipoproteins).
11. Lowers leukotrienes.
12. Stimulate smooth muscle cell K+ channels by increasing cyclic guanosine monophosphate levels (Ascherio et al., 1992; Bao et al., 1998; Mori et al., 1999; Houston, 2016; Alexander, 1998; Houston, 2005).

8.7 CONCLUSION

Hypertension, cardiovascular disease, and target organ damage are all caused by venous pathophysiology, endothelium, vascular smooth muscle failure, and cardiac dysfunction. Interconnection with nutrients and genes, as well as epigenetics, is important elements in determining whether cardiovascular function and hypertension are beneficial or harmful. Through a diversity of mechanisms connected to vascular biology, nutritional content, and micronutrients can help to prevent, regulate, and treat hypertension. High blood pressure and congestive heart failure are initiated and propagated by oxidative stress, inflammation, and immunological dysfunction. Based on scientifically controlled studies, there is a role for the selective use of individual and combination nutraceutical supplements, vitamins, antioxidants, and minerals in the treatment of hypertension, which complements good nutrition and other lifestyle adjustments.

Increased supplementation of certain micronutrients, including vitamin C, D, and B6, could lessen the incidence of hypertension and its related co-morbidities, such as cardiovascular disease, cerebrovascular illnesses, and renal dysfunctions, by positively modulating blood pressure levels. Despite this, the role of different nutrients (vitamins) in the prevention of Hypertension and its consequences has been highlighted in this study. Micronutrients have also been demonstrated to lessen the side effects of antihypertensive drugs. Nonetheless, several micronutrients had a contradictory relationship with blood pressure (neither positive nor negative). As a result, micronutrients could only be used as adjuvant therapy in combination with particular conventional antihypertensive drugs, as well as a change in lifestyle, to optimize their hypotensive properties. However, more depth and huge, brief drug studies (scientific evidence) are required before these nutrients (high precision dose and duration) can be recommended for the therapeutics of hypertension alongside standard antihypertensive drugs.

ACKNOWLEDGMENTS

We thank the Ravindra Vidya Prasarak Mandal Institute of Pharmacy, Dwarka, Nashik, Maharashtra, India, for their constant support and providing all facilities to complete this work. Also, many thanks to all the known and unknowns who helped us right from the writing till the publishing of this chapter.

KEYWORDS

- **ascorbic acid**
- **blood pressure**
- **calciferol**
- **cyanocobalamin**
- **hypertension**
- **nutraceutical**
- **pyridoxine**
- **vitamins**

REFERENCES

Alexander, J. W., (1998). Immunonutrition: The role of ω-3 fatty acids. *Nutrition, 14*(7, 8), 627–633.

Ascherio, A., Rimm, E. B., Giovannucci, E. L., Colditz, G. A., Rosner, B., Willett, W. C., Sacks, F., & Stampfer, M. J., (1992). A prospective study of nutritional factors and hypertension among US men. *Circulation, 86*(5), 1475–1484.

Ashor, A. W., Lara, J., Mathers, J. C., & Siervo, M., (2014). Effect of vitamin C on endothelial function in health and disease: A systematic review and meta-analysis of randomized controlled trials. *Atherosclerosis, 235*(1), 9–20.

Aybak, M., Sermet, A., Ayyildiz, M. O., & Karakilcik, A. Z., (1995). Effect of oral pyridoxine hydrochloride supplementation on arterial blood pressure in patients with essential hypertension. *Arzneimittel-Forschung, 45*(12), 1271–1273.

Aykan, D. A., & Aykan, A. C., (2019). Factors associated with the concomitant use of cardiovascular drugs and dietary herbal products: A cross-sectional study. *Journal of Cardiovascular Pharmacology and Therapeutics, 24*(2), 146–152.

Bao, D. Q., Mori, T. A., Burke, V., Puddey, I. B., & Beilin, L. J., (1998). Effects of dietary fish and weight reduction on ambulatory blood pressure in overweight hypertensives. *Hypertension, 32*(4), 710–717.

Bender, D. A., (1999). Non-nutritional uses of vitamin B6. *British Journal of Nutrition, 81*(1), 7–20.

Benjamin, E. J., Larson, M. G., Keyes, M. J., Mitchell, G. F., Vasan, R. S., Keaney, Jr. J. F., Lehman, B. T., et al., (2004). Clinical correlates and heritability of flow-mediated dilation in the community: The Framingham heart study. *Circulation, 109*(5), 613–619.

Beveridge, L. A., Struthers, A. D., Khan, F., Jorde, R., Scragg, R., Macdonald, H. M., Alvarez, J. A., et al., (2015). Effect of vitamin D supplementation on blood pressure: A systematic review and meta-analysis incorporating individual patient data. *JAMA Internal Medicine, 175*(5), 745–754.

Boshtam, M., Rafiei, M., Sadeghi, K., & Sarraf-Zadegan, N., (2002). Vitamin E can reduce blood pressure in mild hypertensives. *International Journal for Vitamin and Nutrition Research, 72*(5), 309–314.

Boucher, B. J., (1998). Inadequate vitamin D status: Does it contribute to the disorders comprising syndrome 'X'? *British Journal of Nutrition, 79*(4), 315–327.

Broadhurst, C. L., (1997). Balanced intakes of natural triglycerides for optimum nutrition: An evolutionary and phytochemical perspective. *Medical Hypotheses, 49*(3), 247–261.

Bukoski, R. D., & Mccarron, D. A., (1986). Altered aortic reactivity and lowered blood pressure are associated with high calcium intake. *American Journal of Physiology-Heart and Circulatory Physiology, 251*(5), H976–H983.

Burgaz, A., Orsini, N., Larsson, S. C., & Wolk, A., (2011). Blood 25-hydroxyvitamin D concentration and hypertension: A meta-analysis. *Journal of Hypertension, 29*(4), 636–645.

Cain, A. E., & Khalil, R. A., (2002). Pathophysiology of essential hypertension: Role of the pump, the vessel, and the kidney. In: *Seminars in Nephrology* (Vol. 22, No. 1, pp. 3–16). WB Saunders.

Cardillo, C., Kilcoyne, C. M., Quyyumi, A. A., Cannon, III. R. O., & Panza, J. A., (1998). Selective defect in nitric oxide synthesis may explain the impaired endothelium-dependent vasodilation in patients with essential hypertension. *Circulation, 97*(9), 851–856.

Carretero, O. A., & Oparil, S., (2000). Essential hypertension: Part II: Treatment. *Circulation, 101*(4), 446–453.

Chen, J., He, J., Hamm, L., Batuman, V., & Whelton, P. K., (2002). Serum antioxidant vitamins and blood pressure in the United States population. *Hypertension, 40*(6), 810–816.

Chiu, H. F., Venkatakrishnan, K., Golovinskaia, O., & Wang, C. K., (2021). Impact of micronutrients on hypertension: Evidence from clinical trials with a special focus on meta-analysis. *Nutrients, 13*(2), 588.

Christian, P., (2015). Evidence of multiple micronutrient supplementation (MMS) in pregnancy. *Sight and Life, 29*(1), 28–34.

Chumphukam, O., Chaiwangyen, W., Sivamaruthi, B. S., Chaiyasut, C., Natakankitkul, S., Kangwan, N., Tantipaiboonwong, P., et al., (2019). The innovation of functional foods in Asia: IFFA 2018. *Asia Pacific Journal of Clinical Nutrition, 28*(2), 419–426.

Cicero, A. F., Grassi, D., Tocci, G., Galletti, F., Borghi, C., & Ferri, C., (2019). Nutrients and nutraceuticals for the management of high normal blood pressure: An evidence-based consensus document. *High Blood Pressure & Cardiovascular Prevention, 26*(1), 9–25.

Cicero, A. F., Grassi, D., Tocci, G., Galletti, F., Borghi, C., & Ferri, C., (2019). Nutrients and nutraceuticals for the management of high normal blood pressure: An evidence-based consensus document. *High Blood Pressure & Cardiovascular Prevention, 26*(1), 9–25.

Cody, R. J., (1997). The sympathetic nervous system and the renin-angiotensin-aldosterone system in cardiovascular disease. *The American Journal of Cardiology, 80*(9), 9J-14J.

Czernichow, S., Blacher, J., & Hercberg, S., (2004). Antioxidant vitamins and blood pressure. *Current Hypertension Reports, 6*(1), 27–30.

Dakshinamurti, K., & Dakshinamurti, S., (2001). Blood pressure regulation and micronutrients. *Nutrition Research Reviews, 14*(1), 3–44.

Dakshinamurti, K., & Lal, K. J., (1992). Vitamins and hypertension. *World Review of Nutrition and Dietetics.*

Dakshinamurti, K., Jawahar, L. K., & Ganguly, P. K., (1998). Hypertension, calcium channel, and pyridoxine (vitamin B 6). *Molecular and Cellular Effects of Nutrition on Disease Processes*, 137–148.

Dakshinamurti, S., Dakshinamurti, K., Zempleni, J., Suttie, J. W., Gregory, J. F., & Stover, P. J., (2014). Vitamin B6. *Handbook of Vitamins, 4.*

Dandona, P., Ghanim, H., Chaudhuri, A., Dhindsa, S., & Kim, S. S., (2010). Macronutrient intake induces oxidative and inflammatory stress: Potential relevance to atherosclerosis and insulin resistance. *Experimental & Molecular Medicine*, *42*(4), 245–253.

Das, L., Bhaumik, E., Raychaudhuri, U., & Chakraborty, R., (2012). Role of nutraceuticals in human health. *Journal of Food Science and Technology*, *49*(2), 173–183.

Delacroix, S., Chokka, R. G., & Worthley, S. G., (2014). Hypertension: Pathophysiology and treatment. *J. Neurol. Neurophysiol.*, *5*(6), 1–8.

Dillard, C. J., & German, J. B., (2000). Phytochemicals: Nutraceuticals and human health. *Journal of the Science of Food and Agriculture*, *80*(12), 1744–1756.

Donnarumma, E., Trivedi, R. K., & Lefer, D. J., (2011). Protective actions of H2S in acute myocardial infarction and heart failure. *Comprehensive Physiology*, *7*(2), 583–602.

Dozio, E., Briganti, S., Vianello, E., Dogliotti, G., Barassi, A., Malavazos, A. E., Ermetici, F., et al., (2015). Epicardial adipose tissue inflammation is related to vitamin D deficiency in patients affected by coronary artery disease. *Nutrition, Metabolism and Cardiovascular Diseases*, *25*(3), 267–273.

Duffy, S., Gokce, N., Holbrook, M., Huang, A., Frei, B., Keaney, Jr. J. F., & Vita, J. A., (1999). Treatment of hypertension with ascorbic acid. *The Lancet*, *354*(9195), 2048–2049.

Eaton, S. B., & Konner, M. J., (1997). Review paleolithic nutrition revisited: A twelve-year retrospective on its nature and implications. *European Journal of Clinical Nutrition*, *51*(4), 207–216.

Ferrario, C. M., (2006). Role of angiotensin II in cardiovascular disease—Therapeutic implications of more than a century of research. *Journal of the Renin-Angiotensin-ALDOSTERONE SYSTEM*, *7*(1), 3–14.

Giles, T. D., Materson, B. J., Cohn, J. N., & Kostis, J. B., (2009). Definition and classification of hypertension: An update. *The Journal of Clinical Hypertension*, *11*(11), 611–614.

Golzarand, M., Shab-Bidar, S., Koochakpoor, G., & Djafarian, K., (2016). Effect of vitamin D3 supplementation on blood pressure in adults: An updated meta-analysis. *Nutrition, Metabolism and Cardiovascular Diseases*, *26*(8), 663–673.

Gratacós, E., Casals, E., Deulofeu, R., Cararach, V., Alonso, P. L., & Fortuny, A., (1998). Lipid peroxide and vitamin E patterns in pregnant women with different types of hypertension in pregnancy. *American Journal of Obstetrics and Gynecology*, *178*(5), 1072–1076.

Guan, Y., Dai, P., & Wang, H., (2020). Effects of vitamin C supplementation on essential hypertension: A systematic review and meta-analysis. *Medicine*, *99*(8).

He, S., & Hao, X. (2019). The effect of vitamin D3 on blood pressure in people with vitamin D deficiency: A systematic review and meta-analysis. *Medicine*, *98*(19).

Hensley, K., Benaksas, E. J., Bolli, R., Comp, P., Grammas, P., Hamdheydari, L., Mou, S., et al., (2004). New perspectives on vitamin E: γ-tocopherol and carboxyethyl hydroxy chroman metabolites in biology and medicine. *Free Radical Biology and Medicine*, *36*(1), 1–15.

Hickey, K. A., Rubanyi, G. A. B. O. R., Paul, R. J., & Highsmith, R. F., (1985). Characterization of a coronary vasoconstrictor produced by cultured endothelial cells. *American Journal of Physiology-Cell Physiology*, *248*(5), C550–C556.

Houston, M. C., & Harper, K. J., (2008). Potassium, magnesium, and calcium: Their role in both the cause and treatment of hypertension. *The Journal of Clinical Hypertension*, *10*(7), 3–11.

Houston, M. C., (2005). Nutraceuticals, vitamins, antioxidants, and minerals in the prevention and treatment of hypertension. *Progress in Cardiovascular Diseases*, *47*(6), 396–449.

Houston, M. C., (2007). Treatment of hypertension with nutraceuticals, vitamins, antioxidants, and minerals. *Expert Review of Cardiovascular Therapy*, *5*(4), 681–691.

Houston, M. C., (2011). The importance of potassium in managing hypertension. *Current Hypertension Reports*, *13*(4), 309–317.

Houston, M. C., (2016). Utilizing nutrition in treatment. *Food and Nutrients in Disease Management*, 75.

Houston, M. C., (2018). Treatment of hypertension with nutrition and nutraceutical supplements: Part 1. *Alternative and Complementary Therapies*, *24*(6), 260–275.

Houston, M., (2014). The role of nutrition and nutraceutical supplements in the treatment of hypertension. *World Journal of Cardiology*, *6*(2), 38.

Iino, K., Abe, K., Kariya, S., Kimura, H., Kusaba, T., Kusunoki, R., Saku, J., et al., (1977). A controlled, double-blind study of dl-alpha-tocopheryl nicotinate (Juvela-Nicotinate®) for treatment of symptoms in hypertension and cerebral arteriosclerosis. *Japanese Heart Journal*, *18*(3), 277–286.

Judd, S. E., Nanes, M. S., Ziegler, T. R., Wilson, P. W., & Tangpricha, V., (2008). Optimal vitamin D status attenuates the age-associated increase in systolic blood pressure in white Americans: Results from the third national health and nutrition examination survey. *The American Journal of Clinical Nutrition*, *87*(1), 136–141.

Juraschek, S. P., Guallar, E., Appel, L. J., & Miller, III. E. R., (2012). Effects of vitamin C supplementation on blood pressure: A meta-analysis of randomized controlled trials. *The American Journal of Clinical Nutrition*, *95*(5), 1079–1088.

Kailasapathy, K., (2009). Encapsulation technologies for functional foods and nutraceutical product development. *CAB Reviews*.

Katsanos, A. H., Filippatou, A., Manios, E., Deftereos, S., Parissis, J., Frogoudaki, A., Vrettou, A. R., et al., (2017). Blood pressure reduction and secondary stroke prevention: A systematic review and metaregression analysis of randomized clinical trials. *Hypertension*, *69*(1), 171–179.

Keservani, R. K., & Sharma, A. K., (2014). Flavonoids: Emerging trends and potential health benefits. *Journal of Chinese Pharmaceutical Sciences*, *23*(12), 815.

Keservani, R. K., Kesharwani, R. K., Sharma, A. K., & Jarouliya, U., (2015). Dietary supplements, nutraceutical and functional foods in immune response (immunomodulators); Chapter 20. In: Debasis, B., Harry, G. P., & Anand, S., (eds.), *Nutraceutical and Functional Foods in Human Life and Disease Prevention* (pp. 343–358). Boca Raton, Fl. CRC Press, Taylor and Francis, ISBN: 9781482237214.

Keservani, R. K., Kesharwani, R. K., Sharma, A. K., Vyas, N., & Chadoker, A., (2010b). Nutritional supplements: An overview. *International Journal of Current Pharmaceutical Review and Research*, *1*(1), 59–75.

Keservani, R. K., Kesharwani, R. K., Vyas, N., Jain, S., Raghuvanshi, R., & Sharma, A. K., (2010a). Nutraceutical and functional food as future food: A review. *Der Pharmacia Lettre*, *2*(1), 106–116.

Keservani, R. K., Sharma, A. K., & Kesharwani, R. K., (2016a). Nutraceutical and functional foods for cardiovascular health. In: *Food Process Engineering* (pp. 257–278, 291–312). Apple Academic Press, CRC Press. ISBN: 9781771884020.

Keservani, R. K., Sharma, A. K., & Kesharwani, R. K., (2016b). Medicinal effect of nutraceutical fruits for the cognition and brain health. *Scientifica*, 10. Article ID 3109254. doi: 10.1155/2016/3109254.

Keservani, R. K., Sharma, A. K., & Kesharwani, R. K. (2017). An overview and therapeutic applications of nutraceutical and functional foods. *Recent Advances in Drug Delivery Technology*, 160–201. ISBN:9781522507543.

Keservani, R. K., Sharma, A. K., & Kesharwani, R. K. (2020). *Nutraceuticals and Dietary Supplements: Applications in Health Improvement and Disease Management*. CRC Press. ISBN: 9781771888738.

Kim, J. R., Kiefe, C. I., Liu, K., Williams, O. D., Jacobs, Jr. D. R., & Oberman, A., (1999). Heart rate and subsequent blood pressure in young adults: The CARDIA study. *Hypertension, 33*(2), 640–646.

Kim, J. Y., Paik, J. K., Kim, O. Y., Park, H. W., Lee, J. H., Jang, Y., & Lee, J. H., (2011). Effects of lycopene supplementation on oxidative stress and markers of endothelial function in healthy men. *Atherosclerosis, 215*(1), 189–195.

Kokate, C. K., Purohit, A. P., & Gokhale, S. B., (2002). *Nutraceutical and Cosmaceutical. Pharmacognosy,* 21st edition, Pune, India: Nirali Prakashan, 1, 542–549.

Krum, H., Viskoper, R. J., Lacourciere, Y., Budde, M., & Charlon, V., (1998). The effect of an endothelin-receptor antagonist, bosentan, on blood pressure in patients with essential hypertension. *New England Journal of Medicine, 338*(12), 784–791.

Kunutsor, S. K., Apekey, T. A., & Steur, M., (2013). Vitamin D and risk of future hypertension: A meta-analysis of 283,537 participants. *European Journal of Epidemiology, 28*(3), 205–221.

Kurtz, T. W., & Morris, R. C., (1986). Dietary intake of vitamin D is a determinant of deoxycorticosterone (Doc) hypertension (HTN). In: *Hypertension* (Vol. 8, No. 9, pp. 833–833). 7272 Greenville Avenue, Dallas, Tx 75231-4596: Amer Heart Assoc.

Lal, K. J., Dakshinamurti, K., & Thliveris, J., (1996). The effect of vitamin B6 on the systolic blood pressure of rats in various animal models of hypertension. *Journal of Hypertension, 14*(3), 355–363.

Lawson, L. D., (1998). Garlic: A review of its medicinal effects and indicated active compounds. *Blood, 179*, 62.

Layne, J., Majkova, Z., Smart, E. J., Toborek, M., & Hennig, B., (2011). Caveolae: A regulatory platform for nutritional modulation of inflammatory diseases. *The Journal of Nutritional Biochemistry, 22*(9), 807–811.

Lee, J. H., O'Keefe, J. H., Bell, D., Hensrud, D. D., & Holick, M. F., (2008). Vitamin D deficiency: An important, common, and easily treatable cardiovascular risk factor? *Journal of the American College of Cardiology, 52*(24), 1949–1956.

Lind, L., Hänni, A., Lithell, H., Hvarfner, A., Sörensen, O. H., & Ljunghall, S., (1995). Vitamin D is related to blood pressure and other cardiovascular risk factors in middle-aged men. *American Journal of Hypertension, 8*(9), 894–901.

Lundberg, A. M., & Yan, Z. Q., (2011). Innate immune recognition receptors and damage-associated molecular patterns in plaque inflammation. *Current Opinion in Lipidology, 22*(5), 343–349.

Mahajan, A. S., Babbar, R., Kansal, N., Agarwal, S. K., & Ray, P. C., (2007). The antihypertensive and antioxidant action of amlodipine and vitamin C in patients of essential hypertension. *Journal of Clinical Biochemistry and Nutrition, 40*(2), 141–147.

Maqbool, M. A., Aslam, M., Akbar, W., & Iqbal, Z., (2017). Biological importance of vitamins for human health: A review. *J. Agric. Basic. Sci., 2*(3), 50–58.

Margolis, K. L., Ray, R. M., Van, H. L., Manson, J. E., Allison, M. A., Black, H. R., Beresford, S. A., et al., (2008). Effect of calcium and vitamin D supplementation on blood pressure: The women's health initiative randomized trial. *Hypertension, 52*(5), 847–855.

Mark, A. L., (1996). The sympathetic nervous system in hypertension: A potential long-term regulator of arterial pressure. *Journal of Hypertension Supplement: Official Journal of the International Society of Hypertension, 14*(5), S159–165.
Mayet, J., & Hughes, A., (2003). Cardiac and vascular pathophysiology in hypertension. *Heart, 89*(9), 1104–1109.
McRae, M. P., (2006). Is vitamin C an effective antihypertensive supplement? A review and analysis of the literature. *Journal of Chiropractic Medicine, 5*(2), 60–64.
Mori, T. A., & Woodman, R. J., (2006). The independent effects of eicosapentaenoic acid and docosahexaenoic acid on cardiovascular risk factors in humans. *Current Opinion in Clinical Nutrition & Metabolic Care, 9*(2), 95–104.
Morvaridzadeh, M., Sepidarkish, M., Fazelian, S., Rahimlou, M., Omidi, A., Ardehali, S. H., Sanoobar, M., & Heshmati, J., (2020). Effect of calcium and vitamin D co-supplementation on blood pressure: A systematic review and meta-analysis. *Clinical Therapeutics, 42*(3), e45–e63.
Mottram, P., Shige, H., & Nestel, P., (1999). Vitamin E improves arterial compliance in middle-aged men and women. *Atherosclerosis, 145*(2), 399–404.
Ness, A. R., Chee, D., & Elliott, P., (1997). Vitamin C and blood pressure: An overview. *Journal of Human Hypertension, 11*(6), 343–350.
Olas, B. (2018). Dietary supplements with antiplatelet activity: A solution for everyone? *Advances in Nutrition, 9*(1), 51–57.
Palumbo, G., Avanzini, F., Alli, C., Roncaglioni, M. C., Ronchi, E., Cristofari, M., Capra, A., et al., (2000). Effects of vitamin E on clinic and ambulatory blood pressure in treated hypertensive patients. *American Journal of Hypertension, 13*(5), 564–567.
Panza, J. A., Casino, P. R., Kilcoyne, C. M., & Quyyumi, A. A., (1993). Role of endothelium-derived nitric oxide in the abnormal endothelium-dependent vascular relaxation of patients with essential hypertension. *Circulation, 87*(5), 1468–1474.
Panza, J. A., García, C. E., Kilcoyne, C. M., Quyyumi, A. A., & Cannon, III. R. O., (1995). Impaired endothelium-dependent vasodilation in patients with essential hypertension: Evidence that nitric oxide abnormality is not localized to a single signal transduction pathway. *Circulation, 91*(6), 1732–1738.
Panza, J. A., Quyyumi, A. A., Brush, Jr. J. E., & Epstein, S. E., (1990). Abnormal endothelium-dependent vascular relaxation in patients with essential hypertension. *New England Journal of Medicine, 323*(1), 22–27.
Parker, J., Hashmi, O., Dutton, D., Mavrodaris, A., Stranges, S., Kandala, N. B., Clarke, A., & Franco, O. H., (2010). Levels of vitamin D and cardiometabolic disorders: Systematic review and meta-analysis. *Maturitas, 65*(3), 225–236.
Pezeshk, A., & Dalhouse, A. D., (2000). Vitamin E, membrane fluidity, and blood pressure in hypertensive and normotensive rats. *Life Sciences, 67*(15), 1881–1889.
Piepho, R. W., & Beal, J., (2000). An overview of antihypertensive therapy in the 20th century. *The Journal of Clinical Pharmacology, 40*(9), 967–977.
Plantinga, Y., Ghiadoni, L., Magagna, A., Giannarelli, C., Franzoni, F., Taddei, S., & Salvetti, A., (2007). Supplementation with vitamins C and E improves arterial stiffness and endothelial function in essential hypertensive patients. *American Journal of Hypertension, 20*(4), 392–397.
Rizvi, S., Raza, S. T., Faizal, A. A. A., Abbas, S., & Mahdi, F., (2014). The role of vitamin E in human health and some diseases. *Sultan Qaboos University Medical Journal, 14*(2), e157.

Sander, M., Chavoshan, B., & Victor, R. G., (1999). A large blood pressure–raising effect of nitric oxide synthase inhibition in humans. *Hypertension, 33*(4), 937–942.

Sarzani, R., & Salvi, F., (2008). Dessı-Fulgheri P, Cappelli A. Renin-angiotensin system, natriuretic peptides, obesity, metabolic syndrome, and hypertension: An integrated view in humans. *J Hypertens, 26*(5), 831–843.

Simões, E. S. A. C., & Flynn, J. T., (2012). The renin-angiotensin-aldosterone system in 2011: Role in hypertension and chronic kidney disease. *Pediatric Nephrology, 27*(10), 1835–1845.

Singh, P., Kesharwani, R. K., & Keservani, R. K. (2017). Antioxidants and vitamins: Roles in cellular function and metabolism. In: *Sustained Energy for Enhanced Human Functions and Activity* (pp. 385–407). Academic Press. ISBN:9780128054130.

Sirtori, C. R., Arnoldi, A., & Cicero, A. F., (2015). Nutraceuticals for blood pressure control. *Annals of Medicine, 47*(6), 447–456.

Slominski, A. T., Chaiprasongsuk, A., Janjetovic, Z., Kim, T. K., Stefan, J., Slominski, R. M., Hanumanthu, V. S., et al., (2020). Photoprotective properties of vitamin D and lumisterol hydroxyderivatives. *Cell Biochemistry and Biophysics, 78*(2), 165–180.

Somjen, D., Weisman, Y., Kohen, F., Gayer, B., Limor, R., Sharon, O., Jaccard, N., et al., (2005). 25-Hydroxyvitamin D3–1α-hydroxylase is expressed in human vascular smooth muscle cells and is upregulated by parathyroid hormone and estrogenic compounds. *Circulation, 111*(13), 1666–1671.

Sugden, J. A., Davies, J. I., Witham, M. D., Morris, A. D., & Struthers, A. D., (2008). Vitamin D improves endothelial function in patients with type 2 diabetes mellitus and low vitamin D levels. *Diabetic Medicine, 25*(3), 320–325.

Surana, K. R., Ahire, E. D., Sonawane, V. N., & Talele, S. G., (2021). Biomolecular and molecular docking: A modern tool in drug discovery and virtual screening of natural products. In: *Applied Pharmaceutical Practice and Nutraceuticals* (pp. 209–223). Apple Academic Press.

Surana, K. R., Ahire, E. D., Sonawane, V. N., Talele, S. G., & Talele, G. S., (2021). Molecular modeling: Novel techniques in food and nutrition development. *Natural Food Products and Waste Recovery: Healthy Foods, Nutrition Design, and Extraction of Valuable Compounds*, (p. 17).

Surana, K. R., Ahire, E. D., Sonawane, V. N., Talele, S. G., & Talele, G. S., (2021). Informatics and methods in nutrition design and development. *Natural Food Products and Waste Recovery: Healthy Foods, Nutrition Design, and Extraction of Valuable Compounds* (p. 33).

Talmud, P. J., & Waterworth, D. M., (2000). *In-vivo* and *in-vitro* nutrient-gene interactions. *Current Opinion in Lipidology, 11*(1), 31–36.

Venkatakrishnan, K., Chiu, H. F., & Wang, C. K., (2020). Impact of functional foods and nutraceuticals on high blood pressure with a special focus on meta-analysis: Review from a public health perspective. *Food & Function, 11*(4), 2792–2804.

Vierhapper, H. O. P. W., Wagner, O., Nowotny, P., & Waldhäusl, W., (1990). Effect of endothelin-1 in man. *Circulation, 81*(4), 1415–1418.

Wagner, O. F., Christ, G., Wojta, J., Vierhapper, H., Parzer, S., Nowotny, P. J., Schneider, B., et al., (1992). Polar secretion of endothelin-1 by cultured endothelial cells. *Journal of Biological Chemistry, 267*(23), 16066–16068.

Walingo, K. M., (2005). Role of vitamin C (ascorbic acid) on human health-a review. *African Journal of Food, Agriculture, Nutrition and Development, 5*(1).

Weber, J., (2014). *Hypertension and Nutrition: Fat-soluble Vitamins A, D, and E, 1*, 1–89.

Weber, M. A., Schiffrin, E. L., White, W. B., Mann, S., Lindholm, L. H., Kenerson, J. G., Flack, J. M., et al., (2014). Clinical practice guidelines for the management of hypertension in the community: a statement by the American Society of Hypertension and the International Society of Hypertension. *The Journal of Clinical Hypertension, 16*(1), 14.

Wen, Y., Killalea, S., McGettigan, P., & Feely, J., (1996). Lipid peroxidation and antioxidant vitamins C and E in hypertensive patients. *Irish Journal of Medical Science, 165*(3), 210–212.

Williams, B., Mancia, G., Spiering, W., Agabiti, R. E., Azizi, M., & Burnier, M., (2018). ESC/ESH guidelines for the management of arterial hypertension. *European Heart Journal, 39*(33), 3021–3104.

Witham, M. D., Nadir, M. A., & Struthers, A. D., (2009). Effect of vitamin D on blood pressure: A systematic review and meta-analysis. *Journal of Hypertension, 27*(10), 1948–1954.

Yuan, W., Pan, W., Kong, J., Zheng, W., Szeto, F. L., Wong, K. E., Cohen, R., et al., (2007). 1, 25-dihydroxy vitamin D3 suppresses renin gene transcription by blocking the activity of the cyclic AMP response element in the renin gene promoter. *Journal of Biological Chemistry, 282*(41), 29821–29830.

Zhao, L., Lee, J. Y., & Hwang, D. H., (2011). Inhibition of pattern recognition receptor-mediated inflammation by bioactive phytochemicals. *Nutrition Reviews, 69*(6), 310–320.

CHAPTER 9

Vitamins as Nutraceuticals for Neurodegenerative Disease

ABHIJEET G. PARKHE,[1] KHEMCHAND R. SURANA,[2] EKNATH D. AHIRE,[3] SUNIL K. MAHAJAN,[4] DHANANJAY M. PATIL,[5] and RAJ K. KESERVANI[6]

[1]Research Associate, In Vivo Pharmacology Department, Glenmark Pharmaceutical Ltd., Navi Mumbai, Maharashtra, India

[2]Department of Pharmaceutical Chemistry, Shreeshakti Shaikshanik Sanstha, Divine College of Pharmacy, Satana, Nashik, Maharashtra, India

[3]Department of Pharmaceutics, MET's Institute of Pharmacy, Adgaon, Nashik, Maharashtra, India

[4]Department of Pharmaceutical Chemistry, M.G.V's Samajshri Prashant Dada Hiray, College of Pharmacy, Malegaon, Nashik, Maharashtra, India

[5]Department of Pharmaceutics, Shreeshakti Shaikshanik Sanstha, Divine College of Pharmacy, Satana, Nashik, Maharashtra, India

[6]Faculty of B. Pharmacy, CSM Group of Institutions, Prayagraj, Uttar Pradesh, India

ABSTRACT

Vitamins as nutraceuticals are a new concept growing at a rapid pace in a world full of allopathic medicines. Vitamins are mainly organic molecules required by the body for performing normal functions. Vitamins have multiple functions in the body. Vitamins are an essential part of the body and need to be consumed by the body as not all the vitamins are generated in the body, and deficiency of which may cause severe consequences. Vitamin deficiency

Preventive and Therapeutic Role of Vitamins as Nutraceuticals. Khemchand R. Surana, Eknath D. Ahire, Raj K. Keservani, & Rajesh K. Kesharwani (Eds.)

might not affect instantly, but in the long run, it affects human health and, in some cases, somehow causes neuronal diseases. All types of vitamins have some importance for our body, but in combination, it fulfills daily biological needs; each one has a different activity and a significant role in the human body. Vitamin A has antioxidant (Singh et al., 2017a) activity and is responsible for vision, vitamin D helps in improving bone health, vitamin E acts as an immunity modulator, and vitamin K has a role in coagulation. Deficiency or dysfunction of the selective and important nutrients affects neuronal metabolism. Neurodegenerative diseases such as Alzheimer's disease, Parkinson's disease, Huntington's disease, Amyotrophic lateral sclerosis, and Prion disease are main and significant in the contribution of mental as well as physical disability. In this chapter, we have covered some vital vitamins which, indirectly or directly, have neuroprotective roles. It has been reported widely in the literature that lipid and water-soluble vitamins are screened for the neuroprotection and prevention of amyloid and tau protein formation in the brain. This chapter covers each major vitamin with food sources that play a role in neurodegenerative diseases and, in some cases, how it adversely affects human health.

9.1 INTRODUCTION

In the modern world where we human beings touch new heights periodically but at the same time due to negligence of government, common people, & research institutes, facts lagging behind that we as humans need certain nutrients for survival. Some are essential, and some are non-essential. Figure 9.1 illustrates the classification of the fat-soluble and water-soluble vitamins (Heaney, 2012; Shao et al., 2017).

Vitamins are generally considered essential and majorly play a role in the normal development and functioning of the body. Its theoretically and practically proposed vitamins cannot synthesize by the body, if at all, but sometimes not in enough amount which is required by the body's needs. Here is a mind-blowing fact about the fat-soluble vitamins, it usually gets stored in the fatty tissues in the body, but it is not the same for water-soluble vitamins. Water soluble vitamins are continuously removed from the body with water and very much needed to take regularly as supplements or diet (Albahrani & Greaves, 2016; Surana et al., 2021a, b). Coming to the point, neurodegeneration is a spontaneous process once one gets neurodegenerative disease. Overall, in the disease condition, patients suffer from a series of problems and face many symptoms which are specific to the loss of

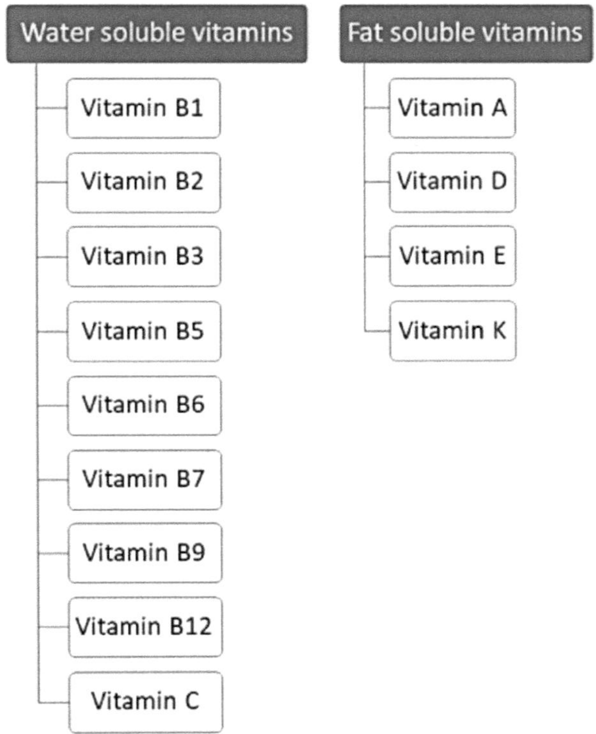

FIGURE 9.1 Classification of the fat-soluble and water-soluble vitamins.

nerve cells/neurons in the different parts of the brain. Neurodegeneration term if we dissect into two it means neuro means nerve cells, and degeneration means decay or slow loss. Many neurodegenerative diseases show different pathology with respect to the disease and affect different parts of the brain. For example, in Alzheimer's disease, all the neurons of the brain start to shrink, and mainly the hippocampus part of the brain gets damaged (Bruno & Ziegenfuss, 2005). Talking about Parkinson's disease, mainly the substantia nigra part of the midbrain gets affected, and mainly neurodegeneration saw in this part. Alzheimer's disease (AD), Parkinson's disease (PD), Huntington's disease (HD), and amyotrophic lateral sclerosis (ALS) are a handful of diseases which was given importance by the researchers due to their prevalence and lack of information on pathology (Surana et al., 2022). Though there is no treatment available for the above-mentioned diseases, only symptomatic treatment can extend the life of the patient. These major diseases cannot be cured, but with the symptomatic treatment, supplementary nutrition (Keservani et al., 2010a, b, 2017, 2020) can be given to the patient to improve their health and lower/reduce side effects of symptomatic relief drugs. In the nutritional supplement, several market products play a major role, but it has been reported that vitamins play a major role in lowering disease progression and getting relief from the severe side effects of the drugs. As vitamins as such have no side/adverse effects on the health of the patient so as a nutritional supplement, it has proven as an effective remedy for tackling disease (Sies et al., 1992; Surana et al., 2021c, d).

9.2 VITAMINS-RICH FOODS FOR THE MANAGEMENT OF NEURODEGENERATIVE DISEASES

It is reported in the literature that mentioned vitamins in Table 9.1 provide significant improvement in the neurodegenerative diseases. Some of them are easily available to common people, which significantly impacts the life of patients with such neurodegenerative diseases (Ahire et al., 2021).

TABLE 9.1 Specific Vitamins Used in the Neurodegenerative Diseases and its Food Source

Sl. No.	Vitamin	Food Source	Disease	References
1.	Vitamin A	Fish, meat, and dairy products	Schizophrenia, depression, Parkinson's disease (PD), and Alzheimer's disease (AD).	Janesick et al. (2015); Tafti & Ghyselinck (2007)
2.	Vitamin D	Fatty fish, dairy products, orange juice, cereals, beef liver, cheese, and egg yolks.	Parkinson disease	Luo et al. (2018); Janjusevic et al. (2022)
3.	Vitamin E	Sunflower seeds, almonds, mango, avocado, and peanuts.	Parkinson's disease, Alzheimer's disease, stroke, and amyotrophic lateral sclerosis.	Kubis & Piwowar (2015); Icer et al. (2021)
4.	Vitamin K	Green leafy vegetables, Soybean, Smaller amounts in meat, cheese, and eggs	Alzheimer's disease	Ferland (2012)
5.	Vitamin B1	Peas, fresh fruits, nuts, and wholegrain bread	Parkinson's disease, Alzheimer's disease, Wernicke's encephalopathy or Wernicke-Korsakoff syndrome, and Huntington's disease.	Bubko et al. (2015); Gibson et al. (2016)

TABLE 9.1 *(Continued)*

Sl. No.	Vitamin	Food Source	Disease	References
6.	Vitamin B2	Milk and dairy products, and dark-green vegetables.	Peripheral nerve demyelination	Johnson & Storts (1988); Jortner et al. (1987)
7.	Vitamin B3	Whole grains, eggs, milk, nuts, and avocados.	Nerve demyelination	Lemprière (2020); Xu et al. (2020)
8.	Vitamin B5	Cereals, mushrooms, avocado, nuts, seeds, dairy milk, yogurt, potatoes, eggs, brown rice, oats, and broccoli	Alzheimer's disease, Huntington's disease, and Parkinson's disease dementia	Patassini et al. (2019); Scholefield et al. (2021)
9.	Vitamin B6	Fish, potatoes, vegetables, and fruit	Parkinson's disease and Alzheimer's disease	Yu et al. (2016); De Lau et al. (2006)
10.	Vitamin B7	Cooked eggs, salmon, avocados, beef liver, pork, sweet potato, and nuts.	Dementia and Alzheimer's disease	Lohr et al. (2020)
11.	Vitamin B9	Dark green leafy vegetables like spinach, asparagus, broccoli, beans, whole grains, sunflower seeds, peanuts, and fresh fruits.	Cognitive decline and dementia	Gómez-Gómez & Zapico (2019)
12.	Vitamin B12	Fish, meat, milk, eggs, and cheese	Parkinson's disease, Alzheimer's disease, and cognitive impairment.	Luthra et al. (2020); Moore et al. (2012)
13.	Vitamin C	Citrus fruit, orange, strawberries, sprouts, broccoli, and potatoes.	Psychiatric disorders and Alzheimer's disease	Kocot et al. (2017); Heo & Lee (2004)

9.2.1 FAT-SOLUBLE VITAMINS REPORTED IN THE LITERATURE COMMONLY USED IN THE TREATMENT OF THE NEURODEGENERATIVE DISEASES

According to the literature, here are some lists of the fat-soluble vitamins actually studied for the treatment of the neurodegenerative disease (Figure 9.2).

9.2.1.1 VITAMIN A

Vitamin A also called Retinol. The main role of this type of vitamin is for the normal functioning of the eye. Apart from the eye, it is also involved in

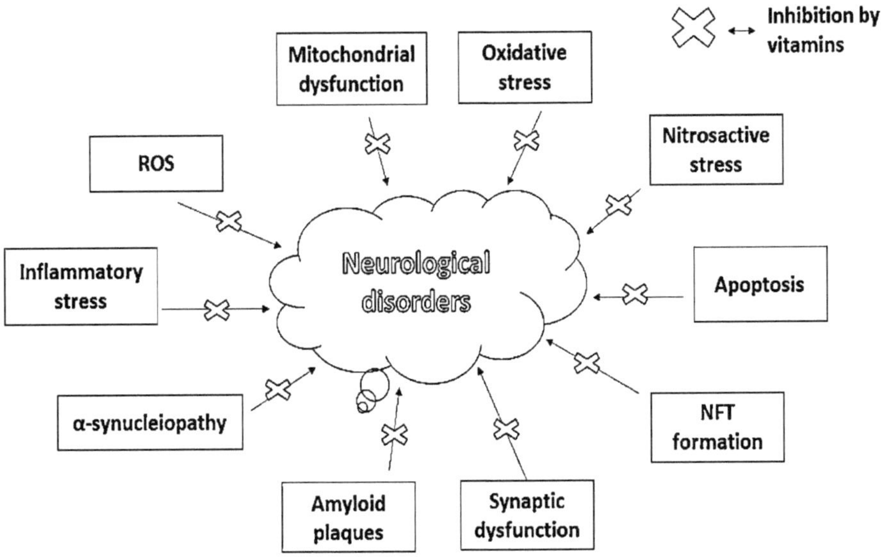

FIGURE 9.2 Role of vitamins in the neurodegenerative disease biomarkers.

the immune system modulation. The normal requirement of vitamin A in children is about 300–700 μg, and in adults, it is 700–900 μg. Other than its basic function in the body, it is involved in the decreasing incidence of neurodegeneration in neurodegenerative disease patients. Studies have been done on vitamin A as having antioxidant activity. Also, in the daily nutrition supplements, vitamin A is present (Huang et al., 2018). It is reported in the scientific journal and several clinical trials that it is safe under the supervision of the medical practitioner and very helpful in tackling neurodegenerative diseases (Dias et al., 2011).

9.2.1.2 VITAMIN D

Cholecalciferol is one of the active forms of Vitamin D. Actually, it's a secondary product from the primary raw material present in the skin with the help of ultraviolet light. The main function of the vitamin is to regulate the levels of calcium and phosphorus in the human body either by mineralization or demineralization. Vitamin D metabolism is mainly mediated by UV B rays/radiation. Hydroxylation of the cholecalciferol in the human liver occurs, which leads to the 25-hydroxyvitamin D formation with a hydroxylation step to produce active form 1,25-dihydroxyvitamin (D3) in the kidneys

(Heidari et al., 2011). In the literature, it is reported that vitamin D levels were significantly low in patients with diseases like Multiple sclerosis (MS), Parkinson's disease, & Alzheimer's disease when compared to the healthy control. As reports suggest that patients with these diseases are having low levels of vitamin D, scientists started thinking about starting vitamin D supplementation in these groups of people (Goldberg, 1974). Also, in the experiments in the rats, it is found that vitamin D increases the activity of the L-type voltage-sensitive calcium channels in the hippocampus of the rat brain. In the literature, it has been reported that vitamin D is also used as prophylactic and as therapeutic in multiple sclerosis. Though it has been elucidated in the preclinical settings in the clinic, if it is planned to be used, then what should be the dose and supplement drug-drug interaction should be taken care of (Camu et al., 2014).

9.2.1.3 VITAMIN E

Vitamin E/Alpha-Tocopherol shows potent cytoprotective (protect cells) and antioxidant (free radical scavenging ability) properties. Apart from the antioxidant property literature reports, it protects reproductive function. All in all, vitamin E has many functions in human life (Ascherio et al., 2005). As mentioned above, vitamin E has antioxidant activity, and, needless to say, free radicals and oxidative stress play a role in neurodegenerative diseases. Apart from the several environmental and genetic factors to cause these diseases but oxidative stress remains prime concern for the factor which worsens the condition of the patient with these diseases (Kašparová et al., 2006). It is reported in the literature that antioxidant properties of vitamin E could be a very interesting idea to adopt for treating neurological diseases. Some literature also depicts vitamin E deficiency in Parkinson's disease, Multiple sclerosis & Alzheimer's disease when compared to healthy individuals (Boccardi et al., 2016).

9.2.1.4 VITAMIN K

There are multiple forms of vitamin K, namely, Vitamin K2 (menaquinone), Vitamin K1 (phytomenadione), and Vitamin K3 (menadione). It is a fat-soluble nutrient with its major role in the blood coagulation explored very well. Apart from this role, it is found that its role in the brain cells/neurons development *in vitro* and *in vivo* (Alisi et al., 2019). One would be amazed to know the fact that vitamin K helps to metabolize sphingolipids. It's a lipid basically involved in the proliferation, differentiation, and survival. Researchers also suggested that through their research sphingolipid profile gets altered in neurodegeneration and neuroinflammation, which is an indicator of its role in neurodegenerative diseases (Josey et al., 2013). Recent trends in cognition and brain research show that vitamin K is gaining importance as a neuroprotective agent. Also, in developing countries, due to environmental factors, cognition-related problems researchers started to face, and in this scenario, vitamin K simply showed a good nutritional supplement as a support to modern medicine (Yagami et al., 2002).

9.2.2 WATER-SOLUBLE VITAMINS REPORTED IN THE LITERATURE COMMONLY USED IN THE TREATMENT OF THE NEURODEGENERATIVE DISEASES

According to the literature, here are some lists of the water-soluble vitamins actually studied for the treatment of neurodegenerative disease. Water-soluble vitamins are mainly responsible for the normal functions of the body, such as growth and development of vital organs of the body. Micronutrients such as water-soluble vitamins are very important. Lack of which may cause acute or severe/chronic diseases such as growth retardation and neurological diseases (Karuppagounder et al., 2009).

9.2.2.1 VITAMIN B1

Thiamine/anti-Beri-Beri factor/Aneurin is the common name for this vitamin B1. A unique complex forms through the reaction between ATP and thiamine. Thiamine pyrophosphate, a phosphatase enzyme with thymine, plays a very important role in carbohydrate metabolism. It is mostly insoluble in the organic solvent but soluble in polar solvents. A great example of such a polar solvent is water. Apart from the main function, thiamine plays a prime role in proper maintenance of the cardiac muscles, nervous system, and digestive (enteral) system. According to the literature, chronic deficiency of thiamine leads to chances of getting neurological disorders. Literature also revealed that vitamin B1 has a neuroprotective effect in several neurological diseases when given supporting vitamin B1 therapy. Some articles also favor vitamin B1 as exerting neuroprotective effects in AD, PD, & ALS. AD is the first ranked killer in history, and to date, there is no definitive treatment for the same, but there are reports wherein vitamin B1 is used as a neuroprotective molecule, and some justifying studies show that less intake by controlled healthy individuals could lead to getting beriberi and Wernicke Korsakoff Syndrome (Victor et al., 1971).

9.2.2.2 VITAMIN B2

Also known by the name riboflavin, it is the precursor of two vital coenzymes, namely flavin mononucleotide and flavin adenine dinucleotide. They are involved in the oxidation or reduction reaction. Mentioned enzymes normally take part in the metabolism of proteins (Singh et al., 2017b) and carbohydrates (Kolbuszewski, 1971). Riboflavin is crucial for healthy hair & skin by modulating glutathione reductase enzymes which thereafter help to increase glutathione levels. It has been proven with sets of experiments showing that riboflavin deficiency causes mainly anorexia and growth-related issues. Moderate deficiency causes paralysis as well (Gries & Scott, 1972).

9.2.2.3 VITAMIN B3

Nicotinic acid/Vitamin B3 is also known as niacin. Lipid content balance in our body is necessary, and this vitamin plays a massive role by reducing the bad cholesterol (Low-Density Lipoprotein) and increasing the good cholesterol (High-Density Lipoprotein) in the body. Dyslipidemia is a major problem in today's world, and vitamin B3 is very good at managing this problem. Enzymes present in the serum called aminotransferases might be responsible for elevating niacin levels in the body, and high doses of which might cause acute liver injury, but the chances are very rare (Lemprière, 2020). Vitamin B3/Niacin is occasionally used as a vasodilator agent, which dilates blood vessels diameter, an antilipemic drug, which decreases blood lipoprotein levels, and an antidote, which blocks the effect of poison or any drug high dose. Reports suggest that axon remyelination is promoted by niacin, and diseases like multiple sclerosis could be treated by this vitamin. Release of growth factors at the site and clearing myelin waste is the best way to promote remyelination. According to the literature, microglia and macrophages derived from the monocytes play a major role in the process of remyelination (Rawji et al., 2020).

9.2.2.4 VITAMIN B5

Pantothenic acid/Vitamin B5 inherently has very strong antioxidative properties, which means it scavenges free radicals in the body, which generates metabolism of different components in the body. It also has several important functions in the body, which are taking part in the synthesis of hormones and involvement in the metabolism of carbohydrates, hemoglobin, neurotransmitters, lipids, and proteins. Researchers found out that vitamin B5 is much needed for the synthesis of coenzyme A, and in neurological disorders' coenzyme A plays a significant role (Venco et al., 2014). It is found that vitamin B5 levels were found very low in the brains of Alzheimer's and Huntington's disease patients. By using these data, scientists have concluded and are trying to treat Alzheimer's and Huntington's disease with vitamin B5 supplements (Hayflick, 2014).

9.2.2.5 VITAMIN B6

Pyridoxine/Vitamin B6/Pyridoxol/Gravidox directly or indirectly plays a crucial role in the synthesis of essential neurochemicals/neurotransmitters like serotonin and norepinephrine. Some glycogen and amino acid synthesis occur in the presence of vitamin B6. As per the existing knowledge of science, vitamin B6's role is well established in research and in clinics, but scientists explored its effect in combination with vitamin B12 and choline (van Wijk et al., 2012). It was hard to distinguish each vitamin's effect on the hypoxia-induced dementia in mice, but it was clear that these multivitamins could reverse disease and prevent further neuronal loss. Some researchers explored this vitamin's activity in Parkinson's disease animal models and found it to have neuroprotective effects by restoring dopamine levels in the brain (Morris, 2012).

9.2.2.6 VITAMIN B7

Biotin/Vitamin B7/Vitamin H is basically an enzyme. For proper growth and metabolism purposes, vitamin B7 is needed. Like other vitamins, biotin also has some neuroprotective effects. specifically speaking, biotin is studied in the Drosophila model by some researchers, and results suggest that by modulating druggable metabolic pathway, biotin has a neuroprotective role in neurodegenerative diseases in humans (Dias-Santagata et al., 2007).

9.2.2.7 VITAMIN B9

Folate/Vitamin B9/vitamin M enzyme plays a crucial role in the metabolism of different amino acids. Vitamin B9 is important in the production of red blood cells (RBC) in the body. There is as such, no reports have been found in the literature that vitamin B9 has a neuroprotective effect, but multivitamin therapy with proper sleep and exercise may help AD & PD patients to get symptomatic relief and improve their quality of life. Medical practitioners also suggest a Mediterranean diet with multivitamin supplements for improving quality of life (Ngandu et al., 2015).

9.2.2.8 VITAMIN B12

Cobalamin/vitamin B12/cyanocobalamin is a cobalt coordination molecule made by intestinal microbes. The important thing is that it needs some intrinsic factors present in the body for its absorption through the enteral system. Deficiency of which causes two types of anemia first megaloblastic anemia and second pernicious anemia. It is repeatedly reported in the literature that vitamin B12 deficiency has a negative effect on human health, and furthermore, it affects cognitive damage (Dietiker et al., 2019). The authors also mentioned that brains of the AD & PD patients have low levels of vitamin B12, and there is scope for AD & PD treatment with vitamin B12 supplements (Boston et al., 2020).

9.2.2.9 VITAMIN C

Vitamin C/ascorbic acid is a potent antioxidant taken through diet. It is found in many citrus fruits, such as lemons and oranges. It is essential and, very importantly, not synthesized by the human body. According to the literature, vitamin C is a vital antioxidant present in nature (Warner et al., 2015). It has different functions in the body. It scavenges most of the reactive oxygen species produced through the metabolic reactions. To date, the mechanism is unknown for neuron protection, maturation, and differentiation, but reports suggest that vitamin C has potent antioxidant activity (Warner et al., 2015).

9.3 CONCLUSION

In conclusion, we have summarized all the vitamins as nutraceuticals and their use in the respective neurological diseases with its proper food source. Further addition to this information and collected data from the literature, it is important to conclude that we as human beings depend on green vegetables and animals to get the required nutrients for the sake of the growth and development of the body. Animals also take their essential nutrition from the vegetables only, so it is simply logical to go for raw materials instead of its derivatives. All green vegetables are full of vitamins and minerals, which are essential for the human body. Vitamins in all nutraceuticals are very important and play an essential role in the body, as mentioned in the introduction part. With this information, we came to the conclusion that these vitamins could be used before any neurological disorder occurs as prophylactic measures. On the other hand, researchers also engaged in studies where they focused on making vitamins as nutraceutical products that would be used as supplements for neurological disorders. In some diseases, as mentioned above, medical practitioners use them as supplementary treatment for better symptomatic relief to patients. As it does not have any side effects in limited quantities for humans, these are safe-to-use supplements in combinations like multivitamins for neurological disease patients.

ACKNOWLEDGMENTS

We thank you to Glenmark Pharmaceuticals Ltd. Mumbai, METs, Institute of Pharmacy, Adgaon, Nashik, and Mahatma Gandhi Vidyamandir's Pharmacy College, Panchavati, Nashik, Maharashtra, India, for their constant support and providing all facilities to complete this work. Also, many thanks to all the known and unknowns who helped us right from the writing till the publishing of this chapter.

KEYWORDS

- **Alzheimer's disease**
- **fat-soluble vitamins**
- **neurodegenerative diseases**
- **Parkinson's disease**
- **prion disease**
- **vitamins**
- **water-soluble vitamins**

REFERENCES

Ahire, E. D., Sonawane, V. N., Surana, K. R., & Talele, G. S., (2021). Drug discovery, drug-likeness screening, and bioavailability: Development of drug-likeness rule for natural products. In: *Applied Pharmaceutical Practice and Nutraceuticals* (pp. 191–208). Apple Academic Press.

Albahrani, A. A., & Greaves, R. F., (2016). Fat-soluble vitamins: Clinical indications and current challenges for chromatographic measurement. *The Clinical Biochemist Reviews, 37*(1), 27.

Alisi, L., Cao, R., De Angelis, C., Cafolla, A., Caramia, F., Cartocci, G., Librando, A., & Fiorelli, M., (2019). The relationships between vitamin K and cognition: A review of current evidence. *Frontiers in Neurology, 10*, 239.

Ascherio, A., Weisskopf, M. G., O'Reilly, E. J., Jacobs, E. J., McCullough, M. L., Calle, E. E., Cudkowicz, M., & Thun, M. J., (2005). Vitamin E intake and risk of amyotrophic lateral sclerosis. *Annals of Neurology: Official Journal of the American Neurological Association and the Child Neurology Society, 57*(1), 104–110.

Boccardi, V., Baroni, M., Mangialasche, F., & Mecocci, P., (2016). Vitamin E family: Role in the pathogenesis and treatment of Alzheimer's disease. *Alzheimer's & Dementia: Translational Research & Clinical Interventions, 2*(3), 182–191.

Boston, P. F., McKirdy, S. J., Al-Turki, M. A., Barker, M. E., & Russell, J. M. (2020). Vitamin B12 and folate levels in progression of Alzheimer's disease–a short report. *International Journal of Psychiatry in Clinical Practice, 24*(1), 68–70.

Bruno, E. J., & Ziegenfuss, T. N., (2005). Water-soluble vitamins: Research update. *Current Sports Medicine Reports, 4*(4), 207–213.

Bubko, I., Gruber, B. M., & Anuszewska, E. L., (2015). The role of thiamine in neurodegenerative diseases. *Postepy Higienyi Medycyny Doswiadczalnej (Online), 69*, 1096–1106.

Camu, W., Tremblier, B., Plassot, C., Alphandery, S., Salsac, C., Pageot, N., Juntas-Morales, R., et al., (2014). Vitamin D confers protection to motoneurons and is a prognostic factor of amyotrophic lateral sclerosis. *Neurobiology of Aging, 35*(5), 1198–1205.

De Lau, L. M. L., Koudstaal, P. J., Witteman, J. C. M., Hofman, A., & Breteler, M. M. B., (2006). Dietary folate, vitamin B12, and vitamin B6 and the risk of Parkinson's disease. *Neurology, 67*(2), 315–318.

Dias, V., Junn, E., & Mouradian, M. M., (2013). The role of oxidative stress in Parkinson's disease. *Journal of Parkinson's Disease, 3*(4), 461–491.

Dias-Santagata, D., Fulga, T. A., Duttaroy, A., & Feany, M. B., (2007). Oxidative stress mediates tau-induced neurodegeneration in *Drosophila*. *The Journal of Clinical Investigation, 117*(1), 236–245.

Dietiker, C., Kim, S., Zhang, Y., Christine, C. W., & NINDS NET-PD Investigators, (2019). Characterization of vitamin B12 supplementation and correlation with clinical outcomes in a large longitudinal study of early Parkinson's disease. *Journal of Movement Disorders, 12*(2), 91.

Ferland, G., (2012). Vitamin K is an emerging nutrient in brain function. *Biofactors, 38*(2), 151–157.

Gibson, G. E., Hirsch, J. A., Fonzetti, P., Jordan, B. D., Cirio, R. T., & Elder, J., (2016). Vitamin B1 (thiamine) and dementia. *Annals of the New York Academy of Sciences, 1367*(1), 21–30.

Goldberg, P., (1974). Multiple sclerosis: Vitamin D and calcium as environmental determinants of prevalence: (A viewpoint) part 2. Biochemical and genetic factors. *International Journal of Environmental Studies, 6*(2, 3), 121–129.

Gómez-Gómez, M. E., & Zapico, S. C., (2019). Frailty, cognitive decline, neurodegenerative diseases, and nutrition interventions. *International Journal of Molecular Sciences, 20*(11), 2842.

Gries, C. L., & Scott, M. L., (1972). The pathology of thiamin, riboflavin, pantothenic acid, and niacin deficiencies in the chick. *The Journal of Nutrition, 102*(10), 1269–1285.

Hayflick, S. J., (2014). Defective pantothenate metabolism and neurodegeneration. *Biochemical Society Transactions, 42*(4), 1063–1068.

Heaney, R. P., (2012). The nutrient problem. *Nutrition Reviews, 70*(3), 165–169.

Heidari, B., Heidari, P., & Hajian-Tilaki, K., (2011). Association between serum vitamin D deficiency and knee osteoarthritis. *International Orthopaedics, 35*(11), 1627–1631.

Heo, H. J., & Lee, C. Y., (2004). Protective effects of quercetin and vitamin C against oxidative stress-induced neurodegeneration. *Journal of Agricultural and Food Chemistry, 52*(25), 7514–7517.

Huang, Z., Liu, Y., Qi, G., Brand, D., & Zheng, S. G. (2018). Role of vitamin A in the immune system. *Journal of Clinical Medicine, 7*(9), 258.

Icer, M. A., Arslan, N., & Gezmen-Karadag, M., (2021). Effects of vitamin E on neurodegenerative diseases: An update. *Acta Neurobiol. Exp., 81*, 21–33.

Janesick, A., Wu, S. C., & Blumberg, B., (2015). Retinoic acid signaling and neuronal differentiation. *Cellular and Molecular Life Sciences, 72*(8), 1559–1576.

Janjusevic, M., Gagno, G., Fluca, A. L., Padoan, L., Beltrami, A. P., Sinagra, G., Moretti, R., & Aleksova, A., (2022). The peculiar role of vitamin D in the pathophysiology of cardiovascular and neurodegenerative diseases. *Life Sciences, 289*, 120193.

Johnson, W. D., & Storts, R. W., (1988). Peripheral neuropathy associated with dietary riboflavin deficiency in the chicken I. Light microscopic study. *Veterinary Pathology, 25*(1), 9–16.

Jortner, B. S., Cherry, J., Lidsky, T. I., Manetto, C., & Shell, L., (1987). Peripheral neuropathy of dietary riboflavin deficiency in chickens. *Journal of Neuropathology & Experimental Neurology, 46*(5), 544–555.

Josey, B. J., Inks, E. S., Wen, X., & Chou, C. J., (2013). Structure–activity relationship study of vitamin K derivatives yields highly potent neuroprotective agents. *Journal of Medicinal Chemistry, 56*(3), 1007–1022.

Karuppagounder, S. S., Xu, H., Shi, Q., Chen, L. H., Pedrini, S., Pechman, D., Baker, H., et al., (2009). Thiamine deficiency induces oxidative stress and exacerbates plaque pathology in Alzheimer's mouse models. *Neurobiology of Aging, 30*(10), 1587–1600.

Kašparová, S., Sumbalová, Z., Bystrický, P., Kucharská, J., Liptaj, T., Mlynárik, V., & Gvozdjáková, A., (2006). Effect of coenzyme Q10 and vitamin E on brain energy metabolism in the animal model of Huntington's disease. *Neurochemistry International, 48*(2), 93–99.

Keservani, R. K., Kesharwani, R. K., Sharma, A. K., Vyas, N., & Chadoker, A., (2010b). Nutritional supplements: An overview. *International Journal of Current Pharmaceutical Review and Research, 1*(1), 59–75.

Keservani, R. K., Kesharwani, R. K., Vyas, N., Jain, S., Raghuvanshi, R., & Sharma, A. K., (2010a). Nutraceutical and functional food as future food: A review. *Der Pharmacia Lettre, 2*(1), 106–116.

Keservani, R. K., Sharma, A. K., & Kesharwani, R. K. (2017). An overview and therapeutic applications of nutraceutical and functional foods. *Recent Advances in Drug Delivery Technology*, 160–201. ISBN:9781522507543.

Keservani, R. K., Sharma, A. K., & Kesharwani, R. K. (2020). *Nutraceuticals and Dietary Supplements: Applications in Health Improvement and Disease Management*. CRC Press. ISBN: 9781771888738.

Kocot, J., Luchowska-Kocot, D., Kiełczykowska, M., Musik, I., & Kurzepa, J., (2017). Does vitamin C influence neurodegenerative diseases and psychiatric disorders? *Nutrients, 9*(7), 659.

Kolbuszewski, T., (1971). Nervous system disturbances in chickens in the background of riboflavin deficiency in the diet. *Pol. Arch. Med. Wewn., 14*, 563–575.

Kubis, A. M., & Piwowar, A., (2015). The new insight on the regulatory role of vitamin D3 in metabolic pathways characteristic for cancerogenesis and neurodegenerative diseases. *Ageing Research Reviews, 24*, 126–137.

Lemprière, S., (2020). Vitamin B3 promotes remyelination. *Nature Reviews Neurology, 16*(4), 184, 185.

Lohr, K. M., Frost, B., Scherzer, C., & Feany, M. B., (2020). Biotin rescues mitochondrial dysfunction and neurotoxicity in a tauopathy model. *Proceedings of the National Academy of Sciences, 117*(52), 33608–33618.

Luo, X., Ou, R., Dutta, R., Tian, Y., Xiong, H., & Shang, H. (2018). Association between serum vitamin D levels and Parkinson's disease: A systematic review and meta-analysis. *Frontiers in Neurology*, 909.

Luthra, N. S., Marcus, A. H., Hills, N. K., & Christine, C. W., (2020). Vitamin B12 measurements across neurodegenerative disorders. *Journal of Clinical Movement Disorders, 7*(1), 1–6.

Mehta, S., & Fawzi, W., (2007). Effects of vitamins, including vitamin A, on HIV/AIDS patients. *Vitamins & Hormones, 75*, 355–383.

Moore, E., Mander, A., Ames, D., Carne, R., Sanders, K., & Watters, D., (2012). Cognitive impairment and vitamin B12: A review. *International Psychogeriatrics, 24*(4), 541–556.

Morris, M. S., (2012). The role of B vitamins in preventing and treating cognitive impairment and decline. *Advances in Nutrition, 3*(6), 801–812.

Ngandu, T., Lehtisalo, J., Solomon, A., Levälahti, E., Ahtiluoto, S., Antikainen, R., Bäckman, L., et al., (2015). A 2-year multidomain intervention of diet, exercise, cognitive training, and vascular risk monitoring versus control to prevent cognitive decline in at-risk elderly people (FINGER): A randomized controlled trial. *The Lancet, 385*(9984), 2255–2263.

Patassini, S., Begley, P., Xu, J., Church, S. J., Kureishy, N., Reid, S. J., Waldvogel, H. J., et al., (2019). Cerebral vitamin B5 (D-pantothenic acid) deficiency is a potential cause of metabolic perturbation and neurodegeneration in Huntington's disease. *Metabolites, 9*(6), 113.

Rawji, K. S., Young, A. M., Ghosh, T., Michaels, N. J., Mirzaei, R., Kappen, J., Kolehmainen, K. L., et al., (2020). Niacin-mediated rejuvenation of macrophage/microglia enhances remyelination of the aging central nervous system. *Acta Neuropathologica, 139*(5), 893–909.

Scholefield, M., Church, S. J., Xu, J., Patassini, S., Hooper, N. M., Unwin, R. D., & Cooper, G. J., (2021). Substantively lowered levels of pantothenic acid (Vitamin B5) in several regions of the human brain in Parkinson's disease dementia. *Metabolites, 11*(9), 569.

Shao, A., Drewnowski, A., Willcox, D. C., Krämer, L., Lausted, C., Eggersdorfer, M., Mathers, J., et al., (2017). Optimal nutrition and the ever-changing dietary landscape: A conference report. *European Journal of Nutrition, 56*(1), 1–21.

Sies, H., Stahl, W., & Sundquist, A. R., (1992). Antioxidant functions of vitamins: Vitamins E and C, Beta-Carotene, and other carotenoids A. *Annals of the New York Academy of Sciences, 669*(1), 7–20.

Singh, P., Kesharwani, R. K., & Keservani, R. K., (2017a). Antioxidants and vitamins: Roles in cellular function and metabolism. In: *Sustained Energy for Enhanced Human Functions and Activity* (pp. 385–407). Academic Press. ISBN:9780128054130.

Singh, P., Kesharwani, R. K., & Keservani, R. K., (2017b). Protein, carbohydrates, and fats: Energy metabolism. In: *Sustained Energy for Enhanced Human Functions and Activity* (pp. 103–115). Academic Press. ISBN:9780128054130.

Surana, K. R., Ahire, E. D., Sonawane, V. N., & Talele, S. G., (2021). Biomolecular and molecular docking: A modern tool in drug discovery and virtual screening of natural products. In: *Applied Pharmaceutical Practice and Nutraceuticals* (pp. 209–223). Apple Academic Press.

Surana, K. R., Ahire, E. D., Sonawane, V. N., Talele, S. G., & Talele, G. S., (2021). Informatics and methods in nutrition design and development. *Natural Food Products and Waste Recovery: Healthy Foods, Nutrition Design, and Extraction of Valuable Compounds* (p. 33).

Surana, K. R., Ahire, E. D., Sonawane, V. N., Talele, S. G., & Talele, G. S., (2021). Molecular modeling: Novel techniques in food and nutrition development. *Natural Food Products and Waste Recovery: Healthy Foods, Nutrition Design, and Extraction of Valuable Compounds*, (p. 17).

Surana, K. R., Parkhe, A. G., Ahire, E. D., Pawar, A. R., Khairnar, S., Mahajan, S. K., Patil, D. M., et al., (2022). Current therapeutic targets for neuropathic pain. *Asian Journal of Pharmaceutical Research, 12*(1), 96–104.

Tafti, M., & Ghyselinck, N. B., (2007). Functional implication of the vitamin A signaling pathway in the brain. *Archives of Neurology, 64*(12), 1706–1711.

Van, W. N., Watkins, C. J., Böhlke, M., Maher, T. J., Hageman, R. J., Kamphuis, P. J., Broersen, L. M., & Wurtman, R. J., (2012). Plasma choline concentration varies with different dietary levels of vitamins B6, B12, and folic acid in rats maintained on choline-adequate diets. *British Journal of Nutrition, 107*(10), 1408–1412.

Venco, P., Dusi, S., Valletta, L., & Tiranti, V., (2014). Alteration of the coenzyme A biosynthetic pathway in neurodegeneration with brain iron accumulation syndromes. *Biochemical Society Transactions, 42*(4), 1069–1074.

Victor, M., Adams, R. D., & Collins, G. H., (1971). The Wernicke-Korsakoff syndrome. A clinical and pathological study of 245 patients, 82 with post-mortem examinations. *Contemporary Neurology Series, 7*, 1–206.

Warner, T. A., Kang, J. Q., Kennard, J. A., & Harrison, F. E. (2015). Low brain ascorbic acid increases susceptibility to seizures in mouse models of decreased brain ascorbic acid transport and Alzheimer's disease. *Epilepsy Research, 110*, 20–25.

Xu, J., Patassini, S., Begley, P., Church, S., Waldvogel, H. J., Faull, R. L., Unwin, R. D., & Cooper, G. J., (2020). Cerebral deficiency of vitamin B5 (d-pantothenic acid; pantothenate) as a potentially-reversible cause of neurodegeneration and dementia in sporadic Alzheimer's disease. *Biochemical and Biophysical Research Communications, 527*(3), 676–681.

Yagami, T., Ueda, K., Asakura, K., Sakaeda, T., Nakazato, H., Kuroda, T., Hata, S., et al., (2002). Gas6 rescues cortical neurons from amyloid β protein-induced apoptosis. *Neuropharmacology, 43*(8), 1289–1296.

Yu, L., Chen, Y., Wang, W., Xiao, Z., & Hong, Y., (2016). Multi-vitamin B supplementation reverses hypoxia-induced tau hyperphosphorylation and improves memory function in adult mice. *Journal of Alzheimer's Disease, 54*(1), 297–306.

CHAPTER 10

Vitamins as Nutraceuticals for Weight Loss and Obesity

PANKAJ R. AHER,[1] KHEMCHAND R. SURANA,[2] EKNATH D. AHIRE,[3] DHANANJAY M. PATIL,[4] SUNIL K. MAHAJAN,[5] and SHIVRAJ P. JADHAV[4]

[1]*Department of Pharmaceutical Chemistry, Loknete Dr. J. D. Pawar College of Pharmacy, Manur, Kalwan, Nashik, Maharashtra, India*

[2]*Department of Pharmaceutical Chemistry, Shreeshakti Shaikshanik Sanstha, Divine College of Pharmacy, Satana, Nashik, Maharashtra, India*

[3]*Department of Pharmaceutics, MET's Institute of Pharmacy, Bhujbal Knowledge City, Adgaon, Nashik, Maharashtra, India*

[4]*Department of Pharmaceutics, Shreeshakti Shaikshanik Sanstha, Divine College of Pharmacy, Satana, Nashik, Maharashtra, India*

[5]*Department of Pharmaceutical Chemistry, M.G.V's Samajshri Prashant Dada Hiray, College of Pharmacy, Malegaon, Nashik, Maharashtra, India*

ABSTRACT

Being overweight and weight gain are properly-established threat elements for cardiovascular disease and several cancers; however, the underlying mechanisms have now no longer been fully elucidated. The prevalence of weight problems has been rising regularly for the past many years everywhere in the world, leading to a growth in the prevalence of many complications of excess weight, a number of that are well acknowledged, such as Type 2 Diabetes (T2D), obstructive sleep apnea syndrome (OSAS), non-alcoholic fatty liver disease (NAFLD), and cardiovascular disease, even as others are emerging and presently being investigated. The recognition of vitamins and

Preventive and Therapeutic Role of Vitamins as Nutraceuticals. Khemchand R. Surana, Eknath D. Ahire, Raj K. Keservani, & Rajesh K. Kesharwani (Eds.)

nutraceuticals for weight management has increased, and a good type of these products is on the market over the counter. The utilization of meals and dietary supplements consisting of dietary products and nutrients rich diet for weight loss functions has quickly gained quality because the prevalence of weight issues increases. Currently a time, weight problems have become increasing health problems for smaller children and additionally in the older age group. Vitamins as nutraceuticals consisting of diet D, C, K, E, B-12 and specific food wealthy sources of calcium utilized for clinical purposes in terms of weight reduction and obesity. The listing of dietary supplements which might be claimed to enhance fats metabolism is long; the most famous dietary supplements encompass caffeine, carnitine, green tea, conjugated linoleic acid, forskolin, chromium, kelp, and fucoxanthin. Obesity frequently coexists with low dietary meal consumption and nutrient insufficiency. There is emerging proof of a role for those vitamins in the law of body weight. However, it miles doubtful whether or not growing intakes of various nutraceuticals and/or nutrients during energy restriction is a better strategy for weight and fat loss.

10.1 INTRODUCTION

The cutting-edge overweight and obesity pandemic and its related troubles concerning adherence to treatment (i.e., lifestyle modification along with a change in nutritional patterns and exercise) have caused different interventional approaches, along with pharmacological therapy, surgery, and the use of nutritional supplements (nutraceuticals) (Keservani et al., 2010a, b, 2017, 2020; Mason et al., 2011). Dietary supplements represent an attractive adjuvant opportunity to standard remedy because of the truth most have a low toxicity profile and are available to the overall population. It is, therefore, now not unexpected that the ones dietary supplements account for more than $37 billion in sales with-in-aspect the USA (Ríos-Hoyo & Gutiérrez-Salmeán, 2016). Nutraceuticals or nutritional supplements are legally defined as products meant to supplement the food plan (i.e., add further nutritional value) as they incorporate one or extra nutritional elements (e.g., vitamins, minerals, amino acids, herbs, metabolite, extract). Moreover, nutritional dietary supplements usually are taken orally; for that reason, they will be found as capsules, tablets, gelatin capsules, liquids, or powders (Soares et al., 2011). Considering the aforementioned definition, nutritional dietary supplements aren't meant to either treat or prevent any disease; in fact, the scientific results of maximum of those dietary supplements have now no longer been evaluated in sufficient double-blinded, randomized clinical trials (Wamberg et al., 2013). Although nutritional elements may have confirmed positive results inside preclinical and small clinical scenarios, the large majority lack proof when thinking about the entire picture, along with the purity grade of the supplement ingested, the general lifestyle (i.e., food plan and exercise), and different health-associated conditions of the patient (e.g., dietary status or concomitant diseases), food–drug interactions, excessive dosing, and potential side effects (Shick et al., 1998). Assessing the clinical effectiveness of nutritional dietary supplements is extremely difficult because the law of these products differs from that of conventional pharmaceuticals. This situation has made nutritional dietary supplements broadly to be had as over-the-counter (OTC) products, for that reason, easily accessible to the overall population. Because dietary supplements are not taken into consideration drugs, policies primarily based totally on their clinical effectiveness are not as strict as those of conventional drugs; consequently, they may be marketed and bought irrespective of scientifically confirmed clinical evidence (Watanabe et al., 2020).

It has been demonstrated currently that overweight people with low calcium and dairy consumption are at an awful lot more danger of developing the metabolic syndrome over a 10-y follow-up than had been overweight people with immoderate calcium and dairy intake (Zittermann et al., 2009). This locating suggests that good enough calcium intake may want to exert a tremendous effect on the predisposition to a healthier metabolic profile, much like that of a macronutrient-balanced weight loss plan and normal physical activity. From a physiologic standpoint, metabolic deteriorations and their capacity relation with calcium or dairy consumption is an area of new interest (MacLean et al., 1983). Figure 10.1 represents (LIPO-MAX Injection) the role of different vitamins, amino acids, and nutraceuticals in the management of weight and fat.

The term dietary supplement is described through the Dietary Supplement Health and Education Act as a product (other than tobacco) supposed to supplement the diet that bears or contains 1 or more of the following dietary substances: (i) a vitamin; (ii) a mineral; (iii) a herb or other botanical; (iv) an amino acid; (v) a nutritional substance to be used by a person to supplement the diet through increasing the total nutritional intake; or (vi) a concentrate, metabolite, constituent, extract, or mixture of any element described in clause (A), (B), (C), (D), or (E) (Pandol et al., 2007). Dietary supplements are, consequently, products supposed to complement the diet, typically taken orally and found as capsules, tablets, liquids, or powders (Gasteyger et al.,

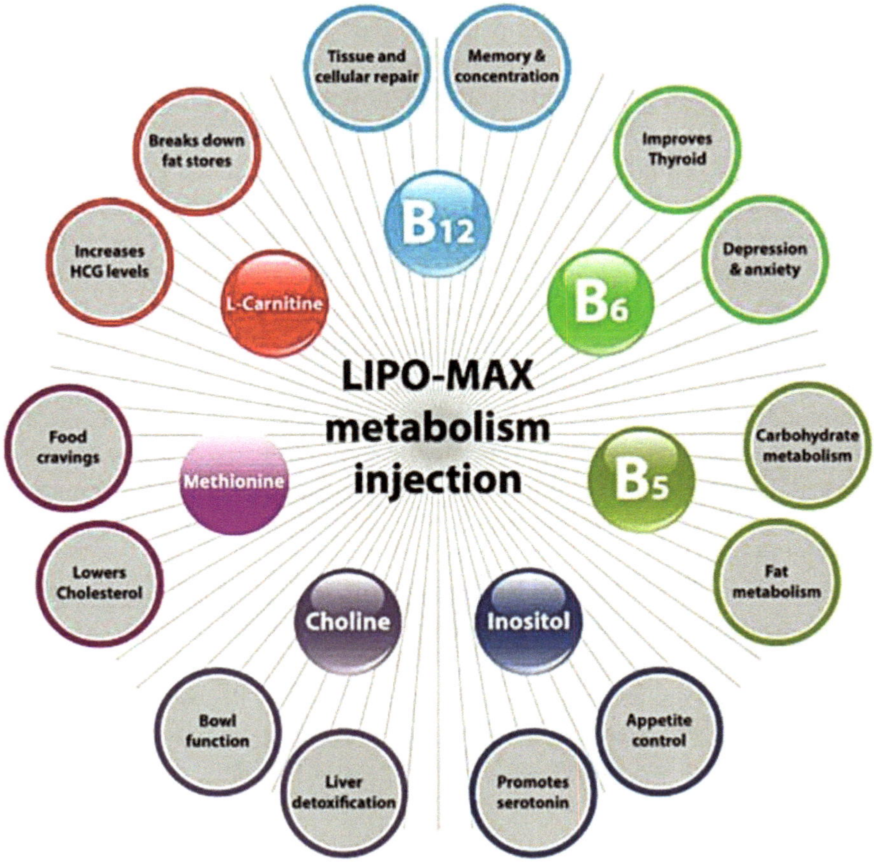

FIGURE 10.1 The image represents (LIPO-MAX injection) the role of different vitamins, amino acids, and nutraceuticals in the management of weight and fat.

2008). Dietary supplements aren't drugs and, consequently, aren't alleged to treat, diagnose, mitigate, prevent, or therapy diseases. Nevertheless, due to their low toxicity profile and clean availability for the overall population, the compounds could probably constitute an appealing adjuvant opportunity to traditional therapies (Major et al., 2007). Therefore, numerous sufferers would possibly flip to nutritional weight loss dietary supplements to attain and keep their weight reduction goals, with the a priori guarantee of protection and efficacy associated with the term 'natural remedy.' Unfortunately, there may be scant records of the interference of components of weight loss dietary with positive medications (Slater et al., 2004). Nevertheless, the thorny troubles that could end result from drug interactions with weight reduction dietary supplements have been now not sufficiently addressed (Jeukendrup & Randell, 2011). Unraveling the efficacy and protection of weight reduction dietary nutritional dietary supplements to grow compliance and adherence to healthy dietary pointers may be of strategic relevance within-aspect the manipulation of obese sufferers (McCarty & Thomas, 2003).

Obesity (Jarouliya & Keservani, 2019a), whose prevalence is tremendously variable all through the world, is concerned with the development of several numbers of communicable diseases, such as coronary heart disease, stroke, some kind of cancer, and chronic respiration disease (Mason et al., 2011). In addition, obesity contributes to lowering the quality of life and increasing mortality and morbidity costs, and, as a result, it ends in high costs for national health services (Ríos-Hoyo & Gutiérrez-Salmeán, 2016). Treatment techniques to acquire superior weight loss consist of each diet and way of life changes. There is an overall agreement that making lifestyle changes, consisting of the advertising of a healthful diet with decreased total energy intake, and engaging in bodily activity, are the basis for accomplishing weight loss (Kral et al., 2006). However, to make sustained healthy way of life changes for coping with frame weight would possibly represent a frustrating revel for some patients, especially considering that a weight-reduction plan consistent with it can result in multiple variations in the homeostatic system that controls frame weight (Bays et al., 2021). Thus, weight regain after weight reduction is probably, unfortunately, a common prevalence in obesity therapeutics. In that respect, dietary weight loss dietary supplements can be perceived to fulfill the common want for a "magic bullet," which is much less demanding than way-of-life modifications (Saper et al., 2004). Despite the reality that many weight loss dietary supplements are costly, during the last 20 years, nutritional complement use, especially as adjuvant therapy for weight reduction and for the prevention of weight regain after weight reduction, has improved greatly, thereby turning into substantial interest amongst consumers and nutritionists (Mason et al., 2014.).

10.2 VITAMINS AND NUTRACEUTICALS (VITAMINS AS NUTRACEUTICALS) FOR THE MANAGEMENT OF WEIGHT LOSS AND OBESITY

10.2.1 VITAMIN D SUPPLEMENT

This vitamin is produced on the skin after exposure to the sun and is also compatible with food, and is contained mainly in other types of fish (Soares et al., 2011). After vitamin D enters the body, it's quickly regenerated into 25-hydroxyvitamin D (25(OH)D), its main current form. D plays a key role in controlling calcium-phosphate physiological conditions and seems to possess anti-inflammatory and anti-inflammatory effects (Melanson et al., 2006).

Various studies recommend that there's a powerful correlation between vitamin D deficiency and cardiovascular disease and describes the negative association between low sun exposure, i.e., low liquid body substance 25 (OH) D levels, and enhanced risk of stroke, cardiac muscle infarction, and peripheral vascular disease and heart condition (Wamberg et al., 2013). In addition, general and native vitamin D deficiency in patients with arterial blood vessel malady (CAD) is related to enhanced regeneration of inflammatory vessels at the extent of epicardial fatty tissue (EAT), and its accumulation could also be a risk issue for CAD (Verreijen et al., 2015). Though Dozio and colleagues are the primary to integrate, in humans, D and EAT-level inflammation in CAD patients, they might not make certain if vitamin D support would be ready to counteract native EAT inflammation in these patients (Shick et al., 1998). Using animal models, Gunasekar and colleagues have shown that vitamin D deficiency increases both the activation of M1 macrophages and the pro-inflammatory expression of adipokine in the EAT, in addition, suggests that vitamin supplementation D reduces inflammatory processes and promotes anti-inflammatory (Pillitteri et al., 2008). Inflammatory responses in EAT (Watanabe et al., 2020). Vitamin D deficiency can also promote the development of atherosclerosis and plasma HDL-C levels, and the addition of vitamin D3 to the diet can significantly increase HDL-C levels, as macrophage pro-inflammatory polarization, in the animal model, leads to immunity in the development of atherosclerosis (Pourshahidi, 2015).

Vitamin D plays an important role in the protective effects of the heart and blood vessels through a variety of mechanisms, such as vascular tone modification, blood pressure control, vascular smooth muscle cell functions, and maintenance of healthy endothelium (McDuffie et al., 2002). Anti-inflammatory and anti-mitotic activities of vitamin D help to strengthen the endothelium, which confirms, at least in part, its cardiovascular effects (Tzotzas et al., 2010). Although much evidence suggests a link between vitamin D deficiency and endothelial dysfunction and CVD, there is no evidence of randomized clinical trials showing that CVDs are prevented by vitamin D supplementation (Aasheim et al., 2008). As well as potential clinical interventions to improve evidence of the effectiveness of vitamin D rejuvenation in cardiovascular health (Zittermann et al., 2009).

10.2.2 VITAMIN C

Several epidemiological research have proven that antioxidant deficiency has been implicated in high blood pressure and cardiovascular diseases (Aills et al., 2008). Considering the epidemiological increase of persistent non-communicable diseases, inclusive of diabetes mellitus and cardiovascular events, selecting meals are of hobby and has been studied because of the antioxidant vitamins which might be contained, inclusive of ascorbic acid (diet C) (MacLean et al., 1983). The significance of diet consumption is widely known and accepted; however, the quantity of how nutrients affect fitness and the cardiovascular machine stays poorly elaborated (Larsen & Astrup, 2003). Several research have proven that decreased ranges of plasma vitamin E have been associated with a boom in cardiovascular chance. Similarly, decreased ascorbic acid or diet C plasma ranges have been related to an elevated chance of cardiovascular events (Papathanasopoulos & Camilleri, 2010).

Higher blood concentrations of diet C in people are related to decrease blood stress. In a 17-week managed-weight loss plan, depletion-repletion of diet c take a look at showed an inverse correlation of plasma ascorbate ranges, diastolic, and systolic blood pressures and affirmed that the efficacy of end result and veggies in lowering blood stress could be associated with diet C (Munro & Garg, 2013). In addition, tissue ascorbic acid ranges can be critical in keeping blood stress low. Thus, so that it will gain a useful impact on blood stress, it's far encouraged to hold a serum degree of plasma ascorbate of at least 100 mcmol/L (Rosenblum et al., 2012). However, extra long-time period intervention research must be completed to verify this finding (DeWind & Payne, 1976). Ascorbic acid decreases the binding affinity of the AT1 receptor without editing its maximal binding ability and without changing the binding affinity of the AT2 receptor for angiotensin II (Earthman et al., 2012). These outcomes offer a mechanistic reason for the pronounced blood stress-reducing impact of ascorbic acid, given that maximum of the angiotensin II prompted cardiovascular results, inclusive of vascular contraction, aldosterone secretion, cardiovascular mobileular increase, and proliferation, amongst others, are mediated with the aid of using AT1 receptor (Surana et al., 2021). This discount of the AT1 receptor affinity for angiotensin II seems to arise with the aid of using disrupting the ATR1 disulfide bridges (Dwyer et al., 2005).

A randomized, double-blind, placebo-controlled factorial trial of vitamin E and vitamin C was completed between 1997 and 2007, which protected 14,641 US male physicians, who were first of all elderly 50 years or older and protected 754 guys with well-known cardiovascular sickness at randomization, changed into completed to confront research suggesting that vitamin E or vitamin C may also lessen the chance of cardiovascular sickness (Finer et al., 2000). According to the authors of this take a look at, few long-time period trials have evaluated guys at a first of all low chance of cardiovascular sickness, and no preceding trial in guys has tested diet C on my own withinside the prevention of cardiovascular sickness (Rössner et al., 2000). Thus, in this large, long-time period trial of male physicians, neither diet E nor diet C supplementation decreased the chance of primary cardiovascular events (Keithley et al., 2013). In middle-elderly and older guys, those facts furnished no assist for the usage of those dietary supplements withinside the prevention of cardiovascular sickness. At any other take a look at, the results of diet C resulted withinside the reduction of blood stress with a boom in nitric oxide, main to a development in endothelial feature and arterial compliance (Amaral et al., 1985). The inverse courting among plasma ascorbic acid and blood stress have been discovered withinside the attenuation of will increase in blood stress in healthful teenagers that decreased the chance of related vascular events (Paccosi et al., 2020). This take a look at indicates that vitamin C can be a critical thing in blood stress regulation, even amongst healthful teenagers. Ingestion of meals wealthy in vitamin C looks critical for reducing blood stress; however, greater long-time period research on sufferers of various ages, in addition to extraordinary levels of high blood pressure want to be completed to make clear which sufferers may also benefit (Hasani-Ranjbar et al., 2009).

10.2.3 VITAMIN B12

Vitamin B12 deficiency impairs fat metabolism and may be associated with obesity during pregnancy, according to the results presented at the annual conference of the Society for Endocrinology (Sugerman et al., 1989). Pregnant women with low levels of vitamin B12 had metabolic symptoms indicating increased fat production and reduced dehydration, suggesting that low levels of vitamin B12 could cause pregnant women to gain weight (Ahuja et al., 2018). These findings highlight the importance of pregnant women eating foods rich in vitamin B12 to help prevent obesity and associated health problems in the long run. Vitamin B12 is a micronutrient found in seafood, meat, and dairy products that are essential for many metabolic reactions that keep our bodies functioning normally (Heber, 2003). High-carbohydrate foods and high-digested foods provide nutritious food and can lead to vitamin B12 deficiency. About 25% of pregnant women worldwide do not have vitamin B12, as an even higher dietary requirement is needed for the baby to grow and develop. Previous research suggests that B12 deficiency increases the risk of metabolic disorders such as obesity or diabetes but existing mechanisms affecting fat metabolism remain poorly understood (Strauss et al., 2001).

Symptoms of fat metabolism in fast-growing lab cells, low vitamin B12, and samples from pregnant women who do not have vitamin B12 indicate that the function of fatty tissue was abnormal, with increased fat production, reduced fat depletion, and increased inflammation, resulting in inflammation. It causes some damage. If all the information gathered together that low B12 levels can damage fat cell metabolism, which can lead to increased fat accumulation, fat metabolism damage, and inflammatory damage, all of these are priorities for weight gain. Although these findings suggest how fat metabolism may be impaired by vitamin B12 deficiency, especially in pregnant women, larger studies are needed to confirm this and further explore basic mechanisms, identify intervention strategies, and help prevent obesity. The team is now planning to investigate genetic factors that affect fat metabolism and how a lack of pregnancy can affect the metabolic health of children. It shows the need for vitamin B12 in pregnancy (Fleischer et al., 2008).

10.3 THE POTENTIAL ROLE OF VITAMIN E AGAINST OBESITY

A viable new manner to fight weight problems-associated illnesses has been found, way to a sad study led by researchers at the Case Western Reserve University School of Medicine. Participants from Case Western Reserve University, the Cleveland Clinic Foundation, and Cornell University found the important factors of vitamin E that may alleviate the signs of weight problems-precipitated liver ailment. As is regularly the case with science, Manor's studies group at Case Western stumbled upon the unsuitable findings. While reading the impact of nutrition E deficiency on the principal frightened system, "We used liver tissue to increase our surgical techniques," recollects Manor, and partner professor of vitamins and pharmacy (Major et al., 2007). To the marvel of the group, they found out that mice have been genuinely in superior ranges of steatohepatitis (NASH), a not unusual place weight problems hassle characterized by gathered fats, oxidative stress, and infection of the liver. It is a completely severe shape of fatty liver ailment and is a prime motive of tissue scars referred to as cirrhosis main to liver failure and might development to liver cancer (Brolin & Leung, 1999). An essential antioxidant, nutrition E has been proven in the latest studies to relieve a number of the signs of NASH in human patients, suggesting that there may be a hyperlink between ok tiers of nutrition E and liver ailment. To check this hypothesis, the group examined a mouse that was designed to be poor in protein (Jarouliya & Keservani, 2019b) that regulates vitamin E tiers withinside the body (Shapses et al., 2004; Surana et al., 2021). As expected, they located a growth in oxidative stress, fat deposits, and different signs of liver harm in mice. Importantly, notes Manor, nutrition E supplementation averted a number of the NASH-associated signs in those animals, confirming the hyperlink between nutrition E deficiency and liver disease (Surana et al., 2021).

10.4 CONCLUSION

Nutraceuticals and vitamins have the most prominent role in the management of weight loss and obesity. Nowadays, it's necessary to mention well-programmed nutraceuticals and vitamins-rich food diets in daily routine to balance weight and fat. In this study, we can conclude how lower levels of some vitamins can affect the functioning of fat cells and their role in pregnant women. Obesity, whose prevalence is tremendously variable all through the world, is concerned with the development of several numbers of metabolic disorders and diseases, such as coronary heart disease and diabetes mellitus. In addition, obesity contributes to lowering the quality of life and increasing mortality and morbidity costs, and, as a result, it ends in high costs for the national health services. In aspects of national and world health, it is most important to control excess weight, and to face such challenges, it's important to follow regular control over vitamins and nutraceuticals.

ACKNOWLEDGMENTS

We thank you to the Dr. J. D. Pawar College of Pharmacy, Manur, METs, Institute of Pharmacy, Adgaon, Nashik, and Mahatma Gandhi Vidyamandir's Pharmacy College, Panchavati, Nashik, Maharashtra, India, for their constant support and providing all facilities to complete this work. Also, many thanks to all the known and unknowns who helped us right from the writing till the publishing of this chapter.

KEYWORDS

- **caffeine**
- **carnitine**
- **fat loss**
- **green tea**
- **metabolism**
- **nutraceuticals**
- **obesity**
- **vitamins (D, C, K, E, B-12)**
- **weight loss**

REFERENCES

Aasheim, E. T., Hofsø, D., Hjelmesæth, J., Birkeland, K. I., & Bøhmer, T., (2008). Vitamin status in morbidly obese patients: A cross-sectional study. *The American Journal of Clinical Nutrition, 87*(2), 362–369.

Ahuja, A., Tantia, O., Goyal, G., Chaudhuri, T., Khanna, S., Poddar, A., Gupta, S., & Majumdar, K. (2018). MGB-OAGB: Effect of biliopancreatic limb length on nutritional deficiency, weight loss, and comorbidity resolution. *Obesity Surgery, 28*(11), 3439–3445.

Aills, L., Blankenship, J., Buffington, C., Furtado, M., & Parrott, J., (2008). ASMBS allied health nutritional guidelines for the surgical weight loss patient. *Surgery for Obesity and Related Diseases, 4*(5), S73–S108.

Amaral, J. F., Thompson, W. R., Caldwell, M. D., Martin, H. F., & Randall, H. T., (1985). Prospective hematologic evaluation of gastric exclusion surgery for morbid obesity. *Annals of Surgery, 201*(2), 186.

Barrea, L., Altieri, B., Polese, B., De Conno, B., Muscogiuri, G., Colao, A., & Savastano, S., (2019). Nutritionist and obesity: Brief overview on efficacy, safety, and drug interactions of the main weight-loss dietary supplements. *International Journal of Obesity Supplements, 9*(1), 32–49.

Bays, H. E., McCarthy, W., Christensen, S., Tondt, J., Karjoo, S., & Davisson, L. (2021). *Obesity Algorithm eBook.* Presented by the Obesity Medicine Association.

Brolin, R. E., & Leung, M., (1999). Survey of vitamin and mineral supplementation after gastric bypass and biliopancreatic diversion for morbid obesity. *Obesity Surgery, 9*(2), 150–154.

DeWind, L. T., & Payne, J. H., (1976). Intestinal bypass surgery for morbid obesity: Long-term results. *JAMA*, *236*(20), 2298–2301.

Dwyer, J. T., Allison, D. B., & Coates, P. M., (2005). Dietary supplements in weight reduction. *Journal of the American Dietetic Association*, *105*(5), 80–86.

Earthman, C. P., Beckman, L. M., Masodkar, K., & Sibley, S. D., (2012). The link between obesity and low circulating 25-hydroxyvitamin D concentrations: Considerations and implications. *International Journal of Obesity*, *36*(3), 387–396.

Finer, N., James, W. P. T., Kopelman, P. G., Lean, M. E. J., & Williams, G., (2000). One-year treatment of obesity: A randomized, double-blind, placebo-controlled, multicenter study of orlistat, a gastrointestinal lipase inhibitor. *International Journal of Obesity*, *24*(3), 306–313.

Fleischer, J., Stein, E. M., Bessler, M., Badia, M. D., Restuccia, N., Olivero-Rivera, L., McMahon, D. J., & Silverberg, S. J., (2008). The decline in hip bone density after gastric bypass surgery is associated with extent of weight loss. *The Journal of Clinical Endocrinology & Metabolism*, *93*(10), 3735–3740.

Gasteyger, C., Suter, M., Gaillard, R. C., & Giusti, V., (2008). Nutritional deficiencies after Roux-en-Y gastric bypass for morbid obesity often cannot be prevented by standard multivitamin supplementation. *The American Journal of Clinical Nutrition*, *87*(5), 1128–1133.

Hasani-Ranjbar, S., Nayebi, N., Larijani, B., & Abdollahi, M., (2009). A systematic review of the efficacy and safety of herbal medicines used in the treatment of obesity. *World Journal of Gastroenterology: WJG*, *15*(25), 3073.

Heber, D., (2003). Herbal preparations for obesity: Are they useful? *Primary Care: Clinics in Office Practice*, *30*(2), 441–463.

Houston, M. C., (2007). Treatment of hypertension with nutraceuticals, vitamins, antioxidants and minerals. *Expert Review of Cardiovascular Therapy*, *5*(4), 681–691.

Jarouliya, U., & Keservani, R. K., (2019a). Pathways leading to child obesity; Chapter 12. In: Debasis, B., (ed.), *Global Perspectives on Childhood Obesity: Current Status, Consequences and Prevention* (2nd edn., pp. 137–146). Academic Press, Elsevier. ISBN: 9780128128404.

Jarouliya, U., & Keservani, R. K., (2019b). "Protein function as cell surface and nuclear receptor in human diseases; Chapter 1. In: Sanjay, B., & Debarshi, K. M., (eds.), *Medicinal Chemistry with Pharmaceutical Product Development* (pp. 1–32). Apple Academic Press, CRC Press, Taylor & Francis Group. ISBN: 9781771887106.

Jeukendrup, A. E., & Randell, R., (2011). Fat burners: Nutrition supplements that increase fat metabolism. *Obesity Reviews*, *12*(10), 841–851.

Josse, A. R., Atkinson, S. A., Tarnopolsky, M. A., & Phillips, S. M., (2011). Increased consumption of dairy foods and protein during diet-and exercise-induced weight loss promotes fat mass loss and lean mass gain in overweight and obese premenopausal women. *The Journal of Nutrition*, *141*(9), 1626–1634.

Keithley, J. K., Swanson, B., Mikolaitis, S. L., DeMeo, M., Zeller, J. M., Fogg, L., & Adamji, J., (2013). Safety and efficacy of glucomannan for weight loss in overweight and moderately obese adults. *Journal of Obesity*, *2013*.

Keservani, R. K., Kesharwani, R. K., Sharma, A. K., Vyas, N., & Chadoker, A., (2010b). Nutritional supplements: An overview. *International Journal of Current Pharmaceutical Review and Research*, *1*(1), 59–75.

Keservani, R. K., Kesharwani, R. K., Vyas, N., Jain, S., Raghuvanshi, R., & Sharma, A. K., (2010a). Nutraceutical and functional food as future food: A review. *Der Pharmacia Lettre, 2*(1), 106–116.

Keservani, R. K., Sharma, A. K., & Kesharwani, R. K. (2017). An overview and therapeutic applications of nutraceutical and functional foods. *Recent Advances in Drug Delivery Technology*, 160–201. ISBN:9781522507543.

Keservani, R. K., Sharma, A. K., & Kesharwani, R. K. (2020). *Nutraceuticals and Dietary Supplements: Applications in Health Improvement and Disease Management*. CRC Press. ISBN: 9781771888738.

Kral, J. G., Biron, S., Simard, S., Hould, F. S., Lebel, S., Marceau, S., & Marceau, P., (2006). Large maternal weight loss from obesity surgery prevents transmission of obesity to children who were followed for 2 to 18 years. *Pediatrics, 118*(6), e1644–e1649.

Larsen, T. M., & Astrup, A., (2003). Efficacy and safety of dietary supplements containing CLA for the treatment of obesity: Evidence from animal and human studies. *Journal of Lipid Research, 44*(12), 2234–2241.

MacLean, L. D., Rhode, B. M., & Shizgal, H. M., (1983). Nutrition following gastric operations for morbid obesity. *Annals of Surgery, 198*(3), 347.

Major, G. C., Alarie, F., Doré, J., Phouttama, S., & Tremblay, A., (2007). Supplementation with calcium+ vitamin D enhances the beneficial effect of weight loss on plasma lipid and lipoprotein concentrations. *The American Journal of Clinical Nutrition, 85*(1), 54–59.

Mason, C., Xiao, L., Imayama, I., Duggan, C. R., Bain, C., Foster-Schubert, K. E., Kong, A., et al., (2011). Effects of weight loss on serum vitamin D in postmenopausal women. *The American Journal of Clinical Nutrition, 94*(1), 95–103.

Mason, C., Xiao, L., Imayama, I., Duggan, C., Wang, C. Y., Korde, L., & McTiernan, A. (2014). Vitamin D3 supplementation during weight loss: A double-blind randomized controlled trial. *The American Journal of Clinical Nutrition, 99*(5), 1015–1025.

McCarty, M. F., & Thomas, C. A., (2003). PTH excess may promote weight gain by impeding catecholamine-induced lipolysis-implications for the impact of calcium, vitamin D, and alcohol on body weight. *Medical Hypotheses, 61*(5, 6), 535–542.

McDuffie, J. R., Calis, K. A., Booth, S. L., Uwaifo, G. I., & Yanovski, J. A., (2002). Effects of orlistat on fat-soluble vitamins in obese adolescents. *Pharmacotherapy: The Journal of Human Pharmacology and Drug Therapy, 22*(7), 814–822.

McDuffie, J. R., Calis, K. A., Booth, S. L., Uwaifo, G. I., & Yanovski, J. A., (2002). Effects of orlistat on fat-soluble vitamins in obese adolescents. *Pharmacotherapy: The Journal of Human Pharmacology and Drug Therapy, 22*(7), 814–822.

Melanson, K. J., Angelopoulos, T. J., Nguyen, V. T., Martini, M., Zukley, L., Lowndes, J., Dube, T. J., et al., (2006). Consumption of whole-grain cereals during weight loss: Effects on dietary quality, dietary fiber, magnesium, vitamin B-6, and obesity. *Journal of the American Dietetic Association, 106*(9), 1380–1388.

Munro, I. A., & Garg, M. L., (2013). Prior supplementation with long chain omega-3 polyunsaturated fatty acids promotes weight loss in obese adults: A double-blinded randomized controlled trial. *Food & Function, 4*(4), 650–658.

Paccosi, S., Cresci, B., Pala, L., Rotella, C. M., & Parenti, A., (2020). Obesity therapy: How and why? *Current Medicinal Chemistry, 27*(2), 174–186.

Pandol, S. J., Saluja, A. K., Imrie, C. W., & Banks, P. A., (2007). Review in basic and clinical Gastroenterology. *Gastroenterology, 132*, 1127–1151.

Papathanasopoulos, A., & Camilleri, M., (2010). Dietary fiber supplements: Effects in obesity and metabolic syndrome and relationship to gastrointestinal functions. *Gastroenterology, 138*(1), 65–72.

Pillitteri, J. L., Shiffman, S., Rohay, J. M., Harkins, A. M., Burton, S. L., & Wadden, T. A., (2008). Use of dietary supplements for weight loss in the United States: Results of a national survey. *Obesity, 16*(4), 790–796.

Poddar, K., Kolge, S., Bezman, L., Mullin, G. E., & Cheskin, L. J., (2011). Nutraceutical supplements for weight loss: A systematic review. *Nutrition in Clinical Practice, 26*(5), 539–552.

Pourshahidi, L. K., (2015). Vitamin D and obesity: Current perspectives and future directions. *Proceedings of the Nutrition Society, 74*(2), 115–124.

Ríos-Hoyo, A., & Gutiérrez-Salmeán, G., (2016). New dietary supplements for obesity: What we currently know. *Current Obesity Reports, 5*(2), 262–270.

Rosenblum, J. L., Castro, V. M., Moore, C. E., & Kaplan, L. M., (2012). Calcium and vitamin D supplementation is associated with decreased abdominal visceral adipose tissue in overweight and obese adults. *The American Journal of Clinical Nutrition, 95*(1), 101–108.

Rössner, S., Sjöström, L., Noack, R., Meinders, A. E., Noseda, G., & European Orlistat Obesity Study, (2000). Weight loss, weight maintenance, and improved cardiovascular risk factors after 2 years of treatment with orlistat for obesity. *Obesity Research, 8*(1), 49–61.

Saper, R. B., Eisenberg, D. M., & Phillips, R. S., (2004). Common dietary supplements for weight loss. *American Family Physician, 70*(9), 1731–1738.

Shapses, S. A., Heshka, S., & Heymsfield, S. B., (2004). Effect of calcium supplementation on weight and fat loss in women. *The Journal of Clinical Endocrinology & Metabolism, 89*(2), 632–637.

Shick, S. M., Wing, R. R., Klem, M. L., McGuire, M. T., Hill, J. O., & Seagle, H., (1998). Persons successful at long-term weight loss and maintenance continue to consume a low-energy, low-fat diet. *Journal of the American Dietetic Association, 98*(4), 408–413.

Slater, G. H., Ren, C. J., Siegel, N., Williams, T., Barr, D., Wolfe, B., Dolan, K., & Fielding, G. A., (2004). Serum fat-soluble vitamin deficiency and abnormal calcium metabolism after malabsorptive bariatric surgery. *Journal of Gastrointestinal Surgery, 8*(1), 48–55.

Soares, M. J., Ping-Delfos, W. C. S., & Ghanbari, M. H., (2011). Calcium and vitamin D for obesity: A review of randomized controlled trials. *European Journal of Clinical Nutrition, 65*(9), 994–1004.

Strauss, R. S., Bradley, L. J., & Brolin, R. E., (2001). Gastric bypass surgery in adolescents with morbid obesity. *The Journal of Pediatrics, 138*(4), 499–504.

Sugerman, H. J., Londrey, G. L., Kellum, J. M., Wolf, L., Liszka, T., Engle, K. M., Birkenhauer, R., & Starkey, J. V., (1989). Weight loss with vertical banded gastroplasty and Roux-Y gastric bypass for morbid obesity with selective versus random assignment. *The American Journal of Surgery, 157*(1), 93–102.

Surana, K. R., Ahire, E. D., Sonawane, V. N., & Talele, S. G., (2021). Biomolecular and molecular docking: A modern tool in drug discovery and virtual screening of natural products. In: *Applied Pharmaceutical Practice and Nutraceuticals* (pp. 209–223). Apple Academic Press.

Surana, K. R., Ahire, E. D., Sonawane, V. N., Talele, S. G., & Talele, G. S., (2021). Molecular modeling: Novel techniques in food and nutrition development. *Natural Food Products and Waste Recovery: Healthy Foods, Nutrition Design, and Extraction of Valuable Compounds*, (p. 17).

Surana, K. R., Ahire, E. D., Sonawane, V. N., Talele, S. G., & Talele, G. S., (2021). Informatics and methods in nutrition design and development. *Natural Food Products and Waste Recovery: Healthy Foods, Nutrition Design, and Extraction of Valuable Compounds* (p. 33).

Tzotzas, T., Papadopoulou, F. G., Tziomalos, K., Karras, S., Gastaris, K., Perros, P., & Krassas, G. E., (2010). Rising serum 25-hydroxy-vitamin D levels after weight loss in obese women correlate with improvement in insulin resistance. *The Journal of Clinical Endocrinology & Metabolism, 95*(9), 4251–4257.

Verreijen, A. M., Verlaan, S., Engberink, M. F., Swinkels, S., De Vogel-Van, D. B. J., & Weijs, P. J., (2015). A high whey protein–, leucine-, and vitamin D–enriched supplement preserves muscle mass during intentional weight loss in obese older adults: A double-blind randomized controlled trial. *The American Journal of Clinical Nutrition, 101*(2), 279–286.

Wamberg, L., Christiansen, T., Paulsen, S. K., Fisker, S., Rask, P., Rejnmark, L., Richelsen, B., & Pedersen, S. B., (2013). Expression of vitamin D-metabolizing enzymes in human adipose tissue—The effect of obesity and diet-induced weight loss. *International Journal of Obesity, 37*(5), 651–657.

Watanabe, M., Risi, R., Masi, D., Caputi, A., Balena, A., Rossini, G., Tuccinardi, D., et al., (2020). Current evidence to propose different food supplements for weight loss: A comprehensive review. *Nutrients, 12*(9), 2873.

Zittermann, A., Frisch, S., Berthold, H. K., Götting, C., Kuhn, J., Kleesiek, K., Stehle, P., et al., (2009). Vitamin D supplementation enhances the beneficial effects of weight loss on cardiovascular disease risk markers. *The American Journal of Clinical Nutrition, 89*(5), 1321–1327.

PART IV
Nutritional Function of Vitamins

CHAPTER 11

Vitamins as a Nutraceutical for Blindness

SHIVRAJ P. JADHAV,[1] DHANANJAY M. PATIL,[1] DEEPAK D. SONAWANE,[1] and KHEMCHAND R. SURANA[2]

[1]*Department of Pharmaceutics, Shreeshakti Shaikshanik Sanstha, Divine College of Pharmacy, Satana, Nashik, Maharashtra, India*

[2]*Department of Pharmaceutical Chemistry, Shreeshakti Shaikshanik Sanstha, Divine College of Pharmacy, Satana, Nashik, Maharashtra, India*

ABSTRACT

A nutraceutical can be called food which provides medical benefits and can be used for the prevention and treatment of disease. Also, the absence of such foods can lead to certain diseases or disorders. Nutraceuticals are composed of a number of bioactive compounds like antioxidants, phytochemicals, fatty acids, amino acids, probiotics, and vitamins. Vitamins, which can be classified as fat-soluble and water-soluble, are essential for various normal body functions. Generally, human beings are not able to synthesize vitamins, and hence humans should rely on an external animal as well as vegetable food sources for daily requirements of vitamins. These vitamins are also required for the normal functioning of human vision. Human vision can be attributed to rod and cone cells. These cells need a regeneration cycle, and for this, vitamin A is required. Lack of Vitamin A can lead to night blindness and dry eyes because of poor regeneration of visual pigment in retinal rods. If the deficiency is continuous, then it can lead to xerophthalmia causing permanent blindness. There is an association between cataract and oxidative damage of the lens, and hence antioxidant supplement is promoted as a strategy to slow down the progression of cataract, which can be given in the form of vitamin C. Vitamin E belongs to fat-soluble antioxidant vitamins

Preventive and Therapeutic Role of Vitamins as Nutraceuticals. Khemchand R. Surana, Eknath D. Ahire, Raj K. Keservani, & Rajesh K. Kesharwani (Eds.)

that protect fatty acids from harmful oxidation. Hence the suitable amount of vitamin E consumption in the diet is significant for the finest eye health as the retina contains a high amount of fatty acids. Apart from these vitamins, vitamins B1, B2, and B12 also play an important role in normal vision. All these vitamins can be obtained from different nutraceuticals.

11.1 INTRODUCTION

"Nutraceutical" term was framed by Dr. Stephen DeFelice in the year 1989 from "Nutrition" and "Pharmaceutical." DeFelice defines nutraceutical as "a part of food or whole food that provides medical or health profits like the prevention and treatment of a disease." But in general term used in the market has no definite definition (Kalra, 2003; Keservani et al., 2017, 2020).

Nutraceuticals are generally present in household foods or plant-based sources known as bioactive materials and can be instilled into the human body in dietary supplement form, which will then supply beneficial effects with the nutritionally essential ingredient (Nasri et al., 2014). Nutraceuticals (Keservani et al., 2010a, b) are composed of a variety of bioactive components derived and segregated in edible sources in the form of amino acids, fatty acids (Singh et al., 2017b), antioxidants (Singh et al., 2017a), probiotics, phytochemicals (Keservani & Sharma, 2014; Keservani et al., 2016a, b) and vitamins (Singh et al., 2017a). Nutraceuticals perform a dynamic part in the treatment and prevention of numerous diseases, have anti-aging properties, and are also used for tumor prevention (Caramia & Silvi, 2011). Nutraceuticals also show antilipidemic, anti-cancer, anti-inflammatory, and antioxidant activity (Affuso et al., 2010; Chen et al., 2016; Pitchaiah et al., 2017; Singla et al., 2014). Nutraceuticals are classified into different groups depending on their source, nature, and application. Table 11.1 represents different classes of nutraceuticals.

Vitamin is one of the classes of nutraceuticals required for the normal functioning of the body. A vitamin is widespread and belongs to the set of organic compounds, normally not produced by the human body but essential for the precise care of the human body's regular functions.

The human body can acquire numerous vitamins from food by taking the right nutrition, but if regular least nutritional supplies are not met, then supplements are necessary to meet the required quantity. The activity of metabolism depends upon vitamins. As well as for the normal development and the proper function of the body also depends upon vitamin. Solitarily, vitamin D is produced by the body; all other vitamins are obtained from food

TABLE 11.1 Different Classes of Nutraceuticals

Sl. No.	Class of Nutraceutical	Examples
1.	Functional foods	Rice, kidney beans, lentils, chocolate, citrus fruits, nuts, soybeans, and fermented milk (Ruchi, 2017; Singh & Sinha, 2012)
2.	Carotenoids	α-Carotene, β-cryptoxanthin, β-carotene, lutein, zeaxanthin, lycopene, fucoxanthin, and astaxanthin (Lee et al., 2019; Hardell et al., 2011)
3.	Collagen hydrolysate	Primary protein obtained from animal connective tissues (Gómez-Guillén et al., 2011; Song & Li, 2017)
4.	Dietary fibers	Diversity of foods like fruits and vegetables, oats, and ispaghula husk (Gidley & Yakubov, 2019; McRorie & McKeown, 2017)
5.	Phytochemicals	Lutein and lycopene (Dhan et al., 2012)
6.	Probiotics	Lactobacillus species, *Bifidobacterium* species, and *Streptococcus* species (Fuller, 2012)
7.	Dietary supplements	Vitamins A, B, C, D, and E, omega-3, folic acid, minerals, and trace elements (Helal et al., 2019; Bailey et al., 2013)

(Amadeo et al., 2017). Vitamins are classified depending on their solubility in water and fat. The first group consists of vitamins that are soluble in water, like vitamin B group, and vitamin C, and the second group compromise vitamins A, D, E, and K, which are fat soluble (Maqbool et al., 2017). The role played by these vitamins in normal body functioning with their source is summarized in Table 11.2.

TABLE 11.2 Vitamins and Their Role in Human Body Functioning

Vitamin	Food Source	Function in the Human Body	References
Vitamin B1 (thiamine)	Tomato, spinach, watermelon, soy milk, sunflower seeds	• Energy metabolism • Maintain nerve function	Haas (1988); Nichols & Basu (1994); Depeint et al. (2006)
Vitamin B2 (riboflavin)	Liver, eggs, spinach, broccoli, mushroom, milk	• Required for normal vision • Maintain skin health	Cardoso et al. (2012); Alhamad et al. (2012)
Vitamin B3 (niacin)	Dairy products, grains, poultry, potatoes, tomato, meat, and fish	• Aids in food digestion • Maintain nerve functioning • Maintain skin health	Jungnickel et al. (1997); Maccubbin et al. (2009)

TABLE 11.2 *(Continued)*

Vitamin	Food Source	Function in the Human Body	References
Vitamin B5 (pantothenic acid)	Chicken, tomato, broccoli, whole grains, avocados	• Support energy metabolism	Depeint et al. (2006)
Vitamin B6 (pyridoxin)	Red meat, beans, chicken, tomato, broccoli.	• Help in red blood cell production • Lowers risk of heart attack • Aids in the metabolism of amino acids and fat.	Depeint et al. (2006); Refsum et al. (1998)
Vitamin B8 (biotin)	Fish, whole fish, grains, egg yolk	• Converts food into energy • Helps in healthy bones and hair • Synthesis of fat and glycogen	Ballard & Hanson (1967)
Vitamin B9 (folic acid)	Tomato, orange juice, broccoli, green beans, black-eyed peas	• Helps in DNA formation • Helps in new cell formation	Refsum et al. (1998); Choi & Mason (2000)
Vitamin B12	Soy milk, eggs, poultry, fish	• Lowers heart attack risk • Helps in new cell production • Support nerve cell	Refsum et al. (1998)
Vitamin C (ascorbic acid)	Kiwis, strawberry, various citrus fruits, spinach, bell peppers.	• New cell synthesis • Metabolism of fat and amino acids • Maintain nerve cell • Antioxidant • Immunomodulator	Kim et al. (2002)
Vitamin A (retinol)	Beef, eggs, shrimp, carrots, cheese, mangoes, spinach, pumpkin, broccoli	• Helps in normal vision • Helps skin, bone, and tooth growth • As an antioxidant	Quadro et al. (1999, 2002)
Vitamin D	Margarine, egg yolk, liver, synthesis in body via sunlight	• Increases bone mineralization • Strengthen bones	Klibanski et al. (2001); Holick (2007)
Vitamin E	Polyunsaturated type plant oils, avocados, grains, nuts, tofu, wheat, sunflower seeds	• Antioxidant • Cell membrane stabilization • Protects vitamin A	Van Den Branden et al. (2002); Buettner (1993)
Vitamin K	Cabbage, spinach, liver, eggs, milk, sprouts	• Help in blood clotting • Regulates blood calcium	Josic et al. (2003)

Lack of specific vitamins can give rise to many diseases. For example, scurvy can be caused due to lack of vitamin C, while beriberi can be caused by a lack of vitamin D.

- Total lack of one or more vitamins is called avitaminosis.
- Partial lack of one or more vitamins is called hypovitaminosis.
- Excess accumulation of one or more vitamins in the human body is called hypervitaminosis.

One of the disease manifestations of certain vitamin deficiency is blindness.

11.2 THE VISION MECHANISM

The vision system of vertebrae works on two sets of light receptors, which are known as rod and cone photoreceptor cells, also called rod and cone. Rod cells are very sensitive to low levels of light such that they will respond to a single photon of light, but their range is very limited. Cones are less sensitive as compared to rods, but their range is wide. Usually, the intensity response curve of these cells will overlap and will generate an impressive visual response. For the normal functioning of the eye, proper working of both rod and cone is required. For proper working, these cells need a regeneration cycle (John, 2016).

The output of absorbed light to the neurotransmitter human vision requires a chromophore substance within the sensory neuron called 11-*cis*-retinal. Isomerization of 11-*cis*-retinal to all-*trans*-retinal is caused by absorption of light, which causes an alteration in the shape of opsin protein. Vitamin A is a form of chromophore 11-*cis*-retinal, and hence there is a huge role of Vitamin A in vision (Lamb & Pugh, 2006). Figure 11.1 represents the vision cycle.

11.2.1 VITAMIN A

Vitamin A deficiency is the most common cause of blindness in the world (DeMaeyer, 1986). Most vitamin A deficiency occurs below the age of five years. This vitamin deficiency accounts for 2% of deaths in this age group (Wirth et al., 2107).

Vitamin A is responsible for maintaining the eye's rod and cone cells which are known as photoreceptors. Vitamin A plays a very significant role in the regeneration of visual pigments, mucosal membrane maintenance, and immunity (Gilbert, 2013).

The daily recommended dietary intake of vitamin A for women is 700 micrograms, while for a man, it is 900 micrograms. While for children, it is

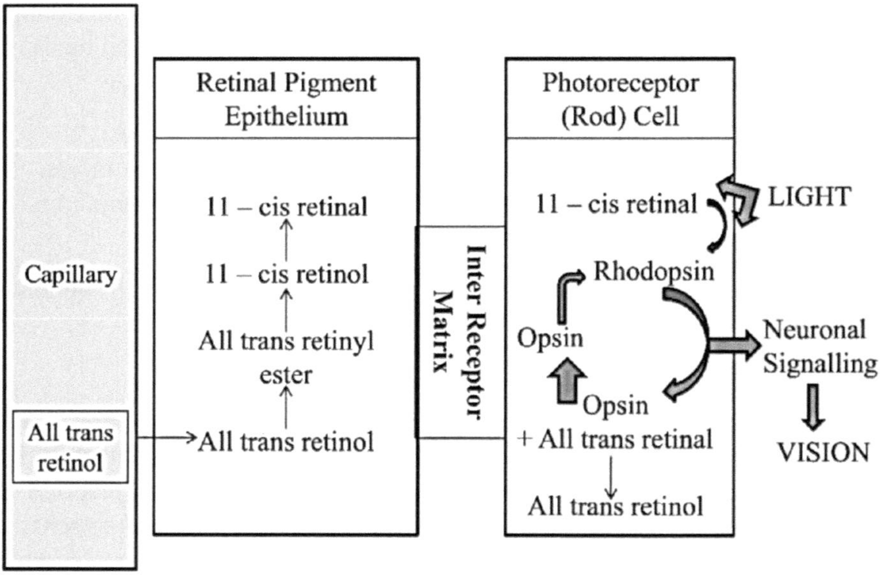

FIGURE 11.1 The vision cycles.

300 to 900 micrograms per day; for a pregnant woman, it is 770 micrograms per day. For a lactating woman, it is slightly higher, 1,300 micrograms per day (Pfeiffer et al., 2013; Fragoso et al., 2012).

Ocular-related deficiency symptoms of vitamin A start to develop when the concentration is less than 10 micrograms per day (Miller et al., 2002).

11.2.1.1 SOURCES OF VITAMIN A

Vitamin A is introduced into the body either in carotenoid form from vegetables or in retinoid form from animals. Carotenoid, beta-carotin, is pro-vitamin A, while retinoid is true vitamin A. About 75 to 100% of retinoid is absorbed while absorption of carotenoid depends upon the dietary source (Pfeiffer et al., 2013).

The high dietary sources of vitamin E are egg yolks, liver, dairy products, and carotenoids. Provitamin A can be obtained from some fruits, kale, spinach, and carrots in beta-carotene form, which provide around 30% of people's vitamin A requirements (Miller et al., 2002).

Provitamin A is converted into vitamin A in the intestine of a human in two steps. In the first stage, beta-carotene gets cleaved into two retinal molecules, which is then reduced to form retinol. In the second step, formed retinol, along with long-chain fatty acids, undergo esterification to form vitamin A (Tang, 2010; Goodman, 1969). Figure 11.2 shows the structure of vitamin A and provitamin A.

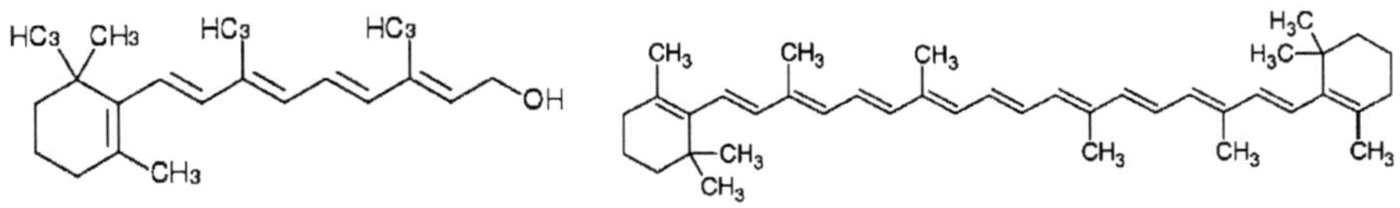

FIGURE 11.2 Structure of vitamin A and provitamin A.

11.2.1.2 SIGNS OF VITAMIN A DEFICIENCY

Some of the signs of vitamin A deficiency include night blindness, corneal xerosis, conjunctivital xerosis, corneal ulcer, keratomalacia, corneal scarring, and Bitot's spot (Gilbert, 2013).

11.2.1.3 ELIMINATION OF VITAMIN A DEFICIENCY

1. **Education About Nutrition:** This method will aim to imbed the importance of vitamin sources in the daily diet of the general public where there is vitamin deficiency. This is the most sustainable method to fight vitamin A deficiency. Schools and primary health care centers can play a crucial role in education along with social marketing of vitamin-rich foods.
2. **Eating Diversified Food:** Diet diversification can help to fulfill all the necessary nutritional requirements. Agricultural research can help to create diversified food sources. Also, genetic engineering can grow crops that are rich in provitamin A (Ye et al., 1997).
3. **Dietary Supplements:** To check existing vitamin A deficiency addition of dietary supplements is an effective way in an emergency situation (Basu et al., 2003). For the production of the adequate liver store of vitamin A, it has been recommended to give 2,00,000 IU at the time of delivery to the mothers and 4 doses of 50,000 IU to the infants at birth, 6, 10, and 14 weeks of age (Humphrey & Rice, 2000).
4. **Food Fortification:** Nutrient-related various deficiencies can be controlled by the addition of minerals and vitamins and other

necessary nutrients in a primary food. This is the safest way of supplementation. This method has several advantages; it is effective, affordable, has high population coverage, and is sustainable (Dary & Mora, 2002).

11.2.2 VITAMIN C

Cataract, also called the clouding of eyes, is the major cause of blindness and account for about 51% of global blindness (WHO, 2022). The only available treatment for cataracts is surgery. There is an association between cataract and oxidative damage of the lens, and hence antioxidant supplement is promoted as a strategy to slow down the progression of cataract (Weikel et al., 2014; Braakhuis et al., 2019; Sella & Afshari, 2019).

Vitamin C, which is also called L-ascorbate or L-ascorbic acid, acts as an antioxidant and is present in the lens and surrounding ocular humor with a concentration 50-fold more than the plasma (Shui et al., 2009; Senthilkumari et al., 2014). Vitamin C acts as a natural sunscreen and protects the lens from UV rays-induced oxidative damage. It also helps to regenerate vitamin E and glutathione to additionally increase the antioxidant capacity. As age increases, there is a decrease in the level of vitamin C in humor which increases the chances of cataracts. People in which a plasma level of vitamin C is lower are more prone to cataracts. This gives evidence that maintaining the vitamin C level in plasma can help to fight cataract-induced blindness (Tessier et al., 1998; Taylor et al., 1991).

Antioxidant activity in vitamin C is due to its ability to donate electrons to free radicles from both second as well as third carbon (Pehlivan et al., 2017). Most animals are capable of synthesizing vitamin C, but humans can't. Conversion of L-gulono-γ-lactone into vitamin C does not function in humans due to the absence of the enzyme gluconolactone oxidase (Corti & Pompella, 2010). Hence humans must rely on the external food source for vitamin C. The levels of vitamin C in humor are related to the amount of vitamin C in the diet. This means the concentration of vitamin C can be increased in humor around the lens by increasing the diet included with vitamin C (Taylor et al., 1991; Linklater et al., 1990).

Experimental studies indicate low antioxidant level is directly related to people with cataracts. This means people who get adequate vitamin C are less prone to cataracts (Leske et al., 1991; Jacques & Chylack, 1991).

The daily recommended intake of vitamin C for an adult man is 90 mg per day, while for women, it is 75 mg per day. In case of pregnancy and lactation, 85 to 120 mg of vitamin C per day is required. Smoking can decrease the level of vitamin C, so an additional 35 mg beyond the daily intake is recommended. The upper limit of vitamin C is 2,000 mg per day. Taking vitamin C beyond this level may cause gastrointestinal distress and diarrhea (German Nutrition Society (DGE), 2015). Figure 11.3 represent the structure of Vitamin C.

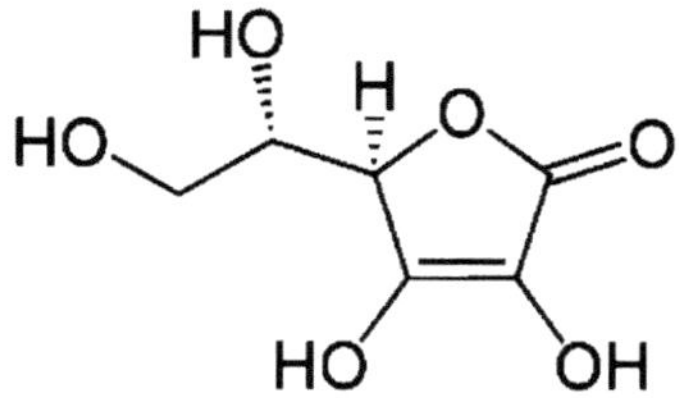

FIGURE 11.3 Structure of vitamin C.

11.2.2.1 SOURCES OF VITAMIN C

Various citrus fruits like oranges, green peppers, broccoli, tomatoes, Brussels sprouts, Indian gooseberry, and leafy vegetables contain high amounts of vitamin C. Animal sources are poor in case of vitamin C content, usually <30–40 mg/100 g. Hence, plants become important as they have a high quantity of vitamin C, up to 5,000 mg/100 g (Chambial et al., 2013).

11.2.2.2 SIGNS OF VITAMIN C DEFICIENCY

- After weeks of dietary deprivation, vitamin C deficiency typically begin and shows irritability, weight loss, and anorexia;
- Gingival swelling;
- Peri-follicular skin hemorrhages;
- Corkscrew hairs;
- Loss of teeth;
- Hyperkeratosis;
- Sternal scorbutic rosary may develop in children.

11.2.2.3 TREATMENT OF VITAMIN C DEFICIENCY

Daily doses of 500 to 1,000 mg per day in adults and 300 mg in children are found to be useful for the treatment of vitamin C deficiencies. When symptoms of deficiency are resolved, treatment is stopped. Alternatively, in adults, 2 gm for 3 days, after that, for a week, 500 mg daily followed by 100 mg daily for up to 3 months can be used for treatment of vitamin C deficiency.

Also, education of patients on lifestyle management, like the inclusion of vitamin C-rich food in the diet and quitting smoking, is necessary.

11.2.3 VITAMIN E

Amongst all the isoforms of vitamin E, α-tocopherol is the most copious in the blood, as it is absorbed within the body, while the remaining forms are excreted through the intestine. Vitamin E belongs to fat-soluble antioxidant vitamins that protect fatty acids from harmful oxidation. And hence, as high amounts of fatty acids are present in the retina, sufficient vitamin E intake is vital for ideal eye health (San & Chew, 2005). The role of additional supplements is unclear in the treatment of retinal degeneration and blindness if a person is getting enough vitamin E from food (Stoyanovsky et al., 1995). Figure 11.4 represents vitamin E structure.

Age-related cataract risk may be reduced by 6% by consuming more than 7 mg of vitamin E daily. Also, some studies suggested that vitamin E supplements do not stop the progression of cataracts (Mathew et al., 2012). Recommended dietary intake in mg for 0 to 13 years of age is 4 to 7 mg per day. In an adult male, it is 15 mg per day; in a lactating woman, it is 19 mg per day and in a pregnant woman, it is 5 mg per day (Rizvi et al., 2014).

11.2.3.1 SOURCES OF VITAMIN E

The key sources of vitamin E are basically planting origin. Coconut, Maize, Palm, Olive, Peanut, Soybean, Wheatgerm, and sunflower are the chief sources of vitamin E (Tokgöz et al., 2018). Figure 11.4 represents vitamin E structure.

11.2.3.2 VITAMIN E DEFICIENCY

Humans rarely show a deficiency of vitamin E. Vitamin E deficiency mainly occurs in people who have a hereditary deficiency in the absorption of vitamin-like cystic fibrosis, bowel syndrome, or bile duct obstruction.

Once the vitamin E deficiency occurs, it shows several symptoms like muscle weakness, vision problems, numbness, changes in the immune system, tremors, and difficulty in walking and maintaining gait. Apart from these, several other problems include spinocerebellar ataxia, myopathies, dysarthria, anemia due to oxidative loss of red blood cells, and retinopathy. If vitamin E deficiency remains untreated, then it can lead to permanent loss of vision, heart disease, permanent damage to nerves, and diminished thinking ability (Tokgöz et al., 2018).

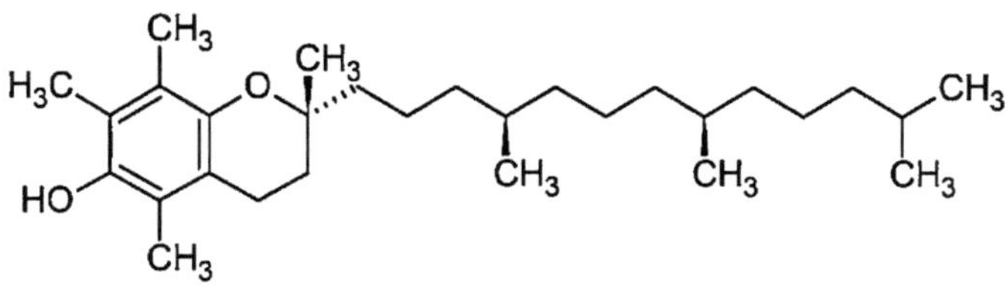

FIGURE 11.4 Vitamin E structure.

11.2.3.3 VITAMIN E DEFICIENCY TREATMENT

Vitamin E deficiency should address the treatment of the underlying cause along with vitamin E supplementation. Modification of diet should be done with vitamin E resources like leafy vegetables, whole grains, nuts, seeds, oils. Vitamin E can be injected intramuscularly if the patient shows poor oral absorption of vitamin E.

11.2.3.4 OTHER VITAMINS NECESSARY FOR VISION

Apart from the above-mentioned vitamins, several other vitamins are also necessary for the normal functioning of the eye.

11.2.4 VITAMIN B12

Vitamin B12 belongs to the vitamin B complex. Vitamin B12 (cobalamin) is essential for neurological function. Optic neuropathy may result due to a deficiency of vitamin B12. Optic neuropathy refers to the damage of optic nerves. In optic neuropathy, slow, bilateral, without pain vision loss occurs, which is associated with reduced color vision along with central scotomas. The key sources of cobalamin are fish, cheese, milk, meat, and poultry. The suggested per-day intake of cobalamin is 6 to 9 micrograms. About 1 mg intramuscular injection of vitamin B12 per week can be given for treatment of deficiency for eight weeks, followed by 1 mg monthly for life or until symptoms are resolved (Amber & Richard, 2017). Figure 11.5 represents the structure of vitamins B12, B1, and B2.

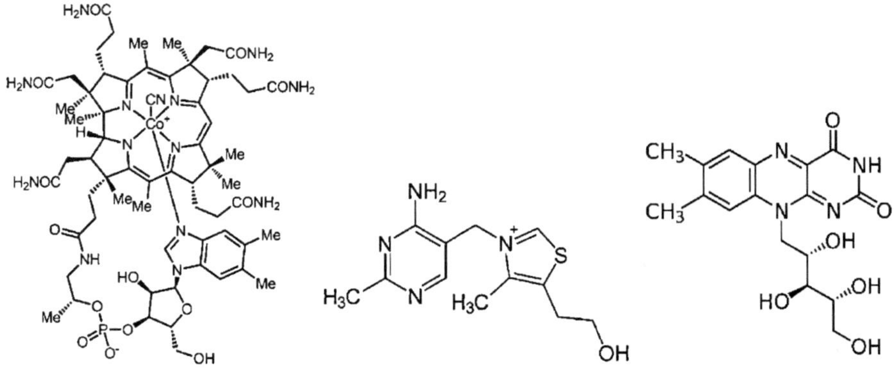

FIGURE 11.5 Structure of vitamins B12, B1, and B2.

11.2.5 VITAMIN B1

Vitamin B1 also called thiamine, is essential for glucose metabolism and the functioning of the central nervous system. Gastric bypass surgery and chronic alcoholism can lead to prolonged dietary deficiency of vitamin B1. Natural sources of thiamine include yeast, whole grains, legumes, and pork. The deficiency of vitamin B1 can lead to optic neuropathy and visual loss (Gratton & Lam, 2014).

11.2.6 VITAMIN B2

Riboflavin is a water-soluble vitamin present in a range of foods. Sources of the vitamin include milk and dairy products, cereals, meats, and dark green vegetables. It has been reported that animals fed with a low riboflavin diet show corneal opacity and corneal vascularization along with cataracts in some cases (Hughes et al., 1981). Deficiency of riboflavin is found to be associated with night blindness (Venkataswamy, 1967).

11.3 CONCLUSION

Vitamins, also called vital amines, are required for various normal body functions. The deficiency of several vitamins can lead to various diseases, including eye disease causing blindness. Lack of these vitamins can lead to night blindness, cataract, optic neuropathy, conjunctival xerosis, corneal ulcer, corneal scarring, and vision problems. These vitamins can be provided in the form of nutraceuticals which are functional food and help to fight with various conditions. Vitamins A, C, E, B1, B2, and B12 can be obtained from various nutraceutical foods to maintain daily diet intake, and problems with vision can be avoided.

ACKNOWLEDGMENTS

We thank the Divine College of Pharmacy Nampur Road, Satana, Nashik, Maharashtra, India, for their constant support and providing all facilities to complete this work. Also, many thanks to all the known and unknowns who helped us right from the writing till the publishing of this chapter.

KEYWORDS

- **corneal scarring**
- **riboflavin**
- **thiamine**
- **vision mechanism**
- **vitamin**
- **water-soluble vitamin**
- **xerosis**

REFERENCES

Affuso, F., Ruvolo, A., Micillo, F., Saccà, L., & Fazio, S., (2010). Effects of a nutraceutical combination (berberine, red yeast rice, and policosanols) on lipid levels and endothelial function randomized, double-blind, placebo-controlled study. *Nutrition, Metabolism and Cardiovascular Diseases, 20*, 656–661.

Alhamad, T. A., O'brart, D. P. S., O'brart, N. A. L., & Meek, K. M., (2012). Evaluation of transepithelial stromal riboflavin absorption with enhanced riboflavin solution using spectrophotometry. *Journal of Cataract and Refractive Surgery, 38*(5), 884–889.

Amadeo, G., Débora, V., Javier, M., Diego, A., & Cristina, G., (2017). Vitamins. In: Charis, M. G., (eds.), *Nutraceutical and Functional Food Components* (pp. 159–201). Academic Press.

Amber, R. S., & Richard, J. Z., (2017). Vitamin B12 deficiency optic neuropathy: A teaching case report. *Optometric Education, 42*(3).

Bailey, R. L., Gahche, J. J., Miller, P. E., Thomas, P. R., & Dwyer, J. T., (2013). Why US adults use dietary supplements. *JAMA Internal Medicine, 173*(5), 355–361.

Ballard, F. J., & Hanson, R. W., (1967). The citrate cleavage pathway and lipogenesis in rat adipose tissue: Replenishment of oxaloacetate. *Journal of Lipid Research, 8*(2), 73–79.

Basu, S., Sengupta, B., & Paladhi, P. K. R., (2003). A single megadose of vitamin A supplementation of Indian mothers and morbidity in breastfeeding young infants. *Postgraduate Medical Journal, 79*, 397–402.

Braakhuis, A. J., Donaldson, C. I., Lim, J. C., & Donaldson, P. J., (2019). Nutritional strategies to prevent lens cataract: Current status and future strategies. *Nutrients, 11*(5), 1186.

Buettner, G. R., (1993). The pecking order of free radicals and antioxidants: Lipid peroxidation, α-tocopherol, and ascorbate. *Archives of Biochemistry and Biophysics, 300*(2), 535–543.

Caramia, G., & Silvi, S., (2011). Probiotics: From the ancient wisdom to the actual therapeutical and nutraceutical perspective. In: *Probiotic Bacteria and Enteric Infections: Cytoprotection by Probiotic Bacteria* (p. 3). Springer: Dordrecht, The Netherlands.

Cardoso, D. R., Libardi, S. H., & Skibsted, L. H., (2012). Riboflavin as a photosensitizer. Effects on human health and food quality. *Food and Function, 3*(5), 487–502.

Chambial, S., Dwivedi, S., Shukla, K. K., John, P. J., & Sharma, P., (2013). Vitamin C in disease prevention and cure: An overview. *Indian Journal of Clinical Biochemistry: IJCB, 28*(4), 314–328.

Chen, G. L., Chen, S. G., Chen, F., Xie, Y. Q., Han, M. D., Luo, C. X., Zhao, Y. Y., & Gaob, Y. Q., (2016). Nutraceutical potential and antioxidant benefits of selected fruit seeds subjected to an *in vitro* digestion. *Journal of Functional Foods, 20*, 317–331.

Choi, S. W., & Mason, J. B., (2000). Folate and carcinogenesis: An integrated scheme. *Journal of Nutrition, 130*(2), 129–132.

Corti, A., & Pompella, A., (2010). Cellular pathways for transport and efflux of ascorbate and dehydroascorbate. *Archives of Biochemistry and Biophysics, 500*(2), 107–115.

Dary, O., & Mora, J. O., (2002). Food fortification to reduce vitamin A deficiency. International vitamin A consultative group recommendations. *Journal of Nutrition, 132*(9 suppli.), 2927–2933.

De Maeyer, E. M., (1986). The WHO program for prevention and control of vitamin A deficiency, xerophthalmia, and nutritional blindness. *Nutrition and Health, 4*(2), 105–112.

Depeint, F., Bruce, W. R., Shangari, N., Mehta, R., & O'Brien, P. J., (2006). Mitochondrial function and toxicity: Role of the B vitamin family on mitochondrial energy metabolism. *Chemico-Biological Interactions, 163*(1, 2), 94–112.

Dhan, P., Gupta, C., & Sharma, G., (2012). Importance of phytochemicals in nutraceuticals. *Journal of Chinese Medicine Research and Development, 1*(3), 70–78.

Fragoso, Y. D., Campos, N. S., Tenrreiro, B. F., & Guillen, F. J., (2012). A systematic review of the literature on vitamin A and memory. *Dementia & Neuropsychologia, 6*(4), 219–222. https://doi.org/10.1590/S1980-57642012DN06040005.

Fuller, R., (2012). *Probiotics: The Scientific Basis* (p. 40). Springer Science & Business Media: Berlin/Heidelberg, Germany.

German Nutrition Society (DGE), (2015). New reference values for vitamin C intake. *Annals of Nutrition & Metabolism, 67*(1), 13–20.

Gidley, M. J., & Yakubov, G. E., (2019). Functional categorization of dietary fiber in foods: Beyond 'soluble' vs. 'insoluble.' *Trends in Food Science & Technology, 86*, 563–568.

Gilbert, C., (2013). The eye signs of vitamin A deficiency. *Community Eye Health, 26*(84), 66, 67.

Gómez-Guillén, M. C., Giménez, B., López-Caballero, M. E., & Montero, M. P., (2011). Functional and bioactive properties of collagen and gelatin from alternative sources: A review. *Food Hydrocolloids, 25*, 1813–1827.

Goodman, D. S., (1969). Biosynthesis of vitamin A from beta-carotene. *American Journal of Clinical Nutrition, 22*(7), 963–965.

Gratton, S. M., & Lam, B. L., (2014). Visual loss and optic nerve head swelling in thiamine deficiency without prolonged dietary deficiency. *Clinical Ophthalmology, 8*, 1021–1024.

Haas, R. H., (1988). Thiamin and the brain. *Annual Review of Nutrition, 8*, 483–515.

Hardell, M. D., Alley, D. E., Hicks, G. E., El-Kamary, S. S., Miller, R. R., Semba, R. D., & Ferrucci, L., (2011). Low-serum carotenoid concentrations and carotenoid interactions predict mortality in US adults: The third national health and nutrition examination survey. *Nutrition Research, 31*, 178–189.

Helal, N. A., Eassa, H. A., Amer, A. M., Eltokhy, M. A., Edafiogho, I., & Nounou, M. I., (2019). Nutraceuticals' novel formulations: The good, the bad, the unknown, and patents involved. *Recent Patents on Drug Delivery & Formulation. 13*(2), 105–156.

Holick, M. F., (2007). Vitamin D deficiency. *New England Journal of Medicine, 357*(3), 266–281.

Hughes, S. G., Rus, R. C., Nickum, J. G., & Rumsey, R., (1981). Biomicroscopic and histologic pathology of the eye in riboflavin-deficient rainbow trout (*Salmo gairdneri*). *The Cornell Veterinarian, 71*, 269–279.

Humphrey, J. H., & Rice, A. L., (2000). Vitamin A supplementation of young infants. *Lancet, 356*, 422–424.

Jacques, P. F., & Chylack, L. T. Jr., (1991). Epidemiologic evidence of a role for the antioxidant vitamins and carotenoids in cataract prevention. *The American Journal of Clinical Nutrition, 53*(1Suppl), 352S–355S.

John, C., (2016). Vitamin A and vision. *Sub-Cellular Biochemistry, 81*, 231–259.

Josic, D., Hoffer, L., & Buchacher, A., (2003). Preparation of vitamin K-dependent proteins, such as clotting factors II, VII, IX, and X and clotting inhibitor protein C. *Journal of Chromatography B: Analytical Technologies in the Biomedical and Life Sciences, 790*(1, 2), 183–197.

Jungnickel, P. W., Maloley, P. A., Vander, T. E. L., Peddicord, T. E., & Campbell, J. R., (1997). Effect of two aspirin pre-treatment regimens on niacin-induced cutaneous reactions. *Journal of General Internal Medicine, 12*(10), 591–596.

Kalra, E. K., (2003). Nutraceutical definition and introduction. *AAPS Pharm Sci., 5*(3), E25.

Keservani, R. K., & Sharma, A. K., (2014). Flavonoids: Emerging trends and potential health benefits. *Journal of Chinese Pharmaceutical Sciences, 23*(12), 815.

Keservani, R. K., Kesharwani, R. K., Sharma, A. K., Vyas, N., & Chadoker, A., (2010b). Nutritional supplements: An overview. *International Journal of Current Pharmaceutical Review and Research, 1*(1), 59–75.

Keservani, R. K., Kesharwani, R. K., Vyas, N., Jain, S., Raghuvanshi, R., & Sharma, A. K., (2010a). Nutraceutical and functional food as future food: A review. *Der Pharmacia Lettre, 2*(1), 106–116.

Keservani, R. K., Sharma, A. K., & Kesharwani, R. K., (2016a). Nutraceutical and functional foods for cardiovascular health. In: *Food Process Engineering* (pp. 257–278, 291–312). Apple Academic Press, CRC Press. ISBN: 9781771884020.

Keservani, R. K., Sharma, A. K., & Kesharwani, R. K., (2016b). Medicinal effect of nutraceutical fruits for the cognition and brain health. *Scientifica*, 10. Article ID 3109254. doi: 10.1155/2016/3109254.

Keservani, R. K., Sharma, A. K., & Kesharwani, R. K. (2017). An overview and therapeutic applications of nutraceutical and functional foods. *Recent Advances in Drug Delivery Technology*, 160–201. ISBN:9781522507543.

Keservani, R. K., Sharma, A. K., & Kesharwani, R. K. (2020). *Nutraceuticals and Dietary Supplements: Applications in Health Improvement and Disease Management*. CRC Press. ISBN: 9781771888738.

Kim, D. O., Lee, K. W., Lee, H. J., & Lee, C. Y., (2002). Vitamin C equivalent antioxidant capacity (VCEAC)of phenolic phytochemicals. *Journal of Agricultural and Food Chemistry, 50*(13), 3713–3717.

Klibanski, A., Adams-Campbell, L., Bassford, T., Blair, S. N., Boden, S. D., Dickersin, K., & Russell, W. E., (2001). Osteoporosis prevention, diagnosis, and therapy. *Journal of the American Medical Association, 285*(6), 785–795.

Lamb T. D., & Pugh, E. N. Jr., (2006). Phototransduction, dark adaptation, and rhodopsin regeneration. The proctor lecture. *Investigative Ophthalmology & Visual Science, 47*, 5138–5152.

Lee, Y., Hu, S., Park, Y. K., & Lee, J. Y., (2019). Health benefits of carotenoids: A role of carotenoids in the prevention of non-alcoholic fatty liver disease. *Preventive Nutrition and Food Science, 24*, 103–113.

Leske, M. C., Chylack, L. T. Jr., & Wu, S. Y., (1991). The lens opacities case-control study. Risk factors for cataracts. *Archives of Ophthalmology, 109*(2), 244–251.

Linklater, H. A., Dzialoszynski, T., McLeod, H. L., Sanford, S. E., & Trevithick, J. R., (1990). Modeling cortical cataractogenesis. XI. Vitamin C reduces gamma-crystallin leakage from lenses in diabetic rats. *Experimental Eye Research, 51*(3), 241–247.

Maccubbin, D., Koren, M. J., Davidson, M., Gavish, D., Pasternak, R. C., Macdonell, G., & Mitchel, Y., (2009). Flushing profile of extended-release niacin/laropiprant versus gradually titrated niacin extended-release in patients with dyslipidemia with and without ischemic cardiovascular disease. *American Journal of Cardiology, 104*(1), 74–81.

Maqbool, M., Muhammad, A., & Waseem, I. (2017). Biological importance of vitamins for human health: A review. *Journal of Agriculture and Basic Science, 2*(3), 50–58.

Mason, C., Xiao, L., Imayama, I., Duggan, C. R., Bain, C., Foster-Schubert, K. E., Kong, A., et al., (2011). Effects of weight loss on serum vitamin D in postmenopausal women. *The American Journal of Clinical Nutrition, 94*(1), 95–103.

Mathew, M. C., Ervin, A. M., Tao, J., & Davis, R. M., (2012). Antioxidant vitamin supplementation for preventing and slowing the progression of age-related cataracts. *The Cochrane Database of Systematic Reviews, 6*(6), CD004567.

McRorie, J. W., & McKeown, N. M., (2017). Understanding the physics of functional fibers in the gastrointestinal tract: An evidence-based approach to resolving enduring misconceptions about insoluble and soluble fiber. *Journal of the Academy of Nutrition and Dietetics, 117*, 251–264.

Miller, M., Humphrey, J., Johnson, E., Marinda, E., Brookmeyer, R., & Katz, J., (2002). Why do children become vitamin A deficient? *Journal of Nutrition, 132*(9 Suppl), 2867S–2880S.

Nasri, H., Baradaran, A., Shirzad, H., & Rafieian-Kopaei, M., (2014). New concepts in nutraceuticals as an alternative to pharmaceuticals. *International Journal of Preventive Medicine, 5*, 1487–1489.

Nichols, H. K., & Basu, T. K., (1994). Thiamin status of the elderly: Dietary intake and thiamin pyrophosphate response. *Journal of the American College of Nutrition, 13*(1), 57–61.

Pehlivan, F. E., (2017). Vitamin C-an antioxidant agent. In: Hamza, A. H., (ed.), *Vitamin C.* Intech Open: London, UK.

Pfeiffer, C. M., Sternberg, M. R., Schleicher, R. L., Haynes, B. M., Rybak, M. E., & Pirkle, J. L., (2013). The CDC's second national report on biochemical indicators of diet and nutrition in the U.S. population is a valuable tool for researchers and policymakers. *Journal of Nutrition, 143*(6), 938S–947S.

Pitchaiah, G., Akula, A., & Chandi, V. (2017). Anticancer potential of nutraceutical formulations in MNU-INDUCED MAMMARY CANCER in Sprague Dawley rats. *Pharmacognosy Magazine, 13*, 46–50.

Quadro, L., Blaner, W. S., Salchow, D. J., Vogel, S., Piantedosi, R., Gouras, P., & Gottesman, M. E., (2002). Muscle expression of human retinol-binding protein (RBP). *The Journal of Biological Chemistry, 277*(33), 30191–30197.

Quadro, L., Blaner, W. S., Salchow, D. J., Vogel, S., Piantedosi, R., Gouras, P., Freeman, S., et al., (1999). Impaired retinal function and vitamin A availability in mice lacking retinol-binding protein. *The EMBO Journal, 18*(17), 4633–4644.

Refsum, H., Ueland, P. M., Nygard, O., & Vollset, S. E., (1998). Homocysteine and cardiovascular disease. *Annual Review of Medicine, 49*, 31–62.

Rizvi, S., Raza, S. T., Ahmed, F., Ahmad, A., Abbas, S., & Mahdi, F., (2014). The role of vitamin E in human health and some diseases. *Sultan Qaboos University Medical Journal, 14*(2), e157–e165.

Ruchi, S. (2017). Role of nutraceuticals in health care: A review. *International Journal of Green Pharmacy, 11*(3), S385–S394.

SanGiovanni, J. P., & Chew, E. Y., (2005). The role of omega-3 long-chain polyunsaturated fatty acids in health and disease of the retina. *Progress in Retinal and Eye Research, 24*(1), 87–138.

Sella, R., & Afshari, N. A., (2019). Nutritional effect on age-related cataract formation and progression. *Current Opinion in Ophthalmology, 30*(1), 63–69.

Senthilkumari, S., Talwar, B., Dharmalingam, K., Ravindran, R. D., Jayanthi, R., Sundaresan, P., Saravanan, C., et al., (2014). Polymorphisms in sodium-dependent vitamin C transporter genes and plasma, aqueous humor, and lens nucleus ascorbate concentrations in an ascorbate-depleted setting. *Experimental Eye Research, 124*, 24–30.

Shui, Y. B., Holekamp, N. M., Kramer, B. C., Crowley, J. R., Wilkins, M. A., Chu, F., Malone, P. E., et al., (2009). The gel state of the vitreous and ascorbate-dependent oxygen consumption: Relationship to the etiology of nuclear cataracts. *Archives of Ophthalmology, 127*(4), 475–482.

Singh, J., & Sinha, S., (2012). Classification, regulatory acts, and applications of nutraceuticals for health. *International Journal of Pharma and Bio Sciences, 2*(1), 177–187.

Singh, P., Kesharwani, R. K., & Keservani, R. K., (2017a). Antioxidants and vitamins: Roles in cellular function and metabolism. In: *Sustained Energy for Enhanced Human Functions and Activity* (pp. 385–407). Academic Press. ISBN:9780128054130.

Singh, P., Kesharwani, R. K., & Keservani, R. K., (2017b). Protein, carbohydrates, and fats: Energy metabolism. In: *Sustained Energy for Enhanced Human Functions and Activity* (pp. 103–115). Academic Press. ISBN:9780128054130.

Singla, V., Pratap, M. V., Garg, S. K., Rai, T., Choudhury, B. N., Verma, P., Deb, R., et al., (2014). Induction with NCB-02 (curcumin) enema for mild-to-moderate distal ulcerative colitis - A randomized, placebo-controlled, pilot study. *Journal of Crohn's and Colitis, 8*, 208–214.

Song, H., & Li, B., (2017). Beneficial effects of collagen hydrolysate: A review on recent developments. *International Journal of Scientific & Technology Research, 1*(2), 458–461.

Stoyanovsky, D. A., Goldman, R., Darrow, R. M., Organisciak, D. T., & Kagan, V. E., (1995). Endogenous ascorbate regenerates vitamin E in the retina directly and in combination with exogenous dihydrolipoic acid. *Current Eye Research, 14*(3), 181–189.

Tang, G., (2010). Bioconversion of dietary provitamin A carotenoids to vitamin A in humans. *The American Journal of Clinical Nutrition, 91*(5), 1468S–1473S.

Taylor, A., Jacques, P. F., Nadler, D., Morrow, F., Sulsky, S. I., & Shepard, D., (1991). Relationship in humans between ascorbic acid consumption and levels of total and reduced ascorbic acid in lens, aqueous humor, and plasma. *Current Eye Research, 10*(8), 751–759.

Tessier, F., Moreaux, V., Birlouez-Aragon, I., Junes, P., & Mondon, H., (1998). Decrease in vitamin C concentration in human lenses during cataract progression. *International Journal for Vitamin and Nutrition Research, 68*(5), 309–315.

Tokgöz, Y., Terlemez, S., & Karul, A., (2018). Fat-soluble vitamin levels in children with newly diagnosed celiac disease, a case-control study. *BMC Pediatric., 18*(1), 130.

Van, D. B. C., Deman, A., Ceyssens, B., Pauwels, M., Empsen, C., & Verbeelen, D., (2002). Vitamin E protects renal antioxidant enzymes and attenuates glomerulosclerosis in adriamycin-treated rats. *Nephron, 91*(1), 129–133.

Venkataswamy, G., (1967). Ocular manifestations of vitamin B complex deficiency. *British Journal of Ophthalmology, 51*, 749–754.

Weikel, K. A., Garber, C., Baburins, A., & Taylor, A., (2014). Nutritional modulation of cataract. *Nutrition Reviews, 72*, 30–47.

Wirth, J. P., Petry, N., Tanumihardjo, S. A., Rogers, L. M., McLean, E., Greig, A., Garrett, G. S., et al., (2107). Vitamin A supplementation programs and country-level evidence of vitamin A deficiency. *Nutrients, 9*(3), 190.

World Health Organization. *Blindness and Vision Impairment Prevention.* Available online: https://www.who.int/blindness/causes/priority/en/index1.html (accessed on 23 July 2023).

Ye, X. S., Al-Babili, A., Kloti, J., Zhang, P., & Lucca, P., (1997). Engineering the provitamin A (beta-carotene) biosynthesis pathway into (carotenoid-free) rice endosperm. *Plant Journal, 11*, 1071–1078.

CHAPTER 12

Vitamins as Nutraceuticals for Baldness

KSHITIJ S. VARMA,[1] TUSHAR N. LOKHANDE,[2] SUPRIYA R. BHAMARE,[3] KHEMCHAND R. SURANA,[4] and SUNIL K. MAHAJAN[5]

[1]*Department of Pharmaceutical Chemistry, Mahatma Gandhi Vidyamandir's Pharmacy College, Panchavati, Nashik, Maharashtra, India*

[2]*Department of Pharmaceutical Chemistry, Maharashtra Educational Society's H. K. College of Pharmacy, Oshiwara, Jogeshwari (W), Maharashtra, India*

[3]*Department of Pharmaceutical Chemistry, Sir Dr. M.S. Gosavi College of Pharmaceutical Education and Research, Nashik, Maharashtra, India*

[4]*Department of Pharmaceutical Chemistry, Shreeshakti Shaikshanik Sanstha, Divine College of Pharmacy, Satana, Nashik, Maharashtra, India*

[5]*Department of Pharmaceutical Chemistry, M.G.V's Samajshri Prashant Dada Hiray, College of Pharmacy, Malegaon, Nashik, Maharashtra, India*

ABSTRACT

Alopecia is normally self-limiting and treatable, although it can also be permanent. A thorough diagnosis of the kind of loss of hair will aid in the selection of the most appropriate treatment. Reassurance is an essential part of any therapy plan. There are several forms of alopecia, each of which requires different therapy. Unfortunately, there is no therapy for alopecia, as most medications are designed to treat the condition. Alopecia areata is a frequent skin condition. Affected patients are frequently upset, and they seek to stop hair loss by using a variety of over-the-counter vitamin

Preventive and Therapeutic Role of Vitamins as Nutraceuticals. Khemchand R. Surana, Eknath D. Ahire, Raj K. Keservani, & Rajesh K. Kesharwani (Eds.)

and mineral supplements. However, the evidence for their effectiveness is minimal. There is other toxicity reported. Low vitamin levels have been linked to androgenic alopecia and alopecia areata (patchy hair loss). Telogen effluvium can be caused by both low and high vitamin A levels, although lower levels are linked to hair breaking. Hair shaft irregularity is caused by a lack of vitamin C.

12.1 INTRODUCTION

Baldness is a state in which the scalp seems to have little or no hair. Alopecia is a problem that involves hair loss on one's head or other places of the body where hair is normally found. Low self-esteem is a result of the distressing disease, which has a psychological and social impact on sufferers (Upton et al., 2015; Falto-Aizpurua et al., 2014).

The diseases can be caused by a variety of factors, including stress, inheritance, hormone imbalances, poor diet, illness, and some drugs, such as those used to treat cancer (Hagenaars et al., 2017; Biran et al., 2015). Even though the FDA has approved only two fortuitous pharmaceuticals to treat alopecia, many unapproved medications claim to reverse the illness. Other hair loss-reversing therapies lack convincing proof from systematic scientific tests, limiting their widespread use and commercialization (Khidhir, 2013). Figure 12.1 represents the factors causing baldness.

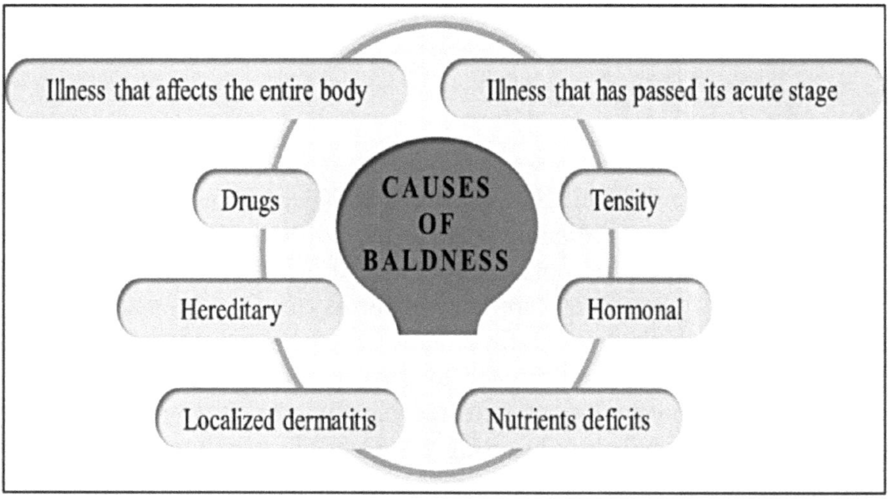

FIGURE 12.1 Factors causing baldness.

Source: Adapted from Hagenaars et al. (2017)

Alopecia is divided into several kinds, the most frequent of which are androgenic alopecia (widespread baldness), alopecia areata, and chemotherapy-induced alopecia (Falto-Aizpurua et al., 2014).

The three types of hair loss are as follows (Figure 12.2):

i. Non-cicatricial;
ii. Cicatricial; and
iii. Due to hair shaft abnormalities.

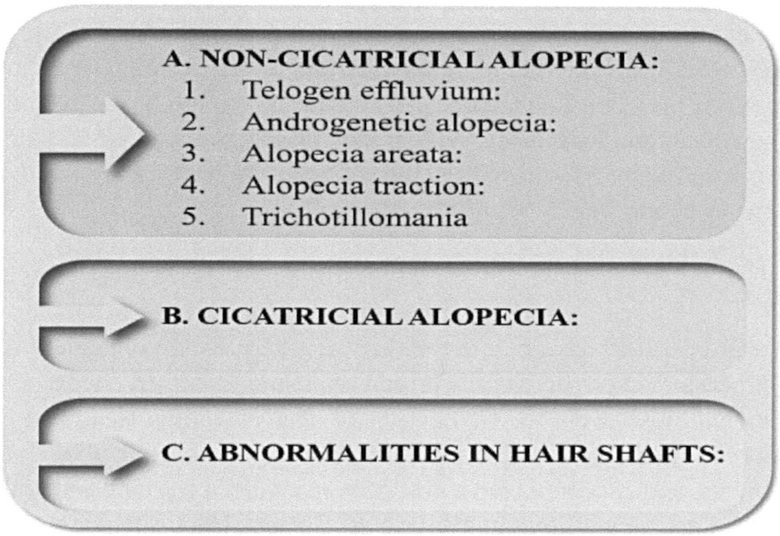

FIGURE 12.2 Types of baldness.

Source: Adapted from Falto-Aizpurua et al. (2014)

12.2 NON-CICATRICIAL ALOPECIA

There are various subtypes of non-cicatricial alopecia:

- Telogen effluvium is a type of telogen effluvium (shedding);
- Alopecia androgenetic (common baldness);
- Alopecia areata (patchy hair loss that is either isolated or recurring);
- Traction alopecia (hair loss caused by tugging);
- Trichotillomania (hair plucking).

Although they produce transient hair loss, trauma to the follicular stem cells or the central region of the hair follicle can induce scarring and lifelong hair loss in chronic situations (Bergfeld & Elston, 1996).

12.2.1 TELOGEN EFFLUVIUM

Telogen effluvium is a type of telogen effluvium that is the most familiar form of hair loss is telogen effluvium or shedding. Hair follicles transition early from the growth stage to the relaxing or shedding (telogen) stage in this disorder.

12.2.1.1 PRESENTATION

The patient's primary symptom is an uptick in the population of hairs they're losing, which can be visible on the shower floor, clothing, or pillow. On days when they don't shampoo, people lose up to 100 hairs; persons with telogen effluvium lose 150 to 400 strands of hair per day. When hair thickness is lowered by 30% to 50%, some patients simply feel a reduction in hair volume (Rebora, 1997).

12.2.1.2 CAUSES

Generally, 90–180 days before the dropping begins, some incident triggers the process. Fever, delivery, chronic systemic illnesses, heparin usage, and mental upset were the first causes of acute shedding (Kligman, 1996). Numerous medicines, endocrine diseases, very restrictive diets, surgical treatments, and anesthesia have also been recognized as acute and long-term causes of telogen effluvium (Pillans & Woods, 1995; Headington, 1993; Goette & Odum, 1976). Telogen effluvium has recently been linked to androgenetic alopecia in both men and women (Whiting, 1996).

- **Diagnosis:** With a comprehensive clinical history, the aim is to determine the trigger. In addition, the doctor should check thyroid function and rule out anemia. Hormonal testing can aid in the detection of perimenopausal alterations as well as androgen excess. Infectious diseases (such as syphilis) and nutrient deficiencies (minerals, vitamins, and protein), which are frequently associated with shedding, should be ruled out during the physical examination.

12.2.1.3 TREATMENT

The origin or causes of telogen effluvium must be identified and treated to treat it. Patients should be convinced that their hairline is being regenerated and that the likelihood of going bald is slim.

12.2.2 ANDROGENETIC ALOPECIA

12.2.2.1 PRESENTATION

Androgenetic alopecia can strike men and women who are genetically susceptible at any age, between puberty to senescence. Hair thinning normally starts from the ages of 12–40, and the majority of people exhibit this feature to some extent by the age of 50 (Price, 1996). The first event could be a telogen loss, though the patient's major symptom is thinning. Both a gradual shrinkage of the hair strand and reduced growth (anagen) phase cause progressive thinning. Hair loss occurs in a variety of patterns. The M-pattern, which is characterized by frontal recession and thinning or missing hair in the temples, is prevalent in both men and women. Another pattern, which is more typical in women, is a decrease in the density of hair.

12.2.2.2 CAUSES

Hair loss is influenced by steroid hormones, including dihydrotestosterone and dehydroepiandrosterone sulfate. The most powerful androgen, dihydrotestosterone, causes the proportion of scalp hair to decrease while increasing the amount of body and genital hair. It's debatable if androgenetic alopecia is inherited; it can be polygenic or autosomal dominant, with varied penetrance. Men and women are both affected by androgenetic alopecia. Regardless of gender, one-third of those with a significant family history should expect to be affected (Kuster & Happle, 1984).

12.2.2.3 DIAGNOSIS

The diagnosis is made based on the patient's symptoms and family history. If androgen oversupply is detected due to acne, hirsutism, or irregular menstrual cycles in women, a hormonal examination is required.

12.2.2.4 TREATMENT

When it comes to treating androgenetic alopecia, one of the main focuses is dihydrotestosterone. The systemic drug, a 5-alpha-reductase inhibitor, reduces this hormone in the hairline follicles locally. Finasteride showed positive outcomes in men but still no change in postmenopausal women experiencing female androgenetic alopecia in studies (Whiting, 1999; Kaufman, 1998).

Topical minoxidil at a concentration of 2%–5% is the first line of defense for women (It's also popular among guys) (Whiting, 1999). When using minoxidil, women should avoid applying it to their faces because it can encourage facial hair growth and aggravate hirsutism.

Spironolactone and flutamide, two systemic therapies in female androgenetic alopecia, are controversial; however, they are recommended to limit androgen consumption by the follicles (Pakinson, 1992). Contraceptives and hormone replacement can be used as adjuvant treatments for the same reason.

12.2.3 ALOPECIA AREATA

12.2.3.1 PRESENTATION

Alopecia areata produces isolated or recurrent spotty hair loss, but alternative clinical manifestations include multiple patches, entire scalp loss of hair (alopecia totalis), and total scalp and body loss of hair (alopecia Universalis). The prognosis is difficult to predict. The thin, light-colored hair regrows initially and is commonly replaced by dense, white-colored hair before the natural hair regrows.

12.2.3.2 CAUSES

A chronic inflammatory reaction around the follicle enhances the shedding phase in alopecia areata (Shapiro & Price, 1998). Although the inflammation is present, the afflicted hair loses, and no replacement is seen. A reason for alopecia areata has yet to be discovered. However, mounting data indicates that it must be a T lymphocyte-mediated autoimmune illness. Alopecia areata can be linked to other autoimmune diseases, including thyroid disease, vitiligo, and atopy, because it is an autoimmune disease (MacDonald, 1999). In the family history, autoimmune diseases like lupus erythematosus, diabetes mellites, and pernicious anemia are widespread. Alopecia areata is caused by genetic causes, and even in 10%–42% of cases, family history is observed (Madani & Shapiro, 2000).

12.2.3.3 TREATMENT

The severity of the ailment and the patient's age determine the treatment. Adults with less than 50% scalp involvement should get intralesional corticosteroid injections as a first-line treatment (Madani & Shapiro, 2000). Corticosteroids are mostly used to reduce inflammation. Minoxidil is a physiological response modifier that promotes hair growth, although it only helps about half of alopecia areata patients achieve cosmetically acceptable results (Price, 1987). In 20% to 25% of individuals, anthralin, a selective immunomodulating drug routinely used in youngsters, results in cosmetically acceptable regrowth (Fiedler & Alaiti, 1996). The most efficient and widely accepted treatment for chronic serious alopecia areata is external immunotherapy with interaction sensitizers (squaric acid dibutyl ester, dinitrochlorobenzene, or diphenylcyclopropenone). The frequency of acceptable regrowth, on the other hand, varies and is dependent on the severity of the alopecia and the type of sensitizer employed (Madani & Shapiro, 2000). The exact mechanism of action of topical sensitizers is unknown; however, they cause mild skin irritation and anaphylaxis by directing T cells aside from the perifollicular area.

12.2.4 ALOPECIA TRACTION

Traction can harm the hair shaft physically and disrupt the new hair growth. Cicatricial alopecia can develop if traction is used repeatedly and for an extended period.

12.2.4.1 PRESENTATION

Hair within the frontal area becomes sparse and breaks due to traction alopecia. This is a typical problem among females with curly hair, particularly African Americans.

12.2.4.2 CAUSES

The majority of instances are caused by tight braids, ponytails, rubber, hair bands, or other devices that impose significant and recurrent stress on the scalp hair.

12.2.4.3 TREATMENT

Traction alopecia is treated by encouraging the patient to modify her hairdo and explaining that even if the traction isn't stopped, the baldness may be irreversible (Whiting, 1999).

12.2.4.4 TRICHOTILLOMANIA

Trichotillomania is a disorder characterized by the obsessive pulling out of one's hair unusually.

12.2.4.5 PRESENTATION

Trichotillomania manifests itself clinically as patches of partial hair loss as well as short hair, most typically on the scalp. Eyelashes, brows, or other hairy parts may be impacted as well. The disorder is common in children who pull because of insecurity rather than a psychiatric disease (Whiting, 1999). The illness can be linked to depression or anxiety both in younger and older women (Muller, 1990). It's worth noting that the patient rarely admits or reports his or her background of hair-pulling.

12.2.4.6 CAUSES

The explanation may be obscure; it could be anything from an internal emotional issue to a diagnosable mental disease.

12.2.4.7 TREATMENT

Psychological examination and counseling are required for trichotillomania patients. Controlling obsessive hair-pulling typically necessitates psychopharmacologic medicines such as fluoxetine (Muller, 1990).

12.3 CICATRICIAL ALOPECIA

Cicatricial alopecia is a type of hair loss that occurs when the stem cell reserve in the center of the follicle is destroyed.

12.3.1 CAUSES

It is affected by a wide variety of cutaneous illnesses that manifest in a variety of ways. Fungi and bacteria folliculitis, bullous lupus erythematosus, as well as lichen planopilaris are all common causes. Trauma, scars bullous disorders, including neoplasms (skin tumors and cutaneous metastatic), are among the others.

12.3.2 DIAGNOSIS

Cicatricial alopecia of uncertain cause begins with fungal and bacterial infection cultures. A scalp biopsy is used to make the diagnosis, and a 4-mm punched biopsy is recommended.

12.3.3 TREATMENT

Treatment is usually prescribed to prevent the condition from expanding to unaffected areas, even though hair loss is permanent. Patients with hair loss should be directed to a dermatologist that specializes in hair loss.

12.4 ABNORMALITIES IN HAIR SHAFTS

Hair that is weak and brittle is caused by irregularities in the hair shaft. Patients may have widespread or patchy regions of short hair, as well as a background of hair not growing past a specific length.

12.5 CAUSES

The most common cause of hair shaft irregularity in adults is repeated stress to the hair strand through traction, bleach, perming, or blow-drying. Inherited illnesses (genodermatoses) and outside hair shaft injury can also alter the structure of the hair shaft. Hair shafts can take on a variety of forms. Trichorrhexis nodosa, a nodal region where the hair breaks into strands, is the most frequent hair shaft abnormality. External injury is the most prevalent cause of trichorrhexis nodosa, although it may also be linked to genetic and metabolic diseases that affect hair keratinization. Patients suffering from these illnesses must be directed to a dermatologist who specializes in hair disorders.

12.6 TREATMENT

If the condition is caused by trauma, treatment focuses on eradicating the source of the problem. Leave-on moisturizers which coat the hair fibers can help to strengthen the hair and prevent breaking (Muller, 1990).

12.7 NUTRACEUTICALS FOR BALDNESS

The term "nutraceutical" is a combination of "nutrient" and "pharmaceutical" (a prescription drug). Nutraceuticals may contain compounds with the "natural" goal of treating or preventing disease (Keservani et al., 2010a, b, 2017, 2020) but which are not universally acknowledged as safe (Ross et al., 2000; Ahire et al., 2021).

"Let diet be the medication and medication be the diet," the Greek physician Sir Hippocrates said approximately 2,500 years ago, and we understand the truth of his words today. Functional foods, dietary supplements, and nutraceuticals are defined as "any ingredient that could be regarded as a food or part of a food that provides health and medical advantages, particularly disease prevention and treatment." Nutraceuticals has to be the most appropriate term used to describe this group (Surana et al., 2021a, b). This title was created by Stephen DeFelice, the chairman and chief executive of a Medicine Research Foundation located in Cranford, New Jersey. Stephen De-Felice created the term nutraceutical in 1979. Nutraceuticals, according to DeFelice, are "foods or components of foods that give medicinal or health advantages, including illness prevention and therapy." Several other terminologies (medical foods, functional food, nutritious supplements) were employed in the succeeding decades (Biesalski, 2001). With these phenomena, ideas like nutraceuticals, nutritional treatment, phytonutrients, and phytotherapy have evolved (Berger & Shenkin, 2006). These active or beneficial foods, phytonutrients, and phytomedicines have been shown to improve health and immunological function, as well as reduce adverse effects and preserve wellness (Ramaa et al., 2006).

A nutrient is a material that an organism consumes in order to grow, reproduce, and survive. Macronutrients and micronutrients are the two major categories of nutrition. Macronutrients are chemicals that the body requires in big amounts, whereas micronutrients are nutrients that the body requires in small amounts. Carbohydrates, proteins (Keservani et al., 2015), and fats are macronutrients that provide molecules for the human body's structural and metabolic functions. They are necessary for the body's correct functioning (Derbyshire, 2018). Because of the growing acceptability of an "inside-out" approach to health, nutraceuticals are an emerging category among health products goods (Farris et al., 2017). Substances, which are biologically derived, biologically active molecules that are progressively being studied and sold to promote health, are found in many nutraceutical goods. Several studies have shown that certain goods, such as vitamins, essential fatty acids, and antioxidants, can help with hair development (Trueb, 2008; Le et al., 2015; Leng et al., 2007; Almohanna et al., 2019).

12.8 VITAMINS

Baldness can occur due to nutrient deficiency, as vitamins play an important part in the hair growth cycle and immunological defense system (Strumia, 2005; Cheung, Sink, & English, 2016):

i. Vitamins A/retinol;
ii. Vitamin D/calciferol;
iii. Vitamin E/tocopherol;
iv. Vitamin B2/riboflavin;
v. Vitamin B7/biotin;
vi. Vitamin B9/folic acid;
vii. Vitamin B12/cobalamin;
viii. Vitamin C/ascorbic acid.

Alopecia patients had a lower extent of endogenous antioxidants and higher amounts of lipid peroxidation metabolites (Naziroglu & Kokcam, 2000). Because of their greater lipid solubility, tocotrienols reduce oxidative risks and stress lipid peroxidation. Although certain vitamin insufficiency has been linked to hair loss, the potential of multivitamin supplements to repair hair is less evident (Almohanna et al., 2019).

12.8.1 VITAMIN A/RETINOL

Vitamin A is made up of retinol, retinal, plus retinyl esters, which are fat-soluble retinoids (Johnson et al., 2010). This vitamin performs a variety of functions in the body, including eyesight, immunological function, and cellular proliferation and differentiation (Ca, 2010). Preformed vitamin A (through animal sources) and provitamin A carotenoids are both found in the diet (sourced from plants). Vitamin A should be processed from both sources to their active versions intracellularly (retinal and retinoic acid). The bulk of vitamin A is deposited as retinyl esters in the liver. Plasma levels of retinol and carotenoids are usually sufficient for assessing retinol and carotenoid levels. Vitamin A deficiency is defined as a plasma retinol content of less than 0.70 mol/L. Supplementing with vitamin A non-central frontal-central baldness as well as a reduction in pubic as well as auxiliary hair.

Dystrophic nail alterations and erythematous dermatitis were also mentioned by the patient. These changes occurred at the same time as medication toxicity, which coincided with the patient's excessive vitamin A use (Cheruvattath et al., 2006).

12.8.2 VITAMIN D/CALCIFEROL

Vitamin D is a type of substance containing fats that regulate calcium and phosphorus balance and immunological function. Osteoarthritis, sclerosis, and systemic lupus erythematosus may all be linked to vitamin D deficiency (Kriegel, Manson, & Costenbader, 2011). Vitamin D receptors are intracellular receptors found in hair follicles that are required for normal hair growth and interfollicular epidermis development. Alopecia and near-total loss of hair were observed in mice with homozygous deletion for vitamin D receptors (Xie et al., 2002).

In comparison to healthy controls, meta-analyzes show that AA patients had a greater association between vitamin D insufficiency and decreased 25-hydroxyvitamin D levels in serum (Tsai & Huang, 2018). Vitamin D insufficiency was found in 39% of AA patients in comparison to 12.79% of healthy controls in one study (Miller et al., 2015). Various research has looked at the efficacy of oral calciferol supplementation for AA therapy because of this link; however, they have found no evidence of its usefulness in alopecia Universalis (AU) and its potential to augment squaric acid-dibutyl-ester (Berth-Jones & Hutchinson, 2009; Orecchia & Rocchetti, 1995). After three months of topical calcipotriol cream 50 g/mL administered once daily, a case report with suspected AA linked with diminished vitamin D receptor activation revealed complete clinical remission (Kim et al., 2012). Around 65% of AA patients who used topical 0.005% calcipotriol cream two times daily over 12 weeks had more than 50% hair regrowth, 62.5% had greater than 75% hair regrowth, and 27.1% had complete regrowth (Cerman et al., 2015). In 22 individuals with patchy AA, twice-daily topical 0.005% calcipotriol resulted in hair growth in 59.1% of patients after 4.21 2.13 weeks. People with low baseline serum calciferol levels healed more quickly and effectively (Narang, Daroach, & Kumaran, 2017). Topical vitamin D studies in alopecia are inconclusive and restricted by a limited sample or a lack of suitable controls. Preliminary findings indicate that topical vitamin D may have a therapeutic advantage with few side effects (Berth-Jones & Hutchinson, 2009; Orecchia & Rocchetti, 1995; Kim et al., 2012; Cerman et al., 2015; Narang, Daroach, & Kumaran, 2017).

12.8.3 VITAMIN E/TOCOPHEROL

Tocotrienols/Tocopherols/Tocopherols are antioxidants that belong to the vitamin E family. Hemolytic anemias, neurologic abnormalities, and skin dryness are all symptoms of deficiency. Vitamin E insufficiency is uncommon; however, it can occur as a result of fat malabsorption problems. There is very little evidence in the literature about the effects of vitamin E treatment on hair loss. When relative to a placebo group, 21 volunteers who obtained tocotrienol treatment (100 milligrams of blended tocotrienols daily) had a substantial rise in hair number (Beoy, Woei, & Hay, 2010). Excessive supplementation, on the other hand, might cause hypervitaminosis E, which can also raise the risk of bleeding and reduce thyroid hormone production. Furthermore, there has been some evidence of a negative influence on hair development, as demonstrated in volunteers who took 600 IU a day for 28 days, which is about 30 times the recommended daily consumption (Rushton, 2002). Thyroid hormone levels in this group were significantly lower (Rushton, 2002).

12.8.4 VITAMIN B COMPLEX

The vitamin B complex contains eight water-soluble vitamin compounds that contribute to cell metabolism:

- Vitamin B1/thiamine;
- Vitamin B2/riboflavin;
- Vitamin B3/niacin (B3);

- Vitamin B5/pantothenic acid (B5);
- Vitamin B6/pyridoxine;
- Vitamin B7/biotin;
- Vitamin B9/folate; and
- Vitamin B12/cobalamin.

Apart from biotin, because that is the only vitamin B body produces, the necessary daily intake of the above vitamins could be met by eating a well-balanced diet. Biotin does not have to be administered to healthy people.

Hair loss has only been linked to vitamin B2/riboflavin, vitamin B7/biotin, vitamin B9/folate, and vitamin B12/cobalamin deficiency.

12.8.5 VITAMIN B2/RIBOFLAVIN

Flavin mononucleotide (FMN), as well as flavin adenine dinucleotide (FAD), as well as flavin adenine dinucleotide (FAD) are two key coenzymes that include vitamin B2. Both FMN and FAD make up 90% of dietary riboflavin and are involved in cell development and function, fat metabolism, and energy production. The heart, kidneys, and liver are the only places in the body where riboflavin is stored at modest levels. Hair loss can be caused by riboflavin insufficiency, which is extremely unusual in the United States (Said & Ross, 2014).

12.8.6 VITAMIN B7/BIOTIN

Vitamin H (also known as Biotin or vitamin B7) is a coenzyme for 5 carboxylases that catalyze processes in the metabolism of fatty acids, glucose, and amino acids. Histone modification, cell signaling, and gene regulation are all influenced by biotin (Zempleni & Kuroishi, 2012). The majority of biotin in the diet is found in proteins. Nutritional protein should be broken down in free biotin before it can be stored in the intestine and liver. Biotin consumption for people in the United States is 30 micrograms per day. Biotin insufficiency is uncommon in Western countries because the typical intake of dietary biotin is acceptable. There has never been a case of severe biotin deficit in healthy people who eat a normal diet (Mock, 2010; Tzellos, 2009). Because there is no evidence of biotin toxicity, there is no upper capacity for biotin intake. However, increased biotin intake can generate an increase in serum or unfairly low laboratory test findings. Many scalp, hair, and nail supplements contain significantly more biotin than is suggested daily basis. Biotin can cause problems with testing that use the biotin-streptavidin technique. Many biotin-based immunoassays are based on the interaction between biotin and streptavidin, and these immunoassays are susceptible to interference when used to test biotin-containing samples. Exogenous biotin interacts with biotinylated reagents for binding on streptavidin reagents, resulting in erroneous positive or negative results (Samarasinghe, 2017). Inpatient samples for thyroid-stimulating hormone, parathyroid hormone, free triiodothyronine (FT3), free thyroxine (FT4), estradiol, testosterone, progesterone, dehydroepiandrosterone sulfate, vitamin B12, luteinizing hormone, prostate-specific antigen, and follicle-stimulating hormone, biotin interference in biotin-streptavidin immunoassay. Cardiovascular and tumor indicators, infectious disease serologies, anemia, and autoimmune disease biomarkers, and immunosuppressive medication concentrations are among the non-hormonal assays (Wijeratne, Doery, & Lu, 2012; Trambas, Sikaris, & Lu, 2016; Batista et al., 2017). Furthermore, biotin interaction (from supplemental biotin) produced a falsely low response in a troponin test, resulting in a missed diagnosis of a cardiac arrest and a patient's death, according to the US Food & Drug Administration. In addition, a recent study found that biotin interference affects various human chorionic gonadotropin (hCG) systems in people who use dietary biotin supplements. As a result, clinicians and laboratory workers should be aware of the possibility of qualitative urine hCG tests interfering with quantitative serum hCG measurements and should recommend quantitative serum hCG measurements instead. Biotin interference does not affect the latter (Williams, Cervinski, & Nerenz, 2018). Biotin deficiencies can be acquired or hereditary. Biotin deficiency can have both neonatal and infantile genetic origins. The neonate type is a life-threatening illness caused by a holocarboxylase enzyme inhibitor that manifests during the first six weeks of life. It usually shows up as acute dermatitis and alopecia, with the removal of vellus and terminal hairs on the scalp, as well as eyebrows, eyelashes, and lanugo hair. Biotin deficit in infants arises after 90 days of birth and is caused by the lack of the enzymes biotinidase. Hair on the scalp, eyebrow, and eyelashes is thin or nonexistent in this variant (Goldberg & Lenzy, 2010). Increased raw egg eating can cause acquired biotin insufficiency, as avidin particles adhere to biotin and prevent it from being absorbed into the intestinal tract. Avidin particles are destroyed in cooked eggs (Durusoy et al., 2009). Malabsorption, drunkenness, pregnancy, prolonged use of medicines that disrupt normal flora, pharmaceuticals like valproic acid, or isotretinoin consumption are some of the other factors of acquired biotin deficiency. Biotinidase activity is inhibited by the aforementioned drugs (Goldberg & Lenzy, 2010). Biotin deficiency is thought to affect 50% of pregnant women (Zempleni, Hassan, & Wijeratne, 2008). Baldness, dermatitis, and brittle nail are all symptoms of biotin insufficiency, yet large-scale studies have found that biotin supplementation for hair, skin, as well as nails are ineffective in treating these disorders (Zempleni & Kuroishi, 2012; Mock, 2010). In fact, through use of biotin tablets for hair development has only been supported by case studies. These case reports in children indicated 3–5 mg of biotin daily improved hair children's health with uncombable hair disorder after 3–4 months (Boccaletti et al., 2007; Shelley & Shelley, 1985).

12.8.7 VITAMIN B9/FOLIC ACID

Folate, which comprises naturally occurring dietary folate and folic acid, is a water-soluble B vitamin (fully oxidized mono glutamate). Folic acid is a coenzyme involved in the production of nucleotides and the metabolism of amino acids. It occurs in the plasma in 5-methyl-tetrahydrofolate, with the liver accounting for nearly half of the entire body content (Carmel et al., 2005). The recommended dietary requirement of food folate for adults is 400 micrograms per day, which is backed by the fact that some foods in the United States are required to be fortified. The maximum amount of folate that can be consumed is 1,000 micrograms. While the majority of people in the United States consume enough folate, certain populations are at risk of deficiencies (In most cases, it's linked to a bad diet, drunkenness, or a malabsorptive disorder). Folic acid insufficiency can lead to changes in hair, skin, and nails (Bailey et al., 2010).

12.8.8 VITAMIN B12/COBALAMIN

Vitamin B12 is required for DNA synthesis, nerve function, and the creation of red blood cells Methyl-cobalamin and 5-deoxy adenosylcobalamin are the active forms of B12. Vitamin B12 functions as a coenzyme for methionine synthase, affecting the synthesis of roughly 100 substrates such as DNA, RNA, as well as proteins. For adults in the United States, the recommended daily intake of cobalamin is 2.4 micrograms. Because vitamin B12 has minimal risk for toxicity, there is no set upper limit for its intake.

As folate and vitamin B12 have a function in nucleic acid synthesis, they may also play a significant role inside the highly proliferative follicle (Gonul et al., 2009). However, just a few research have looked into the link between B vitamins as well as hair loss. Turkish researchers looked examined serum folate and cobalamin levels for 43 patients having AA and 36 normal individuals and reported no difference differences between the AA individuals and the healthy volunteers. Furthermore, the scientists discovered that serum levels were unaffected by the length of illness activity. In a separate trial in Turkey, 75 people having AA and 54 healthy people were enrolled. Serum folate and vitamin B12 concentrations were determined using blood samples. The findings were consistent with those of a recent Turkish study (Gonul et al., 2009), which found no significant variations in cobalamin and folate concentrations between afflicted and normal patients (Ertugrul et al., 2013).

12.8.9 VITAMIN C/ASCORBIC ACID

Vitamin C, also known as ascorbic acid, is just a water-soluble vitamin that is produced as a byproduct of glucose metabolism. It is a powerful antioxidant that protects low-density lipoproteins from oxidation and free radical damage. It also functions as a lowering mediator by hydroxylating lysine and proline, which is required for collagen fiber formation. Due to its chelating and lowering impact, vitamin C aids iron mobilization and intestinal absorption in the intestine (Valdes, 2006). As a result, bioavailability is critical in people who have hair loss due to iron deficiency. Humans are naturally low in an enzyme known as L-gluconolactone oxidase, which is necessary for vitamin C production, and should consequently supplement their diet with vitamin C. Vitamin C levels are particularly high in citrus fruits, potatoes, tomatoes, green peppers, as well as cabbages (Gropper, Smith, & Grodd, 2004). Although vitamin C insufficiency is linked to body hair irregularities, there is no evidence that vitamin C levels are linked to hair loss (Fleming et al., 2013).

12.9 CONCLUSION

Hair loss is a prevalent problem among dermatologists, and it has a serious adverse emotional and psychological impact on patients. Vitamins and other micronutrients play a vital but not completely understood role in optimal hair follicle formation and innate immune activity. Deficiency in certain micronutrients could be a controllable risk factor in the development, management, and intervention of alopecia.

Extensive dual placebo-controlled trials are needed to explore the impact of nutrient supplementation on hair growth in individuals with both micronutrient deficit and non-scarring alopecia to demonstrate any link connecting hair loss and nutrient deficiency.

ACKNOWLEDGMENTS

We thank you to the Ravindra Vidya Prasarak Mandal Institute of Pharmacy, Dwarka, Nashik, Maharashtra, India, and Mahatma Gandhi Vidyamandir's Pharmacy College, Panchavati, Nashik, Maharashtra, India, for their constant support and providing all facilities to complete this work. Also, many thanks to all the known and unknowns who helped us right from the writing till the publishing of this chapter.

KEYWORDS

- **alopecia**
- **baldness**
- **cobalamin**
- **iron deficiency**
- **micronutrient**
- **nutraceutical**
- **telogen effluvium**
- **vitamins**

REFERENCES

Ahire, E. D., Sonawane, V. N., Surana, K. R., & Talele, G. S., (2021). Drug discovery, drug-likeness screening, and bioavailability: Development of drug-likeness rule for natural products. In: *Applied Pharmaceutical Practice and Nutraceuticals* (pp. 191–208). Apple Academic Press.

Akingbola, C., & Vyas, J., (2017). Traction alopecia: A neglected entity in 2017. *Indian Journal of Dermatology, Venereology and Leprology*, *83*(6).

Almohanna, H. M., Ahmed, A. A., Tsatalis, J. P., & Tosti, A., (2019). The role of vitamins and minerals in hair loss: A review. *Dermatology and Therapy*, *9*(1), 51–70.

Bailey, R. L., Dodd, K. W., Gahche, J. J., Dwyer, J. T., McDowell, M. A., Yetley, E. A., Sempos, C. A., et al., (2010). Total folate and folic acid intake from foods and dietary supplements in the United States: 2003–2006. *The American Journal of Clinical Nutrition, 91*(1), 231–237.

Batista, M. C., Ferreira, C. E., Faulhaber, A. C., Hidal, J. T., Lottenberg, S. A., & Mangueira, C. L., (2017). Biotin interference in immunoassays mimicking subclinical graves' disease and hyperestrogenism: A case series. *Clinical Chemistry and Laboratory Medicine (CCLM), 55*(6), e99–e103.

Beoy, L. A., Woei, W. J., & Hay, Y. K., (2010). Effects of tocotrienol supplementation on hair growth in human volunteers. *Tropical Life Sciences Research, 21*(2), 91.

Berger, M. M., & Shenkin, A., (2006). Vitamins and trace elements: Practical aspects of supplementation. *Nutrition, 22*(9), 952–955.

Berth-Jones, J., & Hutchinson, P. E., (1991). Alopecia totalis does not respond to the vitamin-D analogue calcipotriol. *Journal of Dermatological Treatment, 1*(6), 293–294.

Biesalski, H. K., (2001). Nutraceuticals: The link between nutrition and medicine. *Oxidative Stress and Disease, 6*, 1–26.

Biran, R., Zlotogorski, A., & Ramot, Y., (2015). The genetics of alopecia areata: New approaches, new findings, new treatments. *Journal of Dermatological Science, 78*(1), 11–20.

Blume-Peytavi, U., Whiting, D. A., & Trüeb, R. M., (2008). *Hair Growth and Disorders*. Springer Science & Business Media.

Boccaletti, V., Zendri, E., Giordano, G., Gnetti, L., & De Panfilis, G., (2007). Familial uncombable hair syndrome: Ultrastructural hair study and response to biotin. *Pediatric Dermatology, 24*(3), E14–E16.

Cerman, A. A., Solak, S. S., Altunay, İ., & Küçükünal, N., (2015). Topical calcipotriol therapy for mild-to-moderate alopecia areata: A retrospective study. *Journal of Drugs in Dermatology: JDD, 14*(6), 616–620.

Cheruvattath, R., Orrego, M., Gautam, M., Byrne, T., Alam, S., Voltchenok, M., Edwin, M., et al., (2006). Vitamin A toxicity: When one a day doesn't keep the doctor away. *Liver Transplantation, 12*(12), 1888–1891.

Cheung, E. J., Sink, J. R., & JC, E. I., (2016). Vitamin and mineral deficiencies in patients with telogen effluvium: A retrospective cross-sectional study. *Journal of Drugs in Dermatology: JDD, 15*(10), 1235–1237.

Coates, P. M., Betz, J. M., Blackman, M. R., Cragg, G. M., Levine, M., Moss, J., & White, J. D., (2010). *Encyclopedia of Dietary Supplements*. CRC Press.

Coates, P. M., Paul, M. C., Blackman, M., Blackman, M. R., Cragg, G. M., Levine, M., White, J. D., & Moss, J., (2004). *Encyclopedia of Dietary Supplements (Online)*. CRC press.

Derbyshire, E. (2018). Micronutrient intakes of British adults across mid-life: A secondary analysis of the UK national diet and nutrition survey. *Frontiers in Nutrition, 5*, 55.

Durusoy, C., Ozenli, Y., Adiguzel, A., Budakoglu, I. Y., Tugal, O., Arikan, S., Uslu, A., & Gulec, A. T., (2009). The role of psychological factors and serum zinc, folate, and vitamin B12 levels in the etiology of trichodynia: A case–control study. *Clinical and Experimental Dermatology: Clinical Dermatology, 34*(7), 789–792.

Falto-Aizpurua, L., Choudhary, S., & Tosti, A., (2014). Emerging treatments in alopecia. *Expert Opinion on Emerging Drugs, 19*(4), 545–556.

Farris, P. K., Rogers, N., McMichael, A., & Kogan, S. (2017). A novel multi-targeting approach to treating hair loss, using standardized nutraceuticals. *Journal of Drugs in Dermatology, 16*(11 Suppl), s141–148.

Fiedler, V. C., & Alaiti, S., (1996). Treatment of alopecia areata. *Dermatologic Clinics, 14*(4), 733–738.

Fleming, J. D., Martin, B., Card, D. J., & Mellerio, J. E., (2013). Pain, purpura, and curly hairs. *Clin. Exp. Dermatol., 38*(8), 940–942.

Goette, D. K., & Odom, R. B., (1976). Alopecia in crash dieters. *JAMA, 235*(24), 2622–2623.

Goldberg, L. J., & Lenzy, Y., (2010). Nutrition and hair. *Clinics in Dermatology, 28*(4), 412–419.

Gonul, M., Cakmak, S. K., Soylu, S., Kilic, A., & Gul, U., (2009). Serum vitamin B12, folate, ferritin, and iron levels in Turkish patients with alopecia areata. *Indian Journal of Dermatology, Venereology and Leprology, 75,* 552.

Gropper, S. S., & Smith, J. L., (2012). *Advanced Nutrition and Human Metabolism.* Cengage Learning.

Hagenaars, S. P., Hill, W. D., Harris, S. E., Ritchie, S. J., Davies, G., Liewald, D. C., Gale, C. R., et al., (2017). Genetic prediction of male pattern baldness. *PLoS Genetics, 13*(2), e1006594.

Headington, J. T., (1993). Telogen effluvium: New concepts and review. *Archives of Dermatology, 129*(3), 356–363.

Huxley, A., (2004). Require endpoints other than altered perception, 3, 4-methylenedioxymethamphetamine (MDEA; see Chapter 4). *Neurological Aspects of Substance Abuse* (p. 259).

Jang, Y. H., Kim, S. L., Lee, K. C., Kim, M. J., Park, K. H., Lee, W. J., & Lee, S. J., (2016). A comparative study of oral cyclosporine and betamethasone mini pulse therapy in the treatment of alopecia areata. *Annals of Dermatology, 28*(5), 569–574.

Karadag, A. S., Tutal, E., Ertugrul, D. T., Akin, K. O., & Bilgili, S. G., (2012). Serum holotranscobalamine, vitamin B12, folic acid, and homocysteine levels in patients with vitiligo. *Clinical and Experimental Dermatology: Experimental Dermatology, 37*(1), 62–64.

Kaufman, K. D., Olsen, E. A., Whiting, D., Savin, R., DeVillez, R., Bergfeld, W., Price, V. H., et al., (1998). Finasteride in the treatment of men with androgenetic alopecia. *Journal of the American Academy of Dermatology, 39*(4), 578–589.

Keservani, R. K., Kesharwani, R. K., Sharma, A. K., Vyas, N., & Chadoker, A., (2010b). Nutritional supplements: An overview. *International Journal of Current Pharmaceutical Review and Research, 1*(1), 59–75.

Keservani, R. K., Kesharwani, R. K., Vyas, N., Jain, S., Raghuvanshi, R., & Sharma, A. K., (2010a). Nutraceutical and functional food as future food: A review. *Der Pharmacia Lettre, 2*(1), 106–116.

Keservani, R. K., Sharma, A. K., & Jarouliya, U. (2015). Protein and peptide in drug targeting and its therapeutic approach. *Ars Pharmaceutica (Internet), 56*(3), 165–177.

Keservani, R. K., Sharma, A. K., & Kesharwani, R. K. (2017). An overview and therapeutic applications of nutraceutical and functional foods. *Recent Advances in Drug Delivery Technology*, 160–201. ISBN:9781522507543.

Keservani, R. K., Sharma, A. K., & Kesharwani, R. K. (2020). *Nutraceuticals and Dietary Supplements: Applications in Health Improvement and Disease Management.* CRC Press. ISBN: 9781771888738.

Khidhir, K. G., Woodward, D. F., Farjo, N. P., Farjo, B. K., Tang, E. S., Wang, J. W., Picksley, S. M., & Randall, V. A., (2013). The prostamide-related glaucoma therapy, bimatoprost, offers a novel approach for treating scalp alopecias. *The FASEB Journal*, *27*(2), 557–567.

Kim, D. H., Lee, J. W., Kim, I. S., Choi, S. Y., Lim, Y. Y., Kim, H. M., Kim, B. J., & Kim, M. N., (2012). Successful treatment of alopecia areata with topical calcipotriol. *Annals of Dermatology*, *24*(3), 341–344.

Kligman, A. M., (1961). Pathologic dynamics of human hair loss: I. Telogen effluvium. *Archives of Dermatology*, *83*(2), 175–198.

Kriegel, M. A., Manson, J. E., & Costenbader, K. H., (2011). Does vitamin D affect the risk of developing autoimmune disease?: A systematic review. In: *Seminars in Arthritis and Rheumatism* (Vol. 40, No. 6, pp. 512–531). WB Saunders.

Küster, W., & Happle, R., (1984). The inheritance of common baldness: Two B or not two B? *Journal of the American Academy of Dermatology*, *11*(5), 921–926.

Le Floc'h, C., Cheniti, A., Connétable, S., Piccardi, N., Vincenzi, C., & Tosti, A., (2015). Effect of a nutritional supplement on hair loss in women. *Journal of Cosmetic Dermatology*, *14*(1), 76–82.

Lengg, N., Heidecker, B., Seifert, B., & Trüeb, R. M., (2007). Dietary supplement increases anagen hair rate in women with telogen effluvium: Results of a double-blind, placebo-controlled trial. *Clinical Practice*, *4*(1), 59.

Liew, S. C., (2016). Folic acid and diseases-supplement it or not? *Revista da Associacao Medica Brasileira*, *62*, 90–100.

MacDonald, N., (1999). Alopecia areata: Identification and current treatment approaches. *Dermatology Nursing*, *11*(5).

Miller, R., Conic, R. Z., Bergfeld, W., & Mesinkovska, N. A., (2015). November. Prevalence of comorbid conditions and sun-induced skin cancers in patients with alopecia areata. In: *Journal of Investigative Dermatology Symposium Proceedings* (Vol. 17, No. 2, pp. 61–62). Elsevier.

Mulinari-Brenner, F., & Bergfeld, W. F., (2003). Hair loss: Diagnosis and management. *Cleveland Clinic Journal of Medicine*, *70*(8), 705–712.

Muller, S. A., (1990). Trichotillomania: A histopathologic study in sixty–six patients. *Journal of the American Academy of Dermatology*, *23*(1), 56–62.

Narang, T., Daroach, M., & Kumaran, M. S., (2017). Efficacy and safety of topical calcipotriol in management of alopecia areata: A pilot study. *Dermatologic Therapy*, *30*(3), e12464.

Naziroglu, M., & Kokcam, I., (2000). Antioxidants and lipid peroxidation status in the blood of patients with alopecia. *Cell Biochemistry and Function: Cellular Biochemistry and its Modulation by Active Agents or Disease*, *18*(3), 169–173.

Orecchia, G., & Rocchetti, G. A., (1995). Topical use of calcipotriol does not potentiate squaric acid dibutylester effectiveness in the treatment of alopecia areata. *Journal of Dermatological Treatment*, *6*(1), 21–23.

Pillans, P. J., & Woods, D. J., (1995). Drug-associated alopecia. *International Journal of Dermatology*, *34*(3), 149–158.

Price, V. H., (1987). Double-blind, placebo-controlled evaluation of topical minoxidil in extensive alopecia areata. *Journal of the American Academy of Dermatology*, *16*(3), 730–736.

Price, V. H., (1999). Treatment of hair loss. *New England Journal of Medicine*, *341*(13), 964–973.

Ramaa, C. S., Shirode, A. R., Mundada, A. S., & Kadam, V. J., (2006). Nutraceuticals-an emerging era in the treatment and prevention of cardiovascular diseases. *Current Pharmaceutical Biotechnology*, *7*(1), 15–23.

Rebora, A., (1997). Telogen effluvium. *Dermatology*, *195*(3), 209–212.

Ross, S., (2000). Functional foods: The food and drug administration perspective. *The American Journal of Clinical Nutrition*, *71*(6), 1735S–1738S.

Rushton, D. H., (2002). Nutritional factors and hair loss. *Clinical and Experimental Dermatology: Clinical Dermatology*, *27*(5), 396–404.

Samarasinghe, S., Meah, F., Singh, V., Basit, A., Emanuele, N., Emanuele, M. A., Mazhari, A., & Holmes, E. W., (2017). Biotin interference with routine clinical immunoassays: Understand the causes and mitigate the risks. *Endocrine Practice*, *23*(8), 989–998.

Shapiro, J., & Price, V. H., (1998). Hair regrowth: Therapeutic agents. *Dermatologic Clinics*, *16*(2), 341–356.

Shelley, W. B., & Shelley, E. D., (1985). Uncombable hair syndrome: Observations on response to biotin and occurrence in siblings with ectodermal dysplasia. *Journal of the American Academy of Dermatology*, *13*(1), 97–102.

Strumia, R., (2005). Dermatologic signs in patients with eating disorders. *American Journal of Clinical Dermatology*, *6*(3), 165–173.

Surana, K. R., Ahire, E. D., Sonawane, V. N., Talele, S. G., & Talele, G. S., (2021). Informatics and methods in nutrition design and development. *Natural Food Products and Waste Recovery: Healthy Foods, Nutrition Design, and Extraction of Valuable Compounds* (p. 33).

Surana, K. R., Ahire, E. D., Sonawane, V. N., Talele, S. G., & Talele, G. S., (2021). Molecular modeling: Novel techniques in food and nutrition development. *Natural Food Products and Waste Recovery: Healthy Foods, Nutrition Design, and Extraction of Valuable Compounds* (p. 17).

Trambas, C. M., Sikaris, K. A., & Lu, Z. X., (2016). More on biotin treatment mimicking graves' disease. *The New England Journal of Medicine*, *375*(17), 1698.

Tsai, T. Y., & Huang, Y. C., (2018). Vitamin D deficiency in patients with alopecia areata: A systematic review and meta-analysis. *Journal of the American Academy of Dermatology*, *78*(1), 207–209.

Tzellos, T. G., Tahmatzidis, D. K., Lallas, A., Apostolidou, K., & Goulis, D. G., (2009). Pernicious anemia in a patient with type 1 diabetes mellitus and alopecia areata universalis. *Journal of Diabetes and its Complications*, *23*(6), 434–437.

Upton, J. H., Hannen, R. F., Bahta, A. W., Farjo, N., Farjo, B., & Philpott, M. P., (2015). Oxidative stress–associated senescence in dermal papilla cells of men with androgenetic alopecia. *Journal of Investigative Dermatology*, *135*(5), 1244–1252.

Valdés, F., (2006). Vitamina C. *Actas Dermo-sifiliográficas*, *97*(9), 557–568.

Whiting, D. A., (1996). Chronic telogen effluvium. *Dermatologic Clinics*, *14*(4), 723–731.

Whiting, D. A., Waldstreicher, J., Sanchex, M., & Kaufman, K. D., (1999). Measuring reversal of hair miniaturization in androgenetic alopecia by follicular counts in horizontal sections of serial scalp biopsies: Results of finasteride 1 mg treatment of men and postmenopausal women. In: *Journal of Investigative Dermatology Symposium Proceedings* (Vol. 4, No. 3, pp. 282–284). Elsevier.

Wijeratne, N. G., Doery, J. C., & Lu, Z. X., (2012). Positive and negative interference in immunoassays following biotin ingestion: A pharmacokinetic study. *Pathology-Journal of the RCPA*, *44*(7), 674, 675.

Williams, G. R., Cervinski, M. A., & Nerenz, R. D., (2018). Assessment of biotin interference with qualitative point-of-care hCG test devices. *Clinical Biochemistry*, *53*, 168–170.

Xie, Z., Komuves, L., Yu, Q. C., Elalieh, H., Ng, D. C., Leary, C., Chang, S., et al., (2002). Lack of the vitamin D receptor is associated with reduced epidermal differentiation and hair follicle growth. *Journal of Investigative Dermatology*, *118*(1), 11–16.

Zempleni, J. W. S., & Kuroishi, T., (2012). *Biotin. Present Knowledge in Nutrition.* 10th edn. Washington, DC: Wiley-Blackwell; 359–374.

Zempleni, J., Hassan, Y. I., & Wijeratne, S. S., (2008). Biotin and biotinidase deficiency. *Expert Review of Endocrinology & Metabolism*, *3*(6), 715–724.

CHAPTER 13

Vitamins as Nutraceuticals for Skin Care

ADITI M. KOKANDE,[1] KHEMCHAND R. SURANA,[2] EKNATH D. AHIRE,[3] RAJ K. KESERVANI,[4] and SUNIL K. MAHAJAN[5]

[1]*Department of Pharmaceutical Chemistry, Oriental Education Society College of Pharmacy, Navi Mumbai, Maharashtra, India*

[2]*Department of Pharmaceutical Chemistry, Shreeshakti Shaikshanik Sanstha, Divine College of Pharmacy, Satana, Nashik, Maharashtra, India*

[3]*Department of Pharmaceutics, METs, Institute of Pharmacy, BKC, Affiliated to Savitribai Phule Pune University, Adgaon, Nashik, Maharashtra, India*

[4]*Faculty of B. Pharmacy, CSM Group of Institutions, Prayagraj, Uttar Pradesh, India*

[5]*Department of Pharmaceutical Chemistry, M.G.V's Samajshri Prashant Dada Hiray, College of Pharmacy, Malegaon, Nashik, Maharashtra, India*

ABSTRACT

Our skin is the largest organ present all over the body and protects all the internal organs from external damage. As per the study, our skin carries one-sixth of the total body weight. It plays the biggest role in various body functions. It mainly acts as a barrier to many physical and chemical components as they are harmful to the body. It regulates the temperature condition and homeostasis of the body, that is, internal temperature or the environment of the body. The skin is mainly composed of three layers such as epidermis, dermis, and hypodermis which is also called subcutaneous layer. To protect this skin from damage, the term nutraceuticals are come

Preventive and Therapeutic Role of Vitamins as Nutraceuticals. Khemchand R. Surana, Eknath D. Ahire, Raj K. Keservani, & Rajesh K. Kesharwani (Eds.)

into account. Nutraceuticals are nothing but food that provides medical or health benefits, including the prevention and treatment of disease and disorder, and which prevents risk factors. Nutraceuticals may be used for effective health benefits that reduce the aging process and also prevent chronic diseases such as obesity, increase life expectancy, or support the structure or function of the body. Nutraceuticals are marketed names but, in combination with the vitamins which are prevention skin from damage, are useful. Various types of vitamins are used to protect the skin from damage, that as Vitamin A, B3, B5, C, E, and K. Vitamin A is a retinoid and is used for skin rejuvenation and cell growth. Vitamin B3 is a niacinamide, and it is used to remove hyperpigmentation and dark circles. Vitamin B5 is a pantothenic acid and is used to prevent skin from loss of moisture and dehydration. Vitamin C is the most commonly used and mainly acts as an antioxidant to prevent the skin from aging and wrinkles. Vitamin E is tocopherol, and as it contains collagen and elastin, it shows a good building block for the skin. It has moisture-absorbing properties, so, used to make ointment and cream. Vitamin K is phytomenaquinone but commonly known for its function as blood clotting. This vitamin is used to reduce inflammation and is mainly used after surgery to heal damaged skin or to reduce the inflammation. Vitamin D is commonly known as Ergocalciferol, this vitamin boosts immunity, and with this, it also protects the skin from severe disorders of the skin like dry skin, eczema, and psoriasis. Again, some marketed nutraceutical products are there in the market which are prepared in combination with vitamins, and they are Revital, Pediasure, Proteinex, and omega women.

13.1 INTRODUCTION

Our skin is the largest organ of our body, considering an area of 1.5–2.0 square meters. It has 15 to 20 times larger surface area than our small intestine. As per the study, our skin carries one-sixth of the total body weight (Pérez-Sánchez et al., 2018). It plays the biggest role in various body functions. The skin is a very versatile organ as it gives their participation in sensitivity and also in the protection against the microorganism. The main function of the skin is to protect the internal organ of our body. It mainly acts as a barrier to many physical and chemical components as they are harmful to the body. It also acts against ultraviolet radiation such as UV A and UV B (Tambe et al., 2021). Along with this, it opposes the many environmental factors such as pathogens and chemical crises. It regulates the temperature condition and homeostasis of the body, that is, internal temperature or the environment of the body. It also controls the body from dehydration. The skin is mainly composed of three layers such as epidermis, dermis, and hypodermis which is also called subcutaneous layer. The epidermis, which is ectodermal in origin, is the major and shows the body's interaction with the environment (Boelsma et al., 2001). The outermost layer of this epidermis, called the stratum corneum, consists of dead cells or corneocytes, and it has a thickness of 10 um–30 um. After the stratum corneum, the layers of keratinocytes, then melanocytes, and then Langerhans cells. In this, keratinocytes produce keratin in the epidermis, whereas keratin is a quaternary type of protein. Which makes the skin waterproof, as it maintains the skin from water loss. After that, the next group of cells contains the melanocytes, which are a heterogenous group and present in the junction of the epidermis and dermis, belonging to the hair follicles. The melanocytes are the pigment that is responsible for the color of the skin that is the pigmentation of the skin and protection from the rays. Melanin consists of several physical importance like regulatory influence, homeostasis, scavenging of free radicals to protect against oxidative stress, and also antimicrobial properties (Chauhan et al., 2013). After this, the layer of Langerhans cells has generated, which are immune dendritic cells and responsible for protecting against the external microorganism and some outer harmful factors. Here the epidermis layer end and the area of the dermis layer starts. In the dermis layer, which is of mesoderm in origin, provides strength and elasticity to the skin. The dermis layer contains three types of systems that are neuronal, lymphatic, and vascular. Along with this, it is also having with sweat pores and hair follicles. The dermis layer of the skin is primarily composed of complex extracellular matrix proteins and the collagen fiber (DeFelice, 1995). This extracellular matrix protein distinguished as structural collagen and elastin or non-structural collagen that is glycoprotein, which is mainly, depends on their function and working principle. Again, dermal collagen also consists of a vital amount of extracellular proteins, which carry 90% of the total weight of the skin. This dermis layer of the skin functions to provide nutrients to the skin and help to regulate the temperature. The hypodermis or the subcutaneous layer of the skin, which is beneath the dermis, helps to insulate the body from external factors, heat, and also from the cold (Schmitt & Ferro, 2013). Figure 13.1 represents layers of skin.

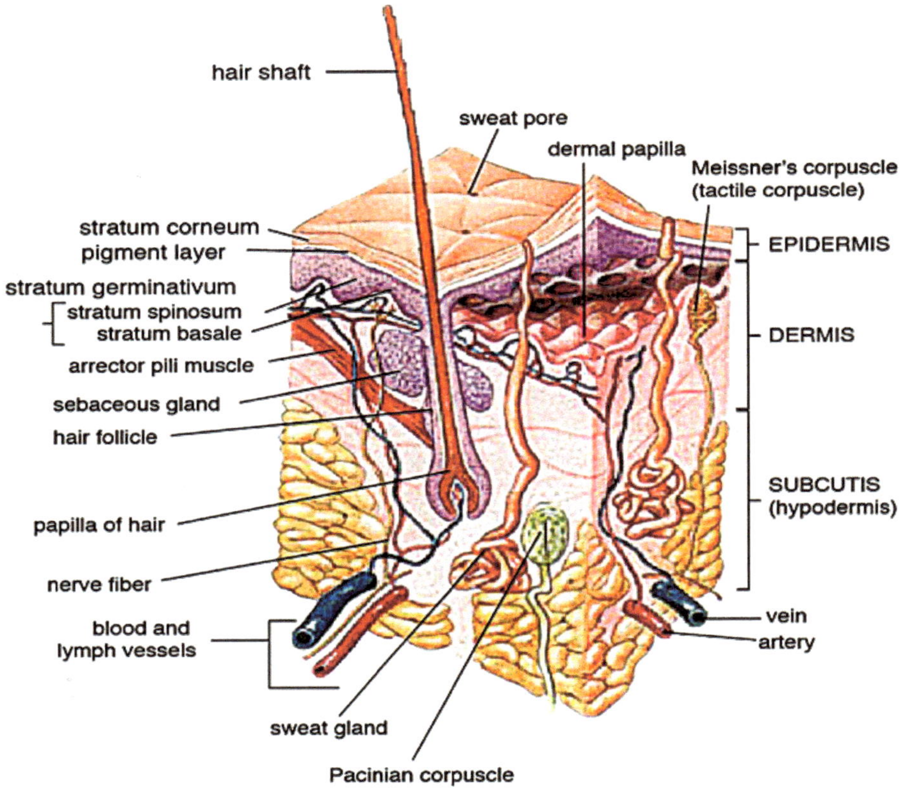

FIGURE 13.1 Layers of skin.

As far as the concerned, skin has to face many challenges about the damage, such as wrinkling, exposure to UV radiation, rough textured appearance, dry skin, pigmentation, and dark spot (Nicoletti, 2012). This type of problem has to face as the increase in age. From the study, carotenoids are the substance that generally helps to reduce these effects. According to the study, carotenoids help with photoprotection against UV radiation by acting as reactive oxygen species. Lycopene which is one type of carotenoid compound helps to reduce photo pigmentation and also the protection against UV radiation (Papandreou & Hamid, 2015).

Nowadays, Food and the cosmetic industry are growing day by day, and their marketing strategies are also changing. From this new change, they are launching their products for skin health with a combination of nutraceuticals (Kosari et al., 2010). As far as it is growing, the use of healthy food and supplements reduces the risk of hazardous skin allergies and skin diseases. These supplements are according to their diet and need the macronutrients like vitamins, minerals, and fatty acids for effective and healthy skin (Graf, 2005). From these bioactive products, the texture of the skin is changing into a good quality and seeing a positive effect. These macronutrients, which are used as nutraceuticals (Keservani et al., 2010a, b, 2017, 2020), are typically from plant sources and some from animal sources (Sunder, 2019).

13.2 NUTRACEUTICAL

The term nutraceutical is developed from the combination of two words named as nutrition and pharmaceuticals. This term was coined by the scientist Stephen DeFelice in the year 1989, which is the chairperson and founder of the Foundation and Innovation in Medicine (Chen & Vissers, 2020). A nutraceutical can be defined as "a food that provides medical or health benefits, including the prevention and treatment of a disease and disorder and which prevents from the risk factors." Nutraceuticals may be used for effective health benefits that reduce the aging process and also prevent chronic diseases such as obesity, increase life expectancy, or support the structure or function of the body (Thiele & Ekanayake-Mudiyanselage, 2007; Ahire et al., 2021). Nowadays, nutraceuticals have much more considerable demand and are of interest to many people due to their nutritional potential, safety, therapeutic effects, and immeasurable health benefits (Shamloul et al., 2019). Although nutraceuticals have shown promising results in various complications, their uncontrolled use may not be devoid of secondary effects, so they should be strictly regulated as prescription drugs. The nutraceutical industry's main segments include dietary supplements, herbal (Sharma et al., 2020; Rane et al., 2020a–c) and the natural products and functional foods. Nutritional supplements value with the macronutrients and herbal or natural products are the most rapidly growing in this new marketed era (Shapiro & Saliou, 2001). A recent study about market research shows that India proposed the global nutraceuticals market is expanding and would reach $340 billion by 2024, growing at a Compound Annual Growth Rate (CAGR) of 7.2% from 2016 to 2024, which is held at Variant Market Research, Pune. Nutraceuticals are mainly categorized on the basis of several criteria, which are the food source, mechanism of action of the product, chemical nature, and positive effect on health (Chiu & Kimball, 2003).

They may be macronutrients (nutrients salts like potassium, magnesium, calcium, and omega 3 fatty acids) and this micronutrient is also available (nutrients salts/chemicals elements required in small quantities, e.g., vitamins and minerals) and phytochemicals. Table 13.1 shows the functional ingredients, their source, and medicinal purpose. Many of the food sources are also used as nutraceuticals which are all of natural origin, like from plants or animals, and these are categorized into some essential food items such as dietary fiber, prebiotics, probiotics, polyunsaturated fatty acids, minerals, vitamins, marine nutrients (Linder, 2012; Surana et al., 2021a, b).

There are various health benefits for nutritional therapy, as it avoids side effects, it improves medical conditions, reduces or minimizes risk, improves diet and the value of health, and increases health benefits. They are readily available everywhere (Ross & Harrison, 2007). Thus, the nutritional therapy is a healing therapy which uses nutritional and pharmaceutical importance and shows many medicinal benefits. This therapy achieves the target by effective nutraceutical in various body functions like as avoiding vitamin, minerals, or other macronutrients deficiency, detoxification of the body, healthy and positive dietary habits, restoring healthy digestion, and increasing gut health and maintaining the intestinal flora as like probiotics (Formelli et al., 1989; Ritter & Smith, 1996).

13.2.1 CATEGORY OF NUTRACEUTICAL

- Substances with established nutritional functions, such as vitamins, minerals, amino acids, and fatty acids – nutrients (Díez-Pérez et al., 2012).
- Herbs or botanical products as concentrates or extracts – herbals (Bouillon et al., 2008).
- Reagents derived from other sources (e.g., pyruvate, chondroitin sulfate, steroid hormone precursors) serving specific functions, such as sports nutrition, weight-loss supplements, fortified conventional foods, and meal replacements – dietary supplements (Jetter et al., 2014).

13.2.1.1 VITAMINS

Vitamins are the essential macronutrient of the body, which is presenting chemically organic in nature. From this, if it is present in small quantities but

TABLE 13.1 Functional Ingredients, Their Source and Medicinal Purpose.

Functional Ingredients	Source	Medicinal Purpose
Carotenoids: Alpha and Beta-carotenoids	Carrots, watermelon, and other fruits.	Neutralize free radicals that cause damage to nerve cells
Lutein	Green vegetables like peas, fenugreek, and spinach.	Reduce the risk of muscle degeneration because they affect oxygen consumption.
Lycopene	Products containing lycopene that is tomato and watermelon.	Reduce the risk of prostate cancer and also related to male hormones defects, which are cured by lycopene.
Dietary fiber, insoluble fiber	Wheat, bran, brown bread.	Reduce the risk of breast, colon cancer, and also relatable female health issues.
Beta-glucan, soluble fiber	Oats, barley, psyllium, and also fiber-containing food.	Reduce the risk of cardiovascular disease and blockage of blood vessels.
Fatty acids: Long-chain omega-3 fatty acid DHA/EPA	Salmon and other fish oil, some marine animals.	Reduce the risk of cardiovascular diseases, improve mental, visual functions because it is loaded with vitamin A.
Minerals: Calcium, selenium, potassium, zinc, copper	Food, rock salt, table salt	An important constituent of a balanced diet and maintaining health.
Conjugated linoleic acid (CLA)	Cheese, meat products, dairy products, and products containing vit B12.	Improve body composition, and decrease the risk of certain cancers.
Phenolics: Anthracyanides, catechins, flavanones, lignans	Fruits, tea, citrus, vegetables.	Prevention of cancer, kidney stone, renal failure.
Tannins	Cranberries, coca, chocolate, mulberries.	Improve the urinary tract, reduce the risk of urinary tract infection, and reduces the risk of cardiac failure.
Plant sterols: Stanol, ester	Corn, soy, green tea	Lower blood cholesterol levels by controlling cholesterol absorption.
Prebiotics/probiotics	Shallots, onion powder	Improve the quality of intestinal microflora and gastrointestinal health.
Soya phytoestrogens: isoflavones, daidzein, genistein	Soybean and other soy-based foods, quinoa.	Protect against heart disease and some cancers, lowers LDL, and increases total cholesterol in HDL.

Source: Adapted from (Lupo, 2001; Tran et al., 2015; Manela-Azulay & Bagatin, 2009; Czajka et al., 2018)

is required for the proper metabolism. This essential macronutrient cannot be synthesized in the human body, so; their external supplementation is the need for every person (Dawson-Hughes et al., 2013). So, everyone needs it from outer sources like diet and fruits. From diet means them animal and plant sources. All the vitamins are discovered in the age of 1931 to 1948. The history behind this tells us that when the intake of vitamins from the diet was reduced, the outcome was a deficiency in vitamins in the human body (Vieth, 1999). Then firstly, Vitamin B complex is discovered, which is a yeast-extracted drug but in tablet form. After that, the Vitamin C ascorbic acid tablet was introduced in semi-synthetic form (Adams & Hewison, 2010). This Vitamin C ascorbic acid tablet is greatly used in this COVID situation to boost the patients' immunity. After this trade from the 1950s, marketing strategies of vitamins changed, and many people started using them as supplements. Because they are not synthesized in the body, their absence can lead to severe health hazardous effects. There are two types of vitamins that have been discovered that is fat-soluble and water-soluble (Holick, 2003). Water-soluble vitamins are vitamin B and Vitamin C., And fat-soluble vitamins are Vitamin A, Vitamin D, Vitamin E, and Vitamin K. There are a total of 13 types of vitamins that exist. And some of them play an essential role in healthy skin purpose, so this nutraceutical came into the market with this combination of vitamins to produce a positive effect on the skin and successfully achieve good results (Lips, 2006). Table 13.2 shows vitamins, their source, and their health benefits.

From Table 13.2, there are various types of vitamins have been displayed, and from this, it also contributes a vital role in skin care and healthy skin benefits. This acts as an anti-acne, antioxidant, antiaging, and glowing effect on the skin, hydration, and many more (Pissios, 2017). So, the nutraceuticals have come forward to market the products for skin care with the help of these seven vitamins in front of the world. These seven vitamins are named as Vitamin A, Vitamin B3, Vitamin B5, Vitamin C, Vitamin E, Vitamin K, and Vitamin D (Williams et al., 2017).

13.2.1.2 VITAMIN A

Vitamin A is commonly known as Retinoid. This vitamin has numerous uses for eye disease but also shows in effective and healthy skin (Jacobson & Jacobson, 2018). This is the only vitamin that is used for reprogramming or regenerating skin cells. It influences the cells to behave in a specific way

TABLE 13.2 Vitamins, Their Source and Health Benefits.

Vitamins	Sources	Health Benefits
Vitamin A1 (retinol)	Fish liver oil, liver	Antioxidants maintenance of healthy skin, vision, and mucous membranes.
Vitamin A2	Cheese, butter carrots, spinach, pumpkins, papaya	Vision
Vitamin B1 (thiamine)	Cereals, pulses	Essential in neurologic
Vitamin B2 (riboflavin)	Nuts, yeast	Helps in energy production
Vitamin B3 (niacin)	Liver, meat, yeast	It helps to convert food into energy and maintain proper brain function.
Vitamin B5 (pantothenic acid)	Yeast, egg, milk	Required for various nervous system functions.
Vitamin B6 (pyridoxine)	Banana, tomato juice	Helps to produce essential proteins and convert protein into energy.
Vitamin B8 (biotin)	Swiss chard	Required for various metabolic functions.
Vitamin B9 (folic acid)	Green vegetables	Essential in pregnancy, it helps in RBC formation.
Vitamin B12 (cyanocobalamin).	Cheese, dairy products.	Formation of RBCs.
Vitamin C (ascorbic acid)	Citrus fruits	Immunity, antiaging, antioxidants.
Vitamin D (calciferol)	Fish liver oil, wheat germ oil, egg yolk, butter.	Essential for the formation of bones and teeth, it helps the body absorb and use calcium.
Vitamin E (tocopherol)	Wheat germ oil, cotton seed oil, peanut oil.	Antioxidant helps form blood cells, muscles, lung, and nerve tissue and boosts the immune system.
Vitamin K (menaquinone)	Cabbage, cauliflower, tomatoes.	Essential for blood clotting.

Source: Adapted from Sauve, 2008; Makarov et al., 2019; Denu, 2005

to reperform the texture of the skin and renewal of the skin and maintains elasticity of the skin (Sheppard et al., 2013). This Vitamin A works by stimulating the fibroblast, collagen, and elastin to give a smooth texture to the skin without generating acne. It also helps to reduce fine lines, dark circle, which is commonly seen as under-eye circles, pigmentation (which is a common problem for Indian skin type that occurs by sun rays), and also the open pores problem. Vitamin A has numerous health benefits but firmly acts against pigmentation and dark spots because it normalizes the action of tyrosinase, which is an enzyme used for nothing but the synthesis of Melanin (Ismail et al., 2020).

13.2.1.3 VITAMIN B3

Vitamin B3 is also known as Niacin. Niacin is a water-soluble vitamin and is used in various body functions (Hennekens et al., 1996). Most commonly, niacin work to boost memory function by regenerating the brain cells, that is, nervous cells; it works to improve the digestive system, and as it regenerates the brain cells, then also helps to reduce severe brain diseases like anxiety and depression. From the pharmaceutical point of view, niacin is available in the market as niacinamide which is used as a topical agent in the form of creams, face serums, and ointments. It has anti-inflammatory and antiaging property, which reduces dark spot, corrects the texture of the skin, and also helps in glowing the skin (Neuhouser et al., 2009). This niacinamide renews the skin cells and removes acne-prone pimples and various skin problems like dark spots, open pores, dullness, and scars. This naturally works with the skin to help out in minimizes the enlarged pores. This also helps to tighten the skin. As this has to minimize the property of the pores, then, it prevents debris from clogging the pores. This niacinamide also helps to restore and renew the skin cells for the smooth skin surface, which avoids moisture loss by improving the production of ceramide. In combination with vitamin C, it strongly acts as an antioxidant and helps to reduce the dark spot and to change skin tone, which results in brighter skin (Watters et al., 2009).

13.2.1.4 VITAMIN B5

This Vitamin B5 is commonly known as Pantothenic acid. This Pantothenic acid prevents water loss or moisture loss from the skin; as we know, water is essential for the body as well as the skin. The main purpose behind this is hydration; thus, it glows the skin. The moisture content in the skin is responsible for dryness and flakiness, and due to this, itching will happen. So, to avoid this, pantothenic acid plays a very important role in controlling moisture loss. Also, the beneficiary effect of this pantothenic acid is it protects the skin from redness and dryness as it happens from the UV exposure (Samuel et al., 2013). It plays a major role in the production of glutathione, which acts as an antioxidant and is responsible for the fighting against free radicals (Sheppard et al., 2013).

13.2.1.5 VITAMIN C

Vitamin C which is commonly known as Ascorbic acid. It has the most widely used vitamin for skin care because of its numerous benefits. The ascorbic acid is strongly acted as antioxidants. It has a photo-protective activity and is used to improve the skin tone against sun damage which is occurred from UV exposure. It also helps to fight or opposes the action against the free radical damage. As it has antioxidants property, it targets acne, fine lines, wrinkles, and, ultimately, aging. It also helps to minimize the risk of oxidative stress and helps to heal the wound and infections as it also has anti-inflammatory action. Along with this beneficiary action, it also helps to control melanin production also helps to lighten hyperpigmentation spots and renew the skin tone (Carr & Maggini, 2017). The face serum of vitamin C, which is available in the market, works to build the skin's immune system and is also used for premature aging, which is further seen as a breakdown of the skin barrier. The high concentration of vitamin C in the skin indicates that it has a number of important biological functions that are responsible for good skin health. Which is based on the function of vitamin C; as we have focused on collagen formation and antioxidant protection, the evidence is found as emerging for other activities. Vitamin C acts as a co-factor for the proline and lysine hydroxylases that stabilize the collagen molecule tertiary structure, and it also promotes collagen gene expression (Evans, 2000). Along with this, zinc, in combination with vitamin C, also shows the best result against aging and prevents skin cells from getting damaged (Bendich et al., 1986).

13.2.1.6 VITAMIN K

Vitamin K is commonly known as phytomenaquione, as it is found in the plant source, and mellaquinone, as it is found in animals. This vitamin K is commonly known for its blood clotting function. But it also shows anti-inflammatory action on the skin and has a good effect on the vasculature of the skin. It helps out in this to induce quick blood clotting. As it has anti-inflammatory action, it helps to reduce swelling and bruising in a very duration of time. It is available in the form of a cream formulation for post-surgery wound healing and also to reduce swelling. It is also used for hyperpigmentation and to remove dark circles, commonly known as under-eye circles (Shearer, 1992, 1995).

13.2.1.7 VITAMIN E

Vitamin E is commonly known as Tocopherol. It also shows strong antioxidant property as like vitamin C. As Vitamin E is fat soluble vitamin so, it shows good moisturizer properties and is mainly used to make soothing creams and ointments as pharmaceutical products (Brigelius-Flohé & Traber, 1999). From the tocopherol, alpha-tocopherol is the most active compound, which provides photoprotection to the skin by absorbing UV rays (Herrera & Barbas, 2001). Vitamin E capsule is the marketed product most widely used for skin and hair. As it increases the texture of the hair. These vitamins E also help in the biosynthesis of elastin and collagen; these two are fibrinogen which maintains skin health and avoids wrinkles and fine lines. Also, this collagen and elastin act as a building block to the skin as this is proteinous in nature, so it helps in rejuvenation. Alpha-tocopherol as it mainly acts antioxidant when in combination with vitamin C because they act upon the formation of free radical. This vitamin E is topically used to clear the scars and the burn and soothes the problem of inflammation on the skin. In addition to the benefit of vitamin E, According to the study, vitamin E directly absorbs the UV B radiation, so mainly used in various sunscreen lotions and creams. As everyone knows that UV B radiation is the most commonly cancer-causing ray. So, this Vitamin E is an essential nutrient that is receiving great attention in effective skincare from the cosmeceutical industry. And this strong antioxidant property is more effective than some human-synthesized antioxidants such as glutathione and ubiquinol. So, nowadays, this has more increasing market than any other antioxidant (Chan, 1993).

13.2.1.8 VITAMIN D

Vitamin D is commonly known as Ergocalciferol. This vitamin is commonly used for bone growth, bone strength, reducing inflammation, and boosting immunity (Adams & Hewison, 2010). But now, a recent study shows that Vitamin D is also useful in skin diseases like allergies, eczema, psoriasis, and for dry skin. It is also used to cure redness and pimple-causing germs on the skin. Table 13.3 represents marketed Preparation of Nutraceuticals. Vitamin D facilitates the function of regulating calcium and phosphorous supplements in combination together in the skin so, to prevent further damage. Another from the skin also helps in mood swings and depression-like psychotic disorders (Lips, 2006).

TABLE 13.3 Marketed Preparation of Nutraceuticals.

Marketed Nutraceutical	Ingredients	Manufacturer	Use
ROX®	Taurine, caffeine	ROX America, SA	Used to relieve pain in joints, used in osteoarthritis.
Omega woman	Antioxidants, vitamins	Wassen, Survey	Reduce the risk of heart disease.
Calcitriol D-3®	Calcium and minerals	Cadilla Healthcare Limited	It maintains the calcium levels in the bone.
Proteinex®	Predigested proteins, vitamins, minerals, and carbohydrates.	Pfizer Limited	It is a protein supplement used to build muscle.
Betafactor® capsules	Beta-glucan	Ameriden® International Inc.	Immunity booster.
5-Hour energy	Taurine, caffeine	Living Essentials, USA	Energy blender.
Pediasure®	Protein, vitamins	Abbott Nutrition	Supplement for protein
Revital®	Vitamins and minerals	Ranbaxy Lab Ltd.	Energy booster
Red Bull®	Taurine, caffeine	Austrian Red Bull Gmbh	Energy booster

Source: Adapted from Holick, 2003; Norman, 2012

13.3 CONCLUSION

From the chapter, we have seen how strongly the vitamin is used for skin care in combination with pharmaceuticals which are commonly known as nutraceuticals nowadays. As these vitamins were used so it will be very beneficial for skin as well as hairs and for other usage also. Vitamins have potential action against various diseases, but for skin, it shows numerous benefits, and nutraceutical is playing a big role in this industry. For example, the Vitamin E capsule for skin care and hair care are most widely used it is the nutraceutical product. Vitamins are very beneficial as it regenerates the cell growth as it contains antioxidants like selenium which helps to maintain the texture of the skin and many more; it also helps the skin to prevent from the sun damage. These antioxidants act with coenzymes to prevent skin from aging. So, these vitamins as nutraceuticals for the skin are becoming important these days.

ACKNOWLEDGMENTS

We thank you to the Oriental Education Society College of Pharmacy, Navi Mumbai, Maharashtra, India, and Mahatma Gandhi Vidyamandir's Pharmacy College, Panchavati, Nashik, Maharashtra, India, for their constant support and for providing all facilities to complete this work. Also, many thanks to all the known and unknowns who helped us right from the writing till the publishing of this chapter.

KEYWORDS

- **collagen**
- **elastin**
- **hyperpigmentation**
- **nutraceuticals**
- **retinoid**
- **tocopherol**
- **vitamins**

REFERENCES

Adams, J. S., & Hewison, M., (2010). Update in vitamin D. *J. Clin. Endocrinol. Metab.*

Adams, J. S., & Hewison, M., (2010). Update in vitamin D. *The Journal of Clinical Endocrinology & Metabolism, 95*(2), 471–478.

Ahire, E. D., Sonawane, V. N., Surana, K. R., & Talele, G. S., (2021). Drug discovery, drug-likeness screening, and bioavailability: Development of drug-likeness rule for natural products. In: *Applied Pharmaceutical Practice and Nutraceuticals* (pp. 191–208). Apple Academic Press.

Bendich, A., Machlin, L. J., Scandurra, O., Burton, G. W., & Wayner, D. D. M., (1986). The antioxidant role of vitamin C. *Advances in Free Radical Biology & Medicine, 2*(2), 419–444.

Boelsma, E., Hendriks, H. F., & Roza, L., (2001). Nutritional skin care: Health effects of micronutrients and fatty acids. *The American Journal of Clinical Nutrition, 73*(5), 853–864.

Bouillon, R., Carmeliet, G., Verlinden, L., Van, E. E., Verstuyf, A., Luderer, H. F., Lieben, L., et al., (2008). Vitamin D and human health: Lessons from vitamin D receptor null mice. *Endocrine Reviews, 29*(6), 726–776.

Brigelius-Flohé, R., & Traber, M. G., (1999). Vitamin E: Function and metabolism. *The FASEB Journal, 13*(10), 1145–1155.

Carr, A. C., & Maggini, S., (2017). Vitamin C and immune function. *Nutrients, 9*(11), 1211.

Chan, A. C., (1993). Partners in defense, vitamin E and vitamin C. *Canadian Journal of Physiology and Pharmacology*, *71*(9), 725–731.

Chauhan, B., Kumar, G., Kalam, N., & Ansari, S. H., (2013). Current concepts and prospects of herbal nutraceutical: A review. *Journal of Advanced Pharmaceutical Technology & Research*, *4*(1), 4.

Chen, Q., & Vissers, M. C., (2020). *Vitamin C: New Biochemical and Functional Insights* (Vol. 1). CRC Press.

Chiu, A., & Kimball, A. B., (2003). Topical vitamins, minerals, and botanical ingredients as modulators of environmental and chronological skin damage. *British Journal of Dermatology*, *149*(4), 681–691.

Czajka, A., Kania, E. M., Genovese, L., Corbo, A., Merone, G., Luci, C., & Sibilla, S., (2018). Daily oral supplementation with collagen peptides combined with vitamins and other bioactive compounds improves skin elasticity and has a beneficial effect on joint and general wellbeing. *Nutrition Research*, *57*, 97–108.

Dawson-Hughes, B., Harris, S. S., Palermo, N. J., Ceglia, L., & Rasmussen, H., (2013). Meal conditions affect the absorption of supplemental vitamin D3 but not the plasma 25-hydroxyvitamin D response to supplementation. *Journal of Bone and Mineral Research*, *28*(8), 1778–1783.

DeFelice, S. L., (1995). The nutraceutical revolution: Its impact on food industry R&D. *Trends in Food Science & Technology*, *6*(2), 59–61.

Denu, J. M., (2005). Vitamin B3 and sirtuin function. *Trends in Biochemical Sciences*, *30*(9), 479–483.

Díez-Pérez, A., Olmos, J. M., Nogués, X., Sosa, M., Díaz-Curiel, M., Pérez-Castrillón, J. L., Pérez-Cano, R., et al., (2012). Risk factors for prediction of inadequate response to antiresorptive. *Journal of Bone and Mineral Research*, *27*(4), 817–824.

Evans, W. J., (2000). Vitamin E, vitamin C, and exercise. *The American Journal of Clinical Nutrition*, *72*(2), 647S-652S.

Formelli, F., Carsana, R., Costa, A., Buranelli, F., Campa, T., Dossena, G., Magni, A., & Pizzichetta, M., (1989). Plasma retinol level reduction by the synthetic retinoid fenretinide: A one-year follow-up study of breast cancer patients. *Cancer Research*, *49*(21), 6149–6152.

Graf, J., (2005). Anti-aging skincare ingredient technologies. In: *Cosmetic Dermatology* (pp. 17–28). Springer, Berlin, Heidelberg.

Hennekens, C. H., Buring, J. E., Manson, J. E., Stampfer, M., Rosner, B., Cook, N. R., Belanger, C., et al., (1996). Lack of effect of long-term supplementation with beta carotene on the incidence of malignant neoplasms and cardiovascular disease. *New England Journal of Medicine*, *334*(18), 1145–1149.

Herrera, E., & Barbas, C., (2001). Vitamin E: Action, metabolism and perspectives. *Journal of Physiology and Biochemistry*, *57*(1), 43–56.

Holick, M. F., (2003). Vitamin D deficiency: What a pain it is. In: *Mayo Clinic Proceedings* (Vol. 78, No. 12, pp. 1457–1459). Elsevier.

Holick, M. F., (2003). Vitamin D: A Millenium perspective. *Journal of Cellular Biochemistry*, *88*(2), 296–307.

Ismail, N., Kureishy, N., Church, S. J., Scholefield, M., Unwin, R. D., Xu, J., Patassini, S., & Cooper, G. J., (2020). Vitamin B5 (d-pantothenic acid) localizes in myelinated structures of the rat brain: Potential role for cerebral vitamin B5 stores in local myelin homeostasis. *Biochemical and Biophysical Research Communications*, *522*(1), 220–225.

Jacobson, M. K., & Jacobson, E. L., (2018). Vitamin B3 in health and disease: Toward the second century of discovery. *ADP-Ribosylation and NAD+ Utilizing Enzymes*, 3–8.

Jetter, A., Egli, A., Dawson-Hughes, B., Staehelin, H. B., Stoecklin, E., Goessl, R., Henschkowski, J., & Bischoff-Ferrari, H. A., (2014). Pharmacokinetics of oral vitamin D3 and calcifediol. *Bone*, *59*, 14–19.

Keservani, R. K., Kesharwani, R. K., Sharma, A. K., Vyas, N., & Chadoker, A., (2010b). Nutritional supplements: An overview. *International Journal of Current Pharmaceutical Review and Research, 1*(1), 59–75.

Keservani, R. K., Kesharwani, R. K., Vyas, N., Jain, S., Raghuvanshi, R., & Sharma, A. K., (2010a). Nutraceutical and functional food as future food: A review. *Der Pharmacia Lettre*, *2*(1), 106–116.

Keservani, R. K., Sharma, A. K., & Kesharwani, R. K. (2017). An overview and therapeutic applications of nutraceutical and functional foods. *Recent Advances in Drug Delivery Technology*, 160–201. ISBN:9781522507543.

Keservani, R. K., Sharma, A. K., & Kesharwani, R. K. (2020). *Nutraceuticals and Dietary Supplements: Applications in Health Improvement and Disease Management*. CRC Press. ISBN: 9781771888738.

Kosari, P., Alikhan, A., Sockolov, M., & Feldman, S. R., (2010). Vitamin E and allergic contact dermatitis. *Dermatitis®*, *21*(3), 148–153.

Linder, J., (2012). The science behind vitamins. *Plastic Surgical Nursing*, *32*(4), 180–181.

Lips, P., (2006). Vitamin D physiology. *Progress in Biophysics and Molecular Biology*, *92*(1), 4–8.

Lupo, M. P., (2001). Antioxidants and vitamins in cosmetics. *Clinics in Dermatology*, *19*(4), 467–473.

Makarov, M. V., Trammell, S. A., & Migaud, M. E., (2019). The chemistry of the vitamin B3 metabolome. *Biochemical Society Transactions*, *47*(1), 131–147.

Manela-Azulay, M., & Bagatin, E., (2009). Cosmeceuticals vitamins. *Clinics in Dermatology*, *27*(5), 469–474.

Neuhouser, M. L., Barnett, M. J., Kristal, A. R., Ambrosone, C. B., King, I. B., Thornquist, M., & Goodman, G. G., (2009). Dietary supplement use and prostate cancer risk in the Carotene and retinol efficacy trial. *Cancer Epidemiology and Prevention Biomarkers*, *18*(8), 2202–2206.

Nicoletti, M., (2012). Nutraceuticals and botanicals: Overview and perspectives. *International Journal of Food Sciences and Nutrition*, *63*(sup1), 2–6.

Norman, A., (2012). *Vitamin D*. Elsevier.

Papandreou, D., & Hamid, Z. T. N., (2015). The role of vitamin D in diabetes and cardiovascular disease: An updated review of the literature. *Disease Markers*, *2015*.

Pérez-Sánchez, A., Barrajón-Catalán, E., Herranz-López, M., & Micol, V., (2018). Nutraceuticals for skin care: A comprehensive review of human clinical studies. *Nutrients*, *10*(4), 403.

Pissios, P., (2017). Nicotinamide N-methyltransferase: More than a vitamin B3 clearance enzyme. *Trends in Endocrinology & Metabolism*, *28*(5), 340–353.

Rane, B. R., Bharath, M. S., Patil, R. R., Keservani, R. K., & Jain, A. S. (2020b). Novel approaches in nutraceuticals; Chapter 11. In: Rajesh, K. K., Raj, K. K., & Anil, K. S., (eds.), *Enhancing the Therapeutic Efficacy of Herbal Formulations Through Novel Drug Delivery Systems* (pp. 241–266). IGI Global International Publisher, Pennsylvania, USA. ISBN13: 9781799844532.

Rane, B. R., Patil, A. S., Keservani, R. K., & Jain, A. S., (2020a). Novel approaches in herbal formulation; Chapter 2. In: Rajesh, K. K., Raj, K. K., & Anil, K. S., (eds.), *Enhancing the Therapeutic Efficacy of Herbal Formulations Through Novel Drug Delivery Systems* (pp. 43–68). IGI Global International Publisher, Pennsylvania, USA. ISBN13: 9781799844532.

Rane, B. R., Tadavi, S. A., & Keservani, R. K., (2020c). Naturopathy; Chapter 12. In: Anil, K. S., Raj, K. K., & Surya, P. G., (eds.), *Herbal Product Development* (pp. 321–347). Apple Academic Press, CRC Press, Taylor & Francis Group. ISBN: 9781771888776.

Ritter, S. J., & Smith, J. E., (1996). Multiple retinoids alter liver bile salt-independent retinyl ester hydrolase activity, serum vitamin A, and serum retinol-binding protein of rats. *Biochimica et Biophysica Acta (BBA)-General Subjects, 1291*(3), 228–236.

Ross, A. C., & Harrison, E. H., (2007). Vitamin A: Nutritional aspects of retinoids and carotenoids. *Handbook of Vitamins* (4th edn.), USA: CRC Press Taylor & Francis Group.

Sauve, A. A., (2008). NAD+ and vitamin B3: From metabolism to therapies. *Journal of Pharmacology and Experimental Therapeutics, 324*(3), 883–893.

Schmitt, J., & Ferro, A., (2013). Nutraceuticals: Is there good science behind the hype? *British Journal of Clinical Pharmacology, 75*(3), 585.

Shamloul, N., Hashim, P. W., Nia, J. J., Farberg, A. S., & Goldenberg, G., (2019). The role of vitamins and supplements on skin appearance. *Cutis, 104*(4), 220–224.

Shapiro, S. S., & Saliou, C., (2001). Role of vitamins in skin care. *Nutrition, 17*(10), 839–844.

Sharma, A. K., Keservani, R. K., & Gautam, S. P., (2020). *Herbal Product Development.* Apple Academic Press, CRC Press, Taylor & Francis Group. ISBN: 9781771888776.

Shearer, M. J., (1992). Vitamin K metabolism and nutriture. *Blood Reviews, 6*(2), 92–104.

Shearer, M. J., (1995). Vitamin K. *The Lancet, 345*(8944), 229–234.

Sheppard, S. K., Didelot, X., Meric, G., Torralbo, A., Jolley, K. A., Kelly, D. J., Bentley, S. D., et al., (2013). Genome-wide association study identifies vitamin B5 biosynthesis as a host specificity factor in *Campylobacter*. *Proceedings of the National Academy of Sciences, 110*(29), 11923–11927.

Sunder, S. (2019). Relevant topical skin care products for prevention and treatment of aging skin. *Facial Plastic Surgery Clinics, 27*(3), 413–418.

Surana, K. R., Ahire, E. D., Sonawane, V. N., Talele, S. G., & Talele, G. S., (2021). Informatics and methods in nutrition design and development. *Natural Food Products and Waste Recovery: Healthy Foods, Nutrition Design, and Extraction of Valuable Compounds* (p. 33).

Surana, K. R., Ahire, E. D., Sonawane, V. N., Talele, S. G., & Talele, G. S., (2021). Molecular MODELING: Novel techniques in food and nutrition development. *Natural Food Products and Waste Recovery: Healthy Foods, Nutrition Design, and Extraction of Valuable Compounds* (p. 17).

Tambe, S., Jain, D., Agarwal, Y., & Amin, P. (2021). Hot-melt extrusion: Highlighting recent advances in pharmaceutical applications. *Journal of Drug Delivery Science and Technology, 63*, 102452.

Thiele, J. J., & Ekanayake-Mudiyanselage, S., (2007). Vitamin E in human skin: Organ-specific physiology and considerations for its use in dermatology. *Molecular Aspects of Medicine, 28*(5, 6), 646–667.

Tran, D., Townley, J. P., Barnes, T. M., & Greive, K. A. (2015). An antiaging skin care system containing alpha hydroxy acids and vitamins improves the biomechanical parameters of facial skin. *Clinical, Cosmetic and Investigational Dermatology, 8*, 9.

Vieth, R., (1999). Vitamin D supplementation, 25-hydroxyvitamin D concentrations, and safety. *The American Journal of Clinical Nutrition, 69*(5), 842–856.

Watters, J. L., Gail, M. H., Weinstein, S. J., Virtamo, J., & Albanes, D., (2009). Associations between α-tocopherol, β-carotene, and retinol and prostate cancer survival. *Cancer Research, 69*(9), 3833–3841.

Williams, P. A., Harder, J. M., Foxworth, N. E., Cochran, K. E., Philip, V. M., Porciatti, V., Smithies, O., & John, S. W., (2017). Vitamin B3 modulates mitochondrial vulnerability and prevents glaucoma in aged mice. *Science, 355*(6326), 756–760.

CHAPTER 14

Overview and Recent Advances of Vitamins

ADITI M. KOKANDE,[1] KHEMCHAND R. SURANA,[2] VANDANA N. JAIN,[3] SUNIL K. MAHAJAN,[4] DHANANJAY M. PATIL,[5] and DEEPAK D. SONAWANE[5]

[1]*Department of Pharmaceutical Chemistry, Oriental Education Society College of Pharmacy, Navi Mumbai, Maharashtra, India*

[2]*Department of Pharmaceutical Chemistry, Shreeshakti Shaikshanik Sanstha, Divine College of Pharmacy, Satana, Nashik, Maharashtra, India*

[3]*Department of Pharmacognosy, Oriental Education Society College of Pharmacy, Navi Mumbai, Maharashtra, India*

[4]*Department of Pharmaceutical Chemistry, M.G.V's Samajshri Prashant Dada Hiray, College of Pharmacy, Malegaon, Nashik, Maharashtra, India*

[5]*Department of Pharmaceutics, Shreeshakti Shaikshanik Sanstha, Divine College of Pharmacy, Satana, Nashik, Maharashtra, India*

ABSTRACT

Proteins, as we all know, are the body's building blocks, and they help to create muscle. Vitamins, on the other hand, are a nutrient supply for the body. They carry out all of the body's functions in accordance with their duties. The fundamental reason for this is that vitamins cannot be manufactured in the body and must be obtained from outside sources. Natural sources such as plants, animals, and other species such as algae, fungi, yeast, and microbes must also be included in this foreign source. Vitamins are not considered to be as important in human diets as they once were. However,

Preventive and Therapeutic Role of Vitamins as Nutraceuticals. Khemchand R. Surana, Eknath D. Ahire, Raj K. Keservani, & Rajesh K. Kesharwani (Eds.)

as the value of nutrition grows in importance, so does the demand for these vitamins. Vitamin A is required for regular cell growth, which includes cell creation, immunity, reproduction, and vision. Vitamin A is associated to the rods and cones of the eyes, which are responsible for the eyes' vision feeling. Synaptic misfortune, variations in glucose digestion, oxidative pressure, and declines in thiamine-subordinate cycles, endosomal anomalies, cholinergic brokenness, and lysosomal inconsistencies are among the many modifications that occur in the cerebrums of patients who succumb to AD. Lucy Wills, a biochemist, developed vitamin B9 in the year 1931. Pernicious anemia is treated with vitamin B12. According to a study on Vitamin C, a lack of L-ascorbic acid is linked to pneumonia. Following its recognizable confirmation, several studies looked into the effects of L-ascorbic acid on various disorders. Vitamin D's task entails covering the fundamentals of production, digestion, and atomic component of activity and then examining the effect of vitamin D and metabolites on tissues. It is not primarily concerned with bone mineral digestion guidelines. Vitamin E refers to a group of tocopherols and tocotrienols, the most important of which is a-tocopherol, which has the most significant organic effect. Vitamin K, also known as phylloquinone, is a fat-soluble nutrient found in plants and supplied by microorganisms as menaquinone.

14.1 INTRODUCTION

Vitamins are compounds that come from a variety of sources, including natural, synthetic, and semi-synthetic sources. The discovery of these vitamins is the scientist's greatest accomplishment. As we all know, proteins are the body's building elements, and they aid in the formation of muscle. Vitamins, on the other hand, supply the organism with nutrients (Mejia, 1994). They perform all physiological functions in accordance with their responsibilities. In the year 1912, "Casmir Funk" created the term "vitamin." Vitamins are commonly referred to as vitamins. Then, as time passes, it is referred to as Vitamin. Vitamin is nothing more than an organic molecule that functions chemically in the body (Semba, 2012). Vitamins are a type of important micronutrients that the body needs in extremely small amounts. However, vitamins are extremely beneficial to the proper functioning of the metabolism. This is due to the fact that vitamins cannot be produced by the body and must be obtained from external sources. This foreign source must also include natural sources such as vegetation, animals, and other species such as algae, fungi, yeast, and microbes. Vitamins are no longer regarded as being as crucial to human nutrition as they once were. However, since the value of nutrition has increased in recent years, the need for these vitamins has increased as well (Gibson et al., 2016). There are currently 13 different types of vitamins available. Vitamins were initially produced in the year 1912, and until 1935, there was not enough demand for them to increase their market, and not enough people used to ingest them (Powers, 2003). However, after 1950, as people became more aware of their benefits, they began to ingest vitamins for their health benefits. And as the marketing approach evolves, vitamins are increasingly marketed in terms of their health benefits, and people have become accustomed to taking supplements and vitamins. Vitamins are now considered a valuable dietary supplement (Keservani et al., 2010a, b, 2017, 2020). Vitamins contain a variety of beneficial microorganisms, important botanicals, and synthetic forms (Jacobson & Jacobson, 2018). Vitamin C is the most ancient vitamin and is widely known for its antioxidant properties. After learning about the rising market for vitamins in 2007, the US Code of federal regulations, Section 21 CFR, which governs GMP in the fields of labeling, packaging, and manufacturing, was created to help dietary supplements run more smoothly (Keservani et al., 2020). The US FDA then establishes guidelines for selling it without a prescription because the health benefits outweigh the risks. And the pharmaceutical sector is in charge of all rules for vitamin development, manufacturing, and marketing (Rumberger et al., 2011). Vitamins, as we all know, are beneficial for a variety of reasons, including skin, hair, and sense organs, as well as internal use. As a result, vitamins have both an essential benefit and a higher marketable worth. Many Nobel Prizes have been awarded in the subject of vitamins, such as the well-known history of thiamine, often known as vitamin B1, which was discovered by Dutch medical practitioner Christian Eijkman. Following that, in 1926, a scientist called George Minot was awarded the Nobel Prize for his discovery of vitamin B12 (Rosenberg, 2012; Irwin, 2012). Pellagra disease has also occurred; thus, to deal with this grave condition, scientist Elmer McCollum has been awarded the Nobel Prize for his discovery of Vitamin B5. Many biochemists received Nobel Prizes for significant discoveries in the field of vitamins in 1937 (György, 1964; Board, 1995).

14.1.1 DISCOVERY OF VITAMINS

The discovery of vitamins is listed in Table 14.1.

TABLE 14.1 Discovery of Vitamins

Vitamins	Year Discovered	Scientist
Vitamin A	1912–1914	Elmer V. McCollum and M. Davis
Vitamin B1	1912	Casimir Funk
Vitamin B2	1926	D. T. Smith and E. G. Hendrick
Vitamin B3	1937	Conard Elvehje
Vitamin B5	1939	Richard Kuhn
Vitamin B6	1941	Paul Gyrogy
Vitamin B8	1934	Paul Gyrogy
Vitamin B9	1933	Lucy Wills
Vitamin B12	1948	Karl A. Folkers and Alexander R. Todd
Vitamin C	1912	A hoist and T. Froelich
Vitamin D	1922	Edward Mellanby
Vitamin E	1922	Herbert Evans and Katherine Bishop
Vitamin K	1929	Henrick Dam

14.1.2 CLASSIFICATIONS OF VITAMINS (FIGURE 14.1)

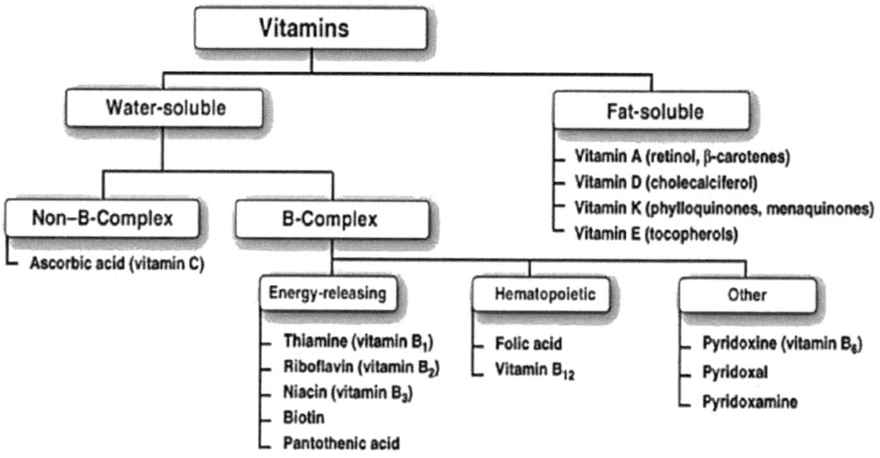

FIGURE 14.1 Classification of vitamins.

14.2 OVERVIEW

14.2.1 VITAMIN A

Vitamin A is also called retinoid, and it is nothing but a fat-soluble vitamin. This vitamin is essential for the normal growth of cells, that is, cell generation, immunity, reproduction, and also the vision. In this case of vision, it is related to the rods and cones of the eyes, which are responsible for the vision sensation of the eyes (Bernstein 1990). In the early days, as if in the 19th century, the scientist belonged to France. After this discovery, a scientist named Nicolai, in the year 1881, he does experiments on mice, and it showed that mice are not able to live only on carbohydrates, fats, minerals, and calcium, but there is another substance that is responsible for their survival of the mice, and that is a vitamin. Vitamin A is responsible for the vision, cell growth, and cell regeneration in the human body. After this experiment which was done by Nicolai again, one experiment was done by a Cambridge biochemist in the year 1906 (Ueland et al., 2017). The results of this experiment were there is a substance that is different from milk, fat, carbohydrates, lipids, and protein (Keservani et al., 2015; Singh et al., 2017b) which protect from eye disease and may help to increase eyesight. Again, one discovery was carried out to prove that vitamin A (Singh et al., 2017a) is a fat-soluble vitamin. As it includes nutritional properties like milk. These were the discoveries that happened to be for vitamin A (Alban, 2011).

14.2.2 VITAMIN B1

Vitamin B1, which is also called thiamine. And which is the first vitamin discovered as B1. The structure of the thiamine includes a pyrimidine rind and a thiazole ring, which is bonded by the methylene group. Thiamine is the term coined by the Dutch medical practitioner named Jacobus Bonitus and which was discovered for the early sign and symptoms of the disease beriberi (Sobczyńska-Malefora & Harrington, 2018). When he used to observe the patients, he notices that the patients are shaking their limbs and can't even walk properly. This is the sign and the symptoms of the disease of beriberi. Then after this, people used to switch on a moderate diet from the source of microorganisms. This shaking of limbs or the tremors which are coming in the hands are now cured. Then scientists discovered the search for thiamine which comes from the source of microorganisms, and people are used to eating it in their diets. To discover this, they first do the experiments on the chicken, but he fails to express whether it is the correct way to express whether it is injecting it by the rice bran or not (Liu, Heying, & Tanumihardjo, 2012). Followed by this, in the year 1936, the scientist named Willaims and Cline established the first formula for the thiamine discovery. And it was the first vitamin discovered as vitamin B1. And which was accepted by the American Chemical Society as a vitamin. Thiamine plays a very vital role in the metabolism of the energy. It also takes part in the catabolism of carbohydrates. If the reduction of thiamine occurred, then the slower of this energy metabolism. This was the early benefits of thiamine when it was discovered (Carr, 2017).

14.2.3 VITAMIN B2

Vitamin B2 is also called riboflavin. This riboflavin was discovered by Richard Kuhn in the year 1922 in Germany. Riboflavin is discovered in a synthetic way and forwarded to the German company. To be followed by this the compound or the molecule was discovered by Kuhn and Paul Gyrogy in the year 1933. In this way, Vitamin B2 is synthesized, which helps to absorb the carbohydrates, fats, proteins, and other nutrients from the body (Mohr, 2009; DeLuca, 2004).

14.2.4 VITAMIN B3

Vitamin B3 is also called nicotinamide. From the early discovery of vitamins in the year 1906, a scientist named Arthur Harden developed the heat-stable heavy molecule, which is required for the fermentation and the production of alcohol. Which is having therapeutic activity? The scientist Joseph Goldberger who is in charge with Unites States Public Health Services, identified that the NAD molecule is present in the molecule, which is responsible for the opposite effects of pellagra (Ferland, 2012). To further discovery, which is observed by Conard Elvehjem from the year 1937, developed two derivatives of nicotinamide which pyridine based. These two derivatives are nothing but the niacin and niacinamide. The bioactive form of nicotinamide is NAD, which is responsible for the therapeutic activity in the disease condition. NAD molecule has a central role in maintaining the homeostasis of the body; along with this, NADP regeneration is used to support cellular reductive needs. This was the early discovery of Vitamin B3 (Gröber et al., 2014; Jacobson et al., 2001).

14.2.5 VITAMIN B5

Vitamin B5 is also called Pantothenic Acid. This vitamin is discovered by Dr. R. J. Willaims in the year 1933 (Bell, 1987). Pantothenic acid is responsible for the synthesis of coenzyme A and also helps to decarboxylating pyruvate in citric acid cycle. According to human biology, this acid is needed for the synthesis of steroids to maintain the metabolism, red blood cells, and neuronal activity, and also induces the production and stimulation of antibodies (Evans, 1962). This pantothenic acid has numerous benefits and has no side effects, so they are useful to cure various diseases, and no such disease condition occurred till this (Zile, 1998).

14.2.6 VITAMIN B6

Pyridoxine is another name for vitamin B6. This pyridoxine was discovered by Rudolf Peters, a scientist. The rats were used in an experiment to synthesize this vitamin in a semi-synthetic form. Scientists conducted this research on rats with the addition of thiamine and riboflavin, but only this pyridoxine treated the disease of rat acrodynia (Zile, 1998). Further research on this pyridoxine has been conducted on dogs, pigs, and rats, with some animals developing anemia-like symptoms. To keep up with the expanding therapeutic activity of pyridoxine research, in the year 1938, scientist Samuel Lepkovsky isolated and crystallized the pyridoxine chemical (Ablin et al., 2015). Many scientists, including Lesile Harris, Karl Folkers, and Richard Kuhn, proposed pyridine derivatives as a pyridine-based pyridoxine derivative. Again, according to this study, the animated pyridoxine product has a more therapeutic effect in animals with varied illness states. Pyridoxal and pyridoxamine are examples of compounds discovered (Sauve, 2008). In 1933, crystalline vitamin B1 became available. The extraction of pure riboflavin provided the key to a genuine breakthrough in the study of the vitamin B2 problem (Denu, 2005).

14.2.7 VITAMIN B8

Vitamin B8 is also called Biotin. This vitamin was discovered by a scientist named Dean Burk, who is an American biochemist who co-founded the biotin. In the early 1900s, biotin was called Vitamin H because it functions as a coenzyme. This coenzyme is involved in the synthesis of fatty acids and amino acids like valine and isoleucine (Sheppard et al., 2013). It also helps in the regeneration of gluconeogenesis. Biotin helps to release carboxylase enzymes. Biotin also helps in some biochemical functions like the formation of malonyl CO A from acetyl CO A and Pyruvate carboxylase reaction, where is from pyruvate forms from oxaloacetate in the mitochondria. It also helps with the formation of beta-methyl carbonyl CO A (Liang et al., 2021). Biotin is a useful component for cell growth, production of fatty acids, metabolism of fats, and synthesis of amino acids. Biotin plays a very important role in the citric acid cycle, which is the process where biochemical energy is generated when in the process of aerobic respiration. Also, another benefit of biotin is that it controls blood sugar levels. Deficiency of biotin is rare and mild and has no more side effects, and it has therapeutic uses in many metabolic functions (Mooney et al., 2009).

14.2.8 VITAMIN B9

Folic Acid is another name for B9. In 1931, biochemist Lucy Wills was the first to find this vitamin. She pointed out that this vitamin has a food source to prevent anemia and meet the needs of a pregnant woman. This folate can help stop a wide range of health problems (Mooney et al., 2009). Most likely in megaloblastic anemia and birth defects of the brain and spinal cord. Chronically low levels of folate may make you more likely to get dementia, depression, neuropathy, and some cancers. But people often forget this. Rarely is the folate status of a patient checked after treatment for a previously known deficiency has ended. People also don't know much about the use of functional markers of folate status and the possible bad effects of taking too much folic acid. Folic acid taken before conception has been shown to protect against spina bifida, which is one of the most important ways folates help keep people healthy (Ueland et al., 2017). Folic acid supplements were given to pregnant women on a regular basis, and in many countries, enriched grain products had to be fortified by law. Folate deficiency is most often caused by not eating enough. Folate deficiency can also be caused by a high turnover of folate. This can happen during pregnancy, breastfeeding, skin diseases like psoriasis and blood disorders. Other major causes include conditions that make it hard for the body to absorb nutrients (Bernstein, 1990).

14.2.9 VITAMIN B12

Vitamin B12 is also called cyanocobalamin. This vitamin is discovered by Folkers scientists in the year 1947. When the synthesis occurred, he found the tiny, bright red crystals of the vitamin. And the scientist tested those crystals on patients who were suffering from anemia, and surprisingly, the effects of those crystals were found on pernicious anemia. The scientist is from a microbiology background, and later on, they worked with the agriculture department (Bikle & Pillai, 1993). And they isolated a bacterium culture from the liver extracts. When after a few days, that culture grows, and it appears in red color. So, that red color compound was nothing but the Vitamin B12 (Cyanocobalamin) compound. As the beneficial growth of vitamin B12 was observed then, it often consumed by animals, and the result was found that the livestock of animal breeds has been increased. The availability of these vitamins results in dietary supplements, and the foods which are rich in vitamins are increased in healthy food habits (Leklem, 1990).

14.2.10 VITAMIN C

Vitamin C is also called citric acid. A scientist named Albert Szent Gyorgyi isolated a substance from the adrenal gland and named it hexuronic acid. After this discovery, followed by this for four years, the scientist named Charles Glen King also separated the same compound that is hexuronic acid which is having same chemical structure; this discovery was made in the year 1933 (Malouf & Grimley, 2003). As the study went further, scientists had been discovered that this compound has a citrus activity which belongs to some citrus fruits. This discovery of fruits is shown in the tropical and subtropical regions of some countries, like in Asia and China. In the year 1965 Florida and in 1769 California, the first production of Vitamin C has been observed there. Then as increased in production, their marketed value also increased (Agnew-Blais et al., 2015). It has a property like an increase in total sugar, and it will decrease in acidity ultimately. It has a high content of ascorbic acid found. Also, it can be identified as a change in the color of the peel and an increase in the size of the fruit. And this will indicate the ripening and malnutrition of the citrus fruit. This newly established citrus fruit has many macronutrients like dietary fiber, sugars, and carbohydrates also (Allen, 2009).

14.2.11 VITAMIN D

Vitamin D is also called Cholecalciferol. This vitamin was isolated by the scientist Elmer V. McCollum who was a chemist from the University of Wisconsin. In the early years that is from 1922, the discovery of a child from the country Poland was detected with rickets disease by the medical practitioner Sniadecki (Allen, 2009). The children who were detected by this disease were from that area where usually not so sunlight is exposed, and their deformed bones are observed due to lack of sunlight. After the discovery of this disease ,medical practitioners observed all the rural areas from that country nearby Poland, and they saw the results of the children suffering from rickets. Followed by this evidence, the molecule Vitamin D, which is a synthetic hormone, has been isolated to cure rickets. This was the early discovery that occurred for Vitamin D, and their beneficiary use was normal but highly effective (Hemilä, 2017).

14.2.12 VITAMIN E

Vitamin E is also called Tocopherol. The beneficial effects of vitamin E were developed by the scientist Herbert McLean Evans in the year 1922. The scientist investigated the antioxidant effects of tocopherol. This vitamin shows the opposite effects on reproduction; it reduces the reproductive capacity of humans when consumed in high amounts. From the early days, the antioxidant inositols were shown to have physical and chemical properties of those inhibitory components from wheat germ, lettuce, palm oils, and cottonseed oil and are separated from this compound (Adams & Hewison, 2010). Tocopherol has strong free radical activity, and this activity serves as an antioxidant property. This several properties of tocopherol group are synthesized from the plant derivatives. Followed by this research also, the chemical properties of tocopherol have been found, and chemically tocopherol has been found in three different forms that are alpha, beta, gamma, and delta. Along with this research about tocopherol, there was a new effect found in the year 1938 that is for infants. This study is all about retinal hemorrhage and intraventricular damage in children. Based upon the severity and the premature birth condition of the infants, vitamin E was helpful for that. These all were the early benefits of vitamin E when there was a discovery and new research was in progress (Holick, 2003).

14.2.13 VITAMIN K

Vitamin K is additionally called Phytomenaquinone. This Vitamin K right off the bat was disconnected by researcher Dam in the year 1929. He observed this nutrient when he was doing the analysis on chicks on a lipid-inadequate eating routine. Dam instituted the term coagulation nutrient to portray this new substance. In the last part of the 1930s, a few gatherings distinguished the causative specialist answerable for the antihemorrhagic properties of hay. Primary assurance of nutrient K1 was the aftereffect of work from a few research facilities. The stereochemical task came a lot later from Mayer. Extra examinations disengaged and portrayed related materials. Nutrient K2 was first found in rotting fish dinner; it is a translucent compound and is recognized by its rehashing isoprenyl units. Nutrient K3 is the most straightforward type of the nutrient (Bikle, 2009). The K nutrients are named after the first nutrient and the quantity of carbon molecules in the side chain. Utilizing this show, nutrient K2 is so named on the grounds that it contains 20 carbon molecules in the chain. In the natural writing, nutrient K2 is often alluded to as menaquinone and is additionally assigned by the quantity of isoprene units in the side chain. Nutrient K1 is insoluble in water and is dissolvable in 70% liquor, chloroform, oil ether, benzene, and hexane. Nutrient K1 is steady in the air yet ought to be safeguarded from light. Albeit unsound in a soluble base, the nutrient is steady in an acidic medium (Brigelius Flohé & Traber, 1999).

14.3 RECENT ADVANCES

14.3.1 VITAMIN A

Higher dietary intakes of retinol, carotenoids, soil products, or a mix of these have been linked to a lower risk of cellular breakdown in the lungs, non-Hodgkin lymphoma, pancreatic disease, oral cavity malignant growth, laryngeal disease, esophageal malignant growth, ovarian malignant growth, glioma, and bladder malignant growth. Even so, other observational studies have found no link between vitamin intake and the risk of liver cancer, non-Hodgkin lymphoma, colorectal disease, prostate cancer, or any cancer (Fritsche et al., 2017).

Some early clinical evidence suggests that taking more vitamin A may lower the risk of some malignant growths but increase the risk of other types of malignant growths, heart disease morbidity and mortality, and death from any cause. The models are listed below (Van Winckel et al., 2009).

The Carotene and Retinol Efficacy Trial (CARET) included 18,314 male and female current and former smokers with a 20 pack-year history of cigarette smoking, which is the same as smoking 1 pack per day for a long time or 2 packs per day for a long time, as well as some men who worked with asbestos and have a higher risk of cellular breakdown in the lungs. The study had people take supplements with 30 mg beta-carotene and 25,000 IU (7,500 mcg RAE) of retinyl palmitate or a placebo every day for six years to find out how likely it was that lung cells would break down (Shearer, 1992).

A follow-up study watched the CARET people for another six years after they stopped taking the review supplements. At this point, the differences between the intercession and false treatment groups in the risk of cellular breakdown in the lungs were not yet big enough to measure. However, women in the mediation group had a 33% higher risk of cellular breakdown in the lungs. A different CARET focus on data study found that men who took the two supplements had a 35% lower risk of nonaggressive prostate cancer during the four-year dynamic preliminary but not during the six-year postintervention period (Vermeer, 2012). The Alpha-Tocopherol, Beta-Carotene (ATBC) Cancer Prevention Study found that beta-carotene supplements made it more likely for smokers' lungs to lose cells. Around 29,133 male smokers between the ages of 50 and 69 who smoked an average of 20.4 cigarettes per day for an average of 35.9 years were given 50 mg/day of alpha-tocopherol, 20 mg/day of beta-carotene, both alpha-tocopherol and beta-carotene, or a placebo for five to eight years. Even though beta-carotene supplements increased the risk of cells breaking down in the lungs by 18%, they had a big effect on how often different cancers happened (van der Wielen et al., 1996). People who took beta-carotene died 8% faster, mostly because their lung cells broke down and they got ischemic heart disease. After that, a report kept track of 25,563 of these members for 18 more years. During this time, members stopped taking the enhancers, but they still smoked. Three other preliminary clinical studies found no link between taking vitamin A or beta-carotene supplements and the number of times cells broke down in the lungs or how many people died from it. In one study, 22,071 male doctors between the ages of 40 and 84 were given either 50 mg of beta carotene every other day or a placebo for a long time. At the start of the review, 11% of the doctors were current smokers, and 38% had smoked in the past. The results showed that there were no differences between the groups in the number of cases of cell death in the lungs, the number of dangerous neoplasms, or the number of people who died from malignant growth. Around 7,627 women, with an average age of 60, 4 years, were given 50 mg beta-carotene every other day, 600 IU of vitamin E every other day, 500 mg of L-ascorbic acid every day, or a placebo for a mean of 9.4 years. At the start of the survey, 15% of the women were current smokers, and 41% had smoked in the past (Eshak et al., 2019).

14.3.2 VITAMIN B1

Nobel Prize-winning research in the 19th and 20th centuries linked to the discovery of thiamine discovered that a lack of thiamine in people causes a common "infection" known as beriberi, which has a large neurological component. By the 1930s, a ternion of gross memory abandons for current occasions, confusion, and confabulation were required for the diagnosis of Korsakoff psychosis (Kalus et al., 2008). Early trials in 1939 used these models to treat KS patients with a good diet and a thiamine supplement and found that those who got a lot of thiamine had a recovery that was nearly multiple times as good as those who didn't. Synaptic misfortune, changes in glucose digestion, oxidative pressure, decreases in thiamine-subordinate cycles, endosomal anomalies, cholinergic brokenness, lysosomal inconsistencies, and modified calcium elements, as well as changes in numerous other factors, occur in the cerebrums of patients who succumb to AD. Any of these disorders could be the cause of Alzheimer's disease (Wang et al., 2018). To be sure, immunocytochemical markers suggest that oxidative pressure is more common in AD than plaques or NFTs, and oxidative pressure markers in the pee of animals hereditarily designed to cause plaques to disappear before plaque development in the cerebrum. The link between cerebrospinal fluids indicators of amyloid and tau, as measured by fluorodeoxyglucose positron emission tomography, and glucose digestion has been studied extensively (Palacios et al., 2014).

14.3.3 VITAMIN B2

Riboflavin is remarkable among the water-dissolvable nutrients in that milk and dairy items make the best commitment to its admission in Western eating regimens. Meat and fish are likewise great wellsprings of riboflavin, and certain leafy foods, particularly dim green vegetables, contain sensibly high fixations. Biochemical indications of exhaustion emerge inside a couple of long stretches of dietary deprivation. Unfortunately, riboflavin status in Western nations is by all accounts of most worry for the old and youth, notwithstanding the variety of riboflavin-rich food sources accessible. Notwithstanding, discrepancies between dietary admission information and biochemical information recommend either that necessities are higher than until recently suspected or that biochemical edges for inadequacy are improper (Astorg, 1997). This chapter audits current proof that diets low in riboflavin present explicit wellbeing gambles. There is sensibly great proof that unfortunate riboflavin status slows down iron taking care of and con recognitions for the etiology of pallor when iron admissions are low. Various systems for this have been proposed, remembering the impacts on the gastrointestinal plot that could think twice about the treatment of different supplements. Riboflavin lack has been ensnared as a gamble factor for malignant growth, albeit this has not been sufficiently settled in people (Stabler, 2013). Momentum interest is centered on the job that riboflavin plays in deciding circling convergences of homocysteine, a gamble factor for cardiovascular illness. Riboflavin inadequacy is endemic in populations drinking little milk or meat items. A decrease in the utilization of endless milk items in Western nations might add to the unfortunate riboflavin status announced in segments of the populace, especially youngsters. Subclinical riboflavin lack might add to expanded groupings of plasma homocysteine, with a related expanded hazard of cardiovascular illness. It might likewise be related to the impeded treatment of iron and night visual deficiency. The significance to people of a portion of the impacts of riboflavin inadequacy seen in animal concentrates still needs to be laid out. Ebb and flow exploration of garlic wellbeing significance connects with the significance of riboflavin as an element in safeguarding against cardiovascular infections and disease. Corneal vascularization and corneal haziness have been portrayed in creatures taken care of diets low in riboflavin. Waterfalls have likewise been depicted in creatures that took care of riboflavin-inadequate weight control plans (Oh & Brown, 2003). The significance of riboflavin lack in the etiology of waterfalls in old people isn't completely perceived. All the more, as of late, it was conjectured that riboflavin deficiency might be related to night visual impairment in some communities and that further developing riboflavin status could upgrade the improvement in night visual impairment evoked by vitamin A. Venkataswamy announced riboflavin-responsive night blindness in India (Baik & Russell, 1999).

14.3.4 VITAMIN B3

Vitamin B3 (niacin) is a water-dissolvable nutrient that happens in two structures: nicotinamide and its corrosive structure, nicotinic corrosive. Cell niacin can be obtained from two unmistakable courses. Niacin can be made in the body from the forerunner tryptophan, which is acquired from food varieties wealthy in this amino corrosive. The novel NADC-subordinate sirtuin response and its aversion to cell nicotinamide levels give an impeccable component to directing the pace of deacetylation and the development of OAADPr. The new examinations featured here have given a sub-atomic comprehension of nicotinamide hindrance and its association with the synergist component of deacetylation (Stabler & Allen, 2004). Along with late cell studies, this information proposes new physiological jobs for niacin and the likelihood that a piece of the medical advantages of niacin feed through pathways interceded by sirtuins. Nonetheless, future investigations are expected to lay out the physiological connection between these medical advantages and sirtuin-managed pathways. Maybe the most telling will be to lay out whether niacin treatment straightforwardly hinders sirtuins or, on the other hand, up-controls these catalysts by means of an expanded NADC blend. It is essential to specify that, albeit just nicotinamide restrains sirtuins, both nicotinic corrosive and nicotinamide lead to expanded cell NADC creation (Sauve, 2008).

14.3.5 VITAMIN B5

Animal pathogens and symbionts can spread more easily when they can live on more than one host species. However, they must quickly adapt to each new host. For organisms like Campylobacter, the genome size isn't very big. Genome-wide association studies could help find the genes that cause important phenotypes, but they haven't been done on bacteria very often. We show an association mapping method that works for both core and accessory genome variation and takes into account how bacteria are made up of clones (Denu, 2005). Campylobacter is a common cause of gastroenteritis in people because it is found in many farm animals and spreads through meat and poultry that has been contaminated. We used our association mapping method to find the factors that helped 192 Campylobacter isolates from cattle, chickens, and other hosts adapt to these hosts. Phylogenetic analysis showed that some lineages were strongly linked to certain hosts but that some lineages switched hosts often. A host association signal was found in a group of seven genes. Genes from this area were almost always found in cattle, but they were often missing in chickens and wild birds. Three of the seven genes tell the body how to make vitamin B5. We found that isolates from cattle were better able to grow in media with fewer vitamins B5. We think this may be because the bacteria have adapted to what the host eats (Ismail et al., 2020).

14.3.6 VITAMIN B6

Vitamin B-6 is a water-solvent nutrient originally found as a figure that restored dermatitis in rodents. There are 6 types of vitamin B-6 found in well-evolved creatures. The normally happening types of the nutrient incorporate pyridoxine, pyridoxal, pyridoxamine, and their individual monophosphorylated subsidiaries (PNP, PLP, and PMP). PN, PL, and PM are switched over completely to pyridoxal 59-phosphate (PLP) through the successive activities of a kinase that phosphorylates the 59 hydroxymethyl gathering and pyridoxamine phosphate oxidase (PNPO), which follows up on PNP and PMP. PLP is a naturally dynamic type of nutrient that capacity as a chemical cofactor as well as a controller for compound-catalyzed responses (Malouf & Evans, 2003). This chapter shows that Gold-standard biomarkers of PLP work are deficient. PLP subordinate pathways contrast in their aversion to changes in vitamin B-6 status, and numerous serum vitamin B-6 practical biomarkers change because of the $1 extra supplement lacks of physiologic states. Current ways to deal with recognizing metabolic/utilitarian biomarkers of vitamin B-6 status include concurrent appraisal of a board of metabolites associated with the PLP-subordinate pathways of tryptophan catabolism, one-carbon digestion, and trans sulfuration including creatine, cystathionine, kynurenic corrosive, and 3-hydroxykynurenine (Leklem, 2001). Supplemental vitamin B-6 has been demonstrated to be advantageous for remedial treatment of specific grown-up beginning clinical circumstances. The mix of supplemental L-methylfolate, methylcobalamin, and PLP increments epidermal nerve fiber thickness in the lower limit of patients with diabetic fringe neuropathy and diminishes the related paresthesias as well as dysesthesias. PN treatment might be useful for kidney relocate beneficiaries with essential hyperoxaluria type 1. In 2014, the FDA endorsed the utilization of doxylamine-pyridoxine treatment for the treatment of sickness and heaving during pregnancy (Mooney et al., 2009).

14.3.7 VITAMIN B8

Biotin, which is also known as nutrient H or B8, is a key cofactor for CO_2-controlling chemicals in all three spaces of life. In the last couple of years, scientists have learned a lot more about how plants digest biotin, both at the atomic and cell levels, and a few unique highlights are coming to light. Biotin synthesis in plants is clearly split between the cytosol and the mitochondria. Compounds that use biotin are also spread out in different parts of the plant cell. The mitochondria are the most important of these parts (Alban, 2011). In this chapter, I'll talk about what we know about how biotin is mixed, controlled, and put into different parts of plant cells. Through a better understanding of how to guide, store, and use the nutrient, these advances make testing possible for plant biotechnology. Understanding how the biotin biosynthetic pathway talks to other metabolic pathways and how the growing role of mitochondria in plant growth and development is linked to the way nutrients are mixed is also very difficult. As scientists learn more about how plants break down biotin, they will be able to control the biotin pathway through genetic engineering in a more focused and coordinated way. Rébeillé et al. (2007) says that biotin is a part of some cycles that make biochemicals that are used for a wide range of good and modern purposes. For example, plant seed oils, which are made with the help of acetyl-CoA carboxylase, are an important source of food for both humans and animals. They are also used in medicine, cosmetics, cleaners, and even biofuels, among other things. Biotin is also added to many foods, feeds, and medicines, but it is mostly made in a lab through a chemical cycle. So, the development of biotin in natural conditions, especially in plants, as opposed to engineered science, may be helpful, especially for getting good public feedback (Sarma, 1944).

14.3.8 VITAMIN B9

Folate is a key part of getting ready for uracil to join DNA and for DNA to become less methylated. Methionine synthase slows down when there isn't enough vitamin B12. This makes it harder for S-adenosyl methionine (SAM) to gather in one spot, which could slow down DNA methylation and make folate unavailable for the conversion of dUMP to dTMP (Sobczyska-Malefora & Harrington, 2018). Most likely, chromosomes break because of unneeded uracil misincorporation into DNA. This is a mutagenic sore that breaks DNA strands when they are being fixed. *In vitro* and *in vivo* tests on human cells show that chromosomal breaks, too much uracil in the DNA, the growth of micronuclei, hypomethylation of the DNA, and the loss of mitochondrial DNA are all caused by not getting enough folate (Guilland & Aimone-Gastin, 2013). *In vivo* studies show that folate, a lack of vitamin B9, and high plasma homocysteine (a metabolic sign of folate deficiency) are all linked to both a higher number of micronuclei and shorter telomeres. Studies done in the lab show that genomic instability in human cells is limited when there is more than 100 nmol/L of folic acid in the culture medium (Kunisawa et al., 2012). Intervention studies on people have shown that (i) DNA hypomethylation, chromosome breaks, uracil consolidation, and micronucleus arrangement are limited when red cell folate concentration is more than 700 nmol/L; and (ii) micronucleus development is limited when plasma concentration of vitamin B9 is more than 300 pmol/L and plasma homocysteine is under 7.5 mol/L. These fixes are possible at folate (e.g., >400 g/day) and vitamin B9 (e.g., >2 g/day) intake levels at or above the current recommended daily allowances, depending on a person's ability to store and use these nutrients, which can vary due to genetic and epigenetic differences (Fenech, 2012). Researchers are writing more and more about how natural differences in folate and vitamin B9 transport and digestion have a big effect on some of the best DNA damage biomarkers used in food concentrates, such as lymphocyte micronuclei, chromosome variations and uracil consolidation, and oxidized guanine (Chapeau et al., 2016).

14.3.9 VITAMIN B12

Vitamin B-12 inadequacy and consumption are normal in more well-off nations, especially among the older, and are most pervasive in less fortunate populations all over the planet. Cobalamin is one of a handful of nutrients that are delivered monetarily by bacterial fermentation. This is on the grounds that the synthetic blend of the nutrient is excessively intricate to consider for industry. There has consequently been some huge examination into exploring the atomic hereditary qualities and organic chemistry of cobalamin biosynthesis with a view towards improving the creation of B12 by microbes (Brown, 2005). Without a doubt, it was this approach created by the Rhone-Poulenc organization that prompted ^ the explanation of the vigorous biosynthetic pathway for nutrient B12 and which permitted the organization to take out a few licenses on augmenting cobalamin union. The examination embraced by Rhone-Poulenc led to a creation type of Pseudomonas denitrificans, which was produced utilizing the obtained data on cobalamin biosynthesis. More than a long-term period, this brought about an expansion in B12 in *P. denitrificans* of roughly 100-crease. There are north of 30 qualities engaged with cobalamin biosynthesis, and the definite licenses recommend that something like 10 of these qualities have had their duplicate number expanded. For example, it was noticed that raising the quality bunch expanded cobalamin creation by 30%, while intensification of cobA and cobE brought about a further 20% upgrade (Baik & Russell, 1999). In addition, almost certainly, quality record and interpretation components were altered to upgrade the creation of the pathway chemicals. The analysts additionally hoped to design the pathway by supplanting one of the vital administrative compounds of the pathway that showed substrate hindrance with a variation that no longer had this undesirable trademark. In this manner, upgraded transition along the pathway could be accomplished by supplanting the uroporphyrinogen methyltransferase with a variation from a methanogen. One of the restricting variables for cobalamin creation is the amalgamation of the lower pivotal ligand, dimethyl benzimidazole (DMB). The Rhone-Poulenc scientists tracked down that overproducing a protein (Hodgkin et al., 1956).

14.3.10 VITAMIN C

In the early review, L-ascorbic acid insufficiency was related to pneumonia. After its recognizable proof, various examinations explored the impacts of L-ascorbic acid on different diseases. A sum of 148 creature concentrates on showed that L-ascorbic acid might lighten or forestall diseases brought about by microscopic organisms, infections, and protozoa. The most broadly concentrated on human disease is the normal virus. The L-ascorbic acid organization doesn't diminish the typical rate of colds in everyone, yet it divides the number of colds in genuinely dynamic individuals. Consistently managed L-ascorbic acid has abbreviated the length of colds, demonstrating an organic impact. In any case, the job of L-ascorbic acid in like manner, cold treatment is hazy (Chan, 1993). L-ascorbic acid seems to apply a large number of gainful consequences for cell elements of both the inborn and versatile resistant framework. Despite the fact that L-ascorbic acid is an intense cancer prevention agent safeguarding the body against endogenous and exogenous oxidative difficulties, almost certainly, its activity as a cofactor for various biosynthetic and quality administrative compounds assumes a key part in its resistant regulating impacts. L-ascorbic acid animates neutrophil relocation to the site of contamination, upgrades phagocytosis and oxidant age, and microbial killing. Simultaneously, it safeguards tissue from unreasonable harm by improving neutrophil apoptosis and leeway by macrophages and diminishing neutrophil corruption and NETosis. In this manner, it is clear that L-ascorbic acid is fundamental for the resistant framework to mount and support a sufficient reaction against microorganisms while keeping away from exorbitant harm to the host (Evans, 2000). L-ascorbic acid has all the earmarks of being ready to both forestall and treat respiratory and foundational contaminations by improving different insusceptible cell capacities. Prophylactic anticipation of contamination requires dietary L-ascorbic acid admissions that give essentially sufficient, in the event that it is not immersing plasma levels (i.e., 100–200 mg/day), which improves cell and tissue levels. Interestingly, treatment of laid-out contaminations requires altogether higher (gram) portions of the nutrient to make up for the expanded metabolic interest. Epidemiological investigations show that hypovitaminosis C is still moderately normal in Western populaces, and L-ascorbic acid insufficiency is the fourth driving supplements lack in the United States. Reasons incorporate diminished consumption joined with restricted body stores. Expanded needs happen because of contamination and smoking, battling diseases, and illnesses with oxidative and provocative parts, e.g., type 2 diabetes, and so on. Guaranteeing satisfactory admission of L-ascorbic acid through the eating regimen or by means of supplementation, particularly in gatherings, for example, the old or in people presented to take a chance with factors for L-ascorbic acid inadequacy, is expected for appropriate insusceptible capacity and protection from contaminations (Carr & Maggini, 2017).

14.3.11 VITAMIN D

There is recharged interest in vitamin D combination, digestion, and activity. The two chief main thrusts for level interest can be followed to:

i. The declining, overall pattern to wholesome vitamin D deficiency; and
ii. New information with respect to the nonhormonal, intracrine, and paracrine activities of 1-hydroxylated vitamin D metabolites in man.

This addresses a multiplying somewhat recently and a 15% increment somewhat recently. In the a couple of years, there has been a developing appreciation for the numerous jobs of vitamin D and its dynamic metabolites in an enormous number of tissues. This has been invigorated by the appreciation that most tissues in the body have receptors for the dynamic type of vitamin D, 1, 25 dihydroxy vitamin D [1,25(OH)2D] or calcitriol. These receptors are named properly vitamin D receptors (VDRs), and tissues with VDR are potential objective tissues. Besides, a large number of these tissues additionally contain the chemical CYP27B1, liable for changing over the major coursing metabolite of vitamin D, 25 hydroxyvitamin D (25OHD), to 1, 25(OH)2D. The guideline of CYP27B1 in these nonrenal tissues, by and large, contrasts from that in the kidney and might be more substrate-subordinate (Adams & Hewison, 2010). This has prompted the idea that support of satisfactory 25OHD levels in the blood is expected for vitamin D guideline of an enormous number of physiologic capacities past that of the exemplary activities engaged with bone mineral digestion. This survey is expected first to cover the rudiments of vitamin D creation, digestion, and atomic component of activity and afterward inspect the effect of vitamin D and metabolites on tissues that are not primarily worried about guidelines of bone mineral digestion (Holick, 2003). Two types of vitamin D exist nutrient D3 or cholecalciferol and nutrient D2 or ergocalciferol. The previous is created in the skin affected by UVB radiation (UVR); the last option is delivered by UVR in an assortment of plant materials and yeast. Contrasts exist in their limiting to the significant vehicle protein in blood, vitamin D restricting protein, and in their digestion due to the distinctions in the science of their side chains, with the outcome that solitary portions of D2 lead to bring down degrees of circling 25OHD than single dosages of D3, albeit everyday organization of D2 and D3 keeps up with tantamount degrees of 25OHD. At the tissue level, these distinctions are minor in that the biological movement of 1, 25(OH)2D2 and 1,25(OH)2D3 give off an impression of being similar, basically regarding restricting to VDR. Subsequently, references to vitamin D or D metabolites will allude to the two structures except if generally demonstrated with a particular addendum (Lips, 2006).

14.3.12 VITAMIN E

Vitamin E has been known as a fundamental supplement for generations, beginning around 1922; we are a long way from figuring out the components of its physiological capacities. Vitamin E is the term for a gathering of tocopherols and tocotrienols, of which a-tocopherol has the most noteworthy organic action. Because of the powerful cell reinforcement properties of tocopherols, the effect of a-tocopherol in the counteraction of ongoing infections accepted to be related with oxidative pressure has frequently been examined, and advantageous impacts have been illustrated. Late perceptions that the a-tocopherol moves protein in the liver explicitly figures out RRR-a-tocopherol from all approaching tocopherols for fusing into plasma lipoproteins and that a-tocopherol has flagging capacities in vascular smooth muscle cells that can't be applied by different types of tocopherols with comparable antioxidative properties, have brought interest up in the jobs of vitamin E past its antioxidative capacity (Niki & Traber, 2012). Additionally, γ-tocopherol could have works separated from being a cancer prevention agent. It is a nucleophile ready to trap electrophilic mutagens in lipophilic compartments and produces a metabolite that works with natriuresis. The digestion of vitamin E is similarly muddled. Abundance a-tocopherol is changed over into a-CEHC and discharged in the pee. Different tocopherols, similar to g-and d-tocopherol, are quantitatively corrupted and discharged in the pee as the related CEHCs. All-rac-α-tocopherol contrasted with RRR-α-tocopherol is specially debased to a-CEHC. Subsequently, there should be a particular sub-atomic job of RRR-a-tocopherol that is directed by a framework that sorts, disseminates, and debases the various types of vitamin E, however, has not yet been distinguished. α-Tocopherol likewise seems remarkable in managing phosphorylation overflows. Such a job might be significant in coronary illness where cell grip, multiplication, and oxidant creation may be generally altered through vitamin E-touchy pathways. γ-Tocopherol is special in being a powerful nucleophile and producing a metabolite, g-CEHC, with a captivating pharmacological capacity, natriuresis (Brigelius-Flohé & Traber, 1999). The previous may add to the rummaging of electrophilic mutagens, the last option to the anticipation of cardiovascular illness by bringing down pulse. Considering the massive contrasts in digestion and, therefore, biopotency of the singular tocopherols, it isn't to be expected that numerous epidemiological and mediation studies meaning to elucidate assumed vitamin E impacts that didn't consider the metabolic contrasts between tocopherols (Chan, 1993).

14.3.13 VITAMIN K

Vitamin K is a fat-soluble nutrient, present in plants as phylloquinone and delivered by microbes as menaquinone. It is going about as a cofactor for γ-glutamyl carboxylase. This compound is answerable for post-translational alteration of some glutamate side chains to γ-carboxyglutamate. Most of the carboxylated proteins work in blood coagulation and in calcium homeostasis. Since its disclosure over a long time back, it has been evident that vitamin K assumes a fundamental part in keeping up with typical coagulation (Shearer, 1995). Ongoing work plays explained its part as a co-factor for GGCX, a significant chemical not just for the enactment of vitamin K-subordinate coagulation factors yet for a scope of other Gla proteins. The capacity of a few of these Gla proteins isn't yet clarified. More essential exploration on the development of these catalysts in the baby and infant and on the movement of their various aggregates still needs to be finished (Stafford, 2005). It isn't clear how menaquinones are ingested from the colon and what their general commitment is to by and large, vitamin K status. Painstakingly led epidemiological investigations utilizing significant libraries have empowered to end a few discussions concerning vitamin K and the infant. It remains, in any case, muddled what the ideal dosing routine is for preterm babies or for patients with cholestasis. Similar remains constant in regards to the job for vitamin K in the anticipation and treatment of osteoporosis (Shearer, 1992).

14.4 CONCLUSION

As the growing market of vitamins reminds us of the early discovery of vitamins, where people are not supposed to use the vitamins on a daily basis. But, as the days and the century go on increasing, people likely to follow a healthy lifestyle the y realizes that vitamins are the supplement which is supporting our body and fulfilling our needs for the body. As followed by this, newer vitamins came into the window, and they are preventing humans from various diseases and disorders. From the early stage to the nowadays, vitamins are becoming the popular supplement. From this vitamin using with suitable plant or animal derivatives are prepared, and this is very useful. Various techniques are also available to check the amount of the vitamin in the body. From this chapter, we concluded that vitamins would be the highest-marketed supplement in the future because of their usage.

KEYWORDS

- **Gla proteins**
- **glutamate side chains**
- **supplement**
- **vitamin A**
- **vitamin B complex**
- **vitamins**
- **γ-carboxyglutamate**

REFERENCES

Ablin, J., Fitzcharles, M. A., Buskila, D., Shir, Y., Sommer, C., & Häuser, W., (2015). Treatment of fibromyalgia syndrome: Recommendations of recent evidence-based interdisciplinary guidelines with special emphasis on complementary and alternative therapies. *Evidence-Based Complementary and Alternative Medicine, 2013.*

Adams, J. S., & Hewison, M., (2010). Update in vitamin D. *The Journal of Clinical Endocrinology & Metabolism, 95*(2), 471–478.

Agnew-Blais, J. C., Wassertheil-Smoller, S., Kang, J. H., Hogan, P. E., Coker, L. H., Snetselaar, L. G., & Smoller, J. W., (2015). Folate, vitamin B-6, and vitamin B-12 intake and mild cognitive impairment and probable dementia in the women's health initiative memory study. *Journal of the Academy of Nutrition and Dietetics, 115*(2), 231–241.

Alban, C., (2011). Biotin (vitamin B8) synthesis in plants. *Advances in Botanical Research, 59*, 39–66.

Allen, L. H., (2009). How common is vitamin B-12 deficiency? *The American Journal of Clinical Nutrition, 89*(2), 693S–696S.

Astorg, P., (1997). Food carotenoids and cancer prevention: An overview of current research. *Trends in Food Science & Technology, 8*(12), 406–413.

Baik, H. W., & Russell, R. M., (1999). Vitamin B12 deficiency in the elderly. *Annual Review of Nutrition, 19*(1), 357–377.

Bell, E. F., (1987). History of vitamin E in infant nutrition. *The American Journal of Clinical Nutrition, 46*(1), 183–186.

Bernstein, A. L., (1990). Vitamin B6 in clinical neurology. *Annals of the New York Academy of Sciences, 585*, 250–260.

Bikle, D. D., & Pillai, S., (1993). Vitamin D, calcium, and epidermal differentiation. *Endocrine Reviews, 14*(1), 3–19.

Bikle, D., (2009). Nonclassic actions of vitamin D. *The Journal of Clinical Endocrinology & Metabolism, 94*(1), 26–34.

Blanck, R. R., Hiatt, J., Hyams, K. C., Kang, H., Mather, S., Murphy, F., Roswell, R., & Thacker, S. B. (1995). Unexplained illnesses among Desert Storm veterans: a search for causes, treatment, and cooperation. *Archives of Internal Medicine. 155*(3), 262–268.

Brigelius-Flohé, R., & Traber, M. G., (1999). Vitamin E: Function and metabolism. *The FASEB Journal, 13*(10), 1145–1155.

Brown, K. L., (2005). Chemistry and enzymology of vitamin B12. *Chemical Reviews, 105*(6), 2075–2150.

Carr, A. C., & Maggini, S., (2017). Vitamin C and immune function. *Nutrients, 9*(11), E1211.

Chan, A. C., (1993). Partners in defense, vitamin E and vitamin C. *Canadian Journal of Physiology and Pharmacology, 71*(9), 725–731.

Chapeau, A. L., Tavares, G. M., Hamon, P., Croguennec, T., Poncelet, D., & Bouhallab, S., (2016). Spontaneous co-assembly of lactoferrin and β-lactoglobulin as a promising carrier for vitamin B9. *Food Hydrocolloids, 57*, 280–290.

DeLuca, H. F., (2004). Overview of general physiologic features and functions of vitamin D. *The American Journal of Clinical Nutrition, 80*(6), 1689S-1696S.

Denu, J. M., (2005). Vitamin B3 and sirtuin function. *Trends in Biochemical Sciences, 30*(9), 479–483.

Eshak, E. S., Iso, H., Muraki, I., & Tamakoshi, A., (2019). Among the water-soluble vitamins, dietary intakes of vitamins C, B2, and folate are associated with the reduced risk of diabetes in Japanese women but not men. *British Journal of Nutrition, 121*(12), 1357–1364.

Evans, H. M., (1962). The pioneer history of vitamin E. In *Vitamins & Hormones* (Vol. 20, pp. 379–387). Academic Press.

Evans, W. J., (2000). Vitamin E, vitamin C, and exercise. *The American Journal of Clinical Nutrition, 72*(2), 647S–652S.

Fenech, M., (2012). Folate (vitamin B9) and vitamin B12 and their function in the maintenance of nuclear and mitochondrial genome integrity. *Mutation Research/Fundamental and Molecular Mechanisms of Mutagenesis, 733*(1, 2), 21–33.

Ferland, G., (2012). The discovery of vitamin K and its clinical applications. *Annals of Nutrition and Metabolism, 61*(3), 213–218.

Fritsche, S., Wang, X., & Jung, C., (2017). Recent advances in our understanding of tocopherol biosynthesis in plants: An overview of key genes, functions, and breeding of vitamin E improved crops. *Antioxidants, 6*(4), 99.

Gibson, G. E., Hirsch, J. A., Fonzetti, P., Jordan, B. D., Cirio, R. T., & Elder, J., (2016). Vitamin B1 (thiamine) and dementia. *Annals of the New York Academy of Sciences, 1367*(1), 21–30.

Gröber, U., Reichrath, J., Holick, M. F., & Kisters, K., (2014). Vitamin K: An old vitamin in a new perspective. *Dermato-Endocrinology, 6*(1), e968490.

Guilland, J. C., & Aimone-Gastin, I., (2013). Vitamin B9. *La Revue du Praticien, 63*(8), 1079–1081.

György, P., (1964). The history of vitamin B6. Introductory remarks. In: *Vitamins & Hormones* (Vol. 22, pp. 361–365). Academic Press.

Hemilä, H., (2017). Vitamin C and infections. *Nutrients, 9*(4), 339.

Hodgkin, D. C., Kamper, J., Mackay, M., Pickworth, J., Trueblood, K. N., & White, J. G., (1956). Structure of vitamin B12. *Nature, 178*(4524), 64–66.

Holick, M. F., (2003). Vitamin D: A Millenium perspective. *Journal of Cellular Biochemistry, 88*(2), 296–307.

Irwin, H. R., (2012). A history of the isolation and identification of vitamin B_6. *Annals of Nutrition & Metabolism, 61*(3), 236–238.

Ismail, N., Kureishy, N., Church, S. J., Scholefield, M., Unwin, R. D., Xu, J., Patassini, S., & Cooper, G. J., (2020). Vitamin B5 (d-pantothenic acid) localizes in myelinated structures of the rat brain: Potential role for cerebral vitamin B5 stores in local myelin homeostasis. *Biochemical and Biophysical Research Communications, 522*(1), 220–225.

Jacobson, J. S., Troxel, A. B., Evans, J., Klaus, L., Vahdat, L., Kinne, D., Lo, K. S., et al., (2001). Randomized trial of black cohosh for the treatment of hot flashes among women with a history of breast cancer. *Journal of Clinical Oncology, 19*(10), 2739–2745.

Jacobson, M. K., & Jacobson, E. L., (2018). Vitamin B3 in health and disease: Toward the second century of discovery. *ADP-ribosylation and NAD+ Utilizing Enzymes*, 3–8.

Kalus, U., Pruss, A., Wodarra, J., Kiesewetter, H., Salama, A., & Radtke, H., (2008). Influence of blood donation on levels of water-soluble vitamins. *Transfusion Medicine, 18*(6), 360–365.

Keservani, R. K., Kesharwani, R. K., Sharma, A. K., Vyas, N., & Chadoker, A., (2010b). Nutritional supplements: An OVERVIEW. *International Journal of Current Pharmaceutical Review and Research, 1*(1), 59–75.

Keservani, R. K., Kesharwani, R. K., Vyas, N., Jain, S., Raghuvanshi, R., & Sharma, A. K., (2010a). Nutraceutical and functional food as future food: A review. *Der Pharmacia Lettre, 2*(1), 106–116.

Keservani, R. K., Sharma, A. K., & Jarouliya, U. (2015). Protein and peptide in drug targeting and its therapeutic approach. *Ars Pharmaceutica (Internet)*, *56*(3), 165–177.

Keservani, R. K., Sharma, A. K., & Kesharwani, R. K. (2017). An overview and therapeutic applications of nutraceutical and functional foods. *Recent Advances in Drug Delivery Technology*, 160–201. ISBN:9781522507543.

Keservani, R. K., Sharma, A. K., & Kesharwani, R. K. (2020). *Nutraceuticals and Dietary Supplements: Applications in Health Improvement and Disease Management*. CRC Press. ISBN: 9781771888738.

Kunisawa, J., Hashimoto, E., Ishikawa, I., & Kiyono, H., (2012). A pivotal role of vitamin B9 in the maintenance of regulatory T cells *in vitro* and *in vivo*. *PloS one*, *7*(2), e32094.

Leklem, J. E., (1990). Vitamin B-6: A status report. *The Journal of Nutrition*, *120*(suppl_11), 1503–1507.

Leklem, J. E., (2001). Vitamin B6. *Handbook of Vitamins*, *3*, 339–396.

Liang, X., Zhang, Q., Zhang, Z., Ding, Q., & Mei, X. (2021). Improving the stability of vitamin B5 through the double salt formation. *Crystal Growth & Design*, *21*(9), 4997–5005.

Lips, P., (2006). Vitamin D physiology. *Progress in Biophysics and Molecular Biology*, *92*(1), 4–8.

Liu, Y., Heying, E., & Tanumihardjo, S. A., (2012). History, global distribution, and nutritional importance of citrus fruits. *Comprehensive Reviews in Food Science and Food Safety*, *11*(6), 530–545.

Malouf, R., & Evans, J. G., (2003). Vitamin B6 for cognition. *Cochrane Database of Systematic Reviews*, (4).

Mejia, L. A., (1994). Fortification of foods: Historical development and current practices. *Food and Nutrition Bulletin*, *15*(4), 1–4.

Mohr, S. B., (2009). A brief history of vitamin D and cancer prevention. *Annals of Epidemiology*, *19*(2), 79–83.

Mooney, S., Leuendorf, J. E., Hendrickson, C., & Hellmann, H., (2009). Vitamin B6: A long-known compound of surprising complexity. *Molecules*, *14*(1), 329–351.

Niki, E., & Traber, M. G., (2012). A history of vitamin E. *Annals of Nutrition and Metabolism*, *61*(3), 207–212.

Oh, R. C., & Brown, D. L., (2003). Vitamin B12 deficiency. *American Family Physician*, *67*(5), 979–986.

Palacios, O. A., Bashan, Y., & de-Bashan, L. E., (2014). Proven and potential involvement of vitamins in interactions of plants with plant growth-promoting bacteria—An overview. *Biology and Fertility of Soils*, *50*(3), 415–432.

Powers, H. J., (2003). Riboflavin (vitamin B-2) and health. *The American Journal of Clinical Nutrition*, *77*(6), 1352–1360.

Rébeillé, F., Ravanel, S., Marquet, A., Mendel, R. R., Smith, A. G., & Warren, M. J., (2007). Roles of vitamins B5, B8, B9, B12, and molybdenum cofactor at cellular and organismal levels. *Natural Product Reports*, *24*(5), 949–962.

Rosenberg, I. H., (2012). A history of the isolation and identification of vitamin B6. *Annals of Nutrition and Metabolism*, *61*(3), 236–238.

Rumberger, J. A., Napolitano, J., Azumano, I., Kamiya, T., & Evans, M., (2011). Pantethine, a derivative of vitamin B5 used as a nutritional supplement, favorably alters low-density lipoprotein cholesterol metabolism in low–to moderate–cardiovascular risk North American subjects: A triple-blinded placebo and diet-controlled investigation. *Nutrition Research*, *31*(8), 608–615.

Sarma, P. S., (1944). The estimation of pyridoxine (vitamin B8) in foods using rice-moth larvae (*Corcyra cephalonica* St.). *Indian Journal of Medical Research, 32*(2), 117–122.

Sauve, A. A., (2008). NAD+ and vitamin B3: from metabolism to therapies. *Journal of Pharmacology and Experimental Therapeutics, 324*(3), 883–893.

Semba, R. D., (2012). On the 'discovery' of vitamin A. *Annals of Nutrition and Metabolism, 61*(3), 192–198.

Shearer, M. J., (1992). Vitamin K metabolism and nutriture. *Blood Reviews, 6*(2), 92–104.

Shearer, M. J., (1995). Vitamin K. *The Lancet, 345*(8944), 229–234.

Sheppard, S. K., Didelot, X., Meric, G., Torralbo, A., Jolley, K. A., Kelly, D. J., Bentley, S. D., et al., (2013). Genome-wide association study identifies vitamin B5 biosynthesis as a host specificity factor in *Campylobacter*. *Proceedings of the National Academy of Sciences, 110*(29), 11923–11927.

Singh, P., Kesharwani, R. K., & Keservani, R. K., (2017a). Antioxidants and vitamins: Roles in cellular function and metabolism. In: *Sustained Energy for Enhanced Human Functions and Activity* (pp. 385–407). Academic Press. ISBN:9780128054130.

Singh, P., Kesharwani, R. K., & Keservani, R. K., (2017b). Protein, carbohydrates, and fats: Energy metabolism. In: *Sustained Energy for Enhanced Human Functions and Activity* (pp. 103–115). Academic Press. ISBN:9780128054130.

Sobczyńska-Malefora, A., & Harrington, D. J., (2018). Laboratory assessment of folate (vitamin B9) status. *Journal of Clinical Pathology, 71*(11), 949–956.

Stabler, S. P., & Allen, R. H., (2004). Vitamin B12 deficiency is a worldwide problem. *Annu. Rev. Nutr., 24*, 299–326.

Stabler, S. P., (2013). Vitamin B12 deficiency. *New England Journal of Medicine, 368*(2), 149–160.

Stafford, D. W., (2005). The vitamin K cycle. *Journal of Thrombosis and Haemostasis, 3*(8), 1873–1878.

Ueland, P. M., McCann, A., Midttun, Ø., & Ulvik, A. (2017). Inflammation, vitamin B6 and related pathways. *Molecular Aspects of Medicine, 53*, 10–27.

Van, D. W. R. P., De Wild, G. M., De Groot, L. C., Hoefnagels, W. H., & Van, S. W. A., (1996). Dietary intakes of energy and water-soluble vitamins in different categories of aging. *The Journals of Gerontology Series A: Biological Sciences and Medical Sciences, 51*(1), B100–B107.

Van, W. M., De Bruyne, R., Van De, V. S., & Van, B. S., (2009). Vitamin K, an update for the pediatrician. *European Journal of Pediatrics, 168*(2), 127–134.

Vermeer, C. V., (2012). Vitamin K: The effect on health beyond coagulation–an overview. *Food & Nutrition Research, 56*(1), 5329.

Wang, X., Li, K., Yao, L., Wang, C., & Van, S. A., (2018). Recent advances in vitamin analysis by capillary electrophoresis. *Journal of Pharmaceutical and Biomedical Analysis, 147*, 278–287.

Zile, M. H., (1998). Symposium: Functional metabolism of vitamin A in embryonic development. *J. Nutr., 128*, 453S–454S.

Zile, M. H., (1998). Vitamin A and embryonic development: An overview. *The Journal of Nutrition, 128*(2), 455S–458S.

CHAPTER 15

Vitamins as Nutraceuticals for Human Nutrition

VIJAYRAJ N. SONAWANE,[1] KHEMCHAND R. SURANA,[1] EKNATH D. AHIRE,[2] DHANANJAY M. PATIL,[3] and DEEPAK D. SONAWANE[3]

[1]Department of Pharmaceutical Chemistry, Shreeshakti Shaikshanik Sanstha, Divine College of Pharmacy, Satana, Nashik, Maharashtra, India

[2]Department of Pharmaceutics, MET's Institute of Pharmacy, BKC, SPPU, Adgaon, Nashik, Maharashtra, India

[3]Department of Pharmaceutics, Shreeshakti Shaikshanik Sanstha, Divine College of Pharmacy, Satana, Nashik, Maharashtra, India

ABSTRACT

The early 20th century turned into a vital length for the identity and biological chemical-physical characterization of nutrients. From then till now, much research has tried to make clear into element the organic position of the nutrients in human beings and their direct reference to positive sicknesses, both in a negative way (look of deficiency sicknesses because of vitamin deficiency) or a high-quality way (use of nutrients to deal with sicknesses and/or to enhance human fitness). This study aims to identify direct relationships between those substances and fitness by conducting an integrated analysis of the records of nutrition and its effects on human fitness. The outcomes of vitamins and dietary supplements on weight-reduction plans also are explored. The evaluation of the outcomes indicates that it's far not possible to set up strong and popular conclusions approximately the gain of nutrition supplementation on human health past the prevention and/or

Preventive and Therapeutic Role of Vitamins as Nutraceuticals. Khemchand R. Surana, Eknath D. Ahire, Raj K. Keservani, & Rajesh K. Kesharwani (Eds.)

remedy of deficiency states. Nutraceutical is the hybrid of nutrients and pharmaceuticals. Nutraceuticals, in broad, are meals or a part of meals gambling an extensive position in editing and keeping ordinary physiological characteristic that continues wholesome human beings. The meal products used as nutraceuticals may be classified as nutritional prebiotics, probiotics, fiber, antioxidants, polyunsaturated fatty acids different unique sorts of natural herbal foods. These nutraceuticals are utilized in diverse sicknesses, inclusive of obesity, cardiovascular sicknesses, cancer, osteoporosis, arthritis, diabetes, LDL cholesterol, etc. On the whole, nutraceutical" has because of the brand-new generation of drugs and health, wherein the meals enterprise has grown to be a study-orientated sector. This chapter's purpose is to offer the expertise of nutrients as nutraceuticals with its makes use in diverse sicknesses. Vitamins are important meal ingredients that offer dietary blessings in addition to medicinal effects. The blessings of those ingredients are because of the presence of energetic compounds, including carotenoids, collagen hydrolysate, and nutritional fibers. Vitamins may be classified into exclusive, less, on primarily based totally on their nature and mode of action.

15.1 INTRODUCTION

Low-molecular-weight natural substances known as vitamins are required in trace levels for critical metabolic processes. A lack of a vitamin can cause a specific symptom of a disease. Vitamins don't consist of other important vitamins like nutritional minerals, important fatty acids, or important amino acids. It also doesn't consist of a wide range of different vitamins that promote health but don't provide cell structure and energy. Plants and microorganisms gave animals vitamins. Vitaminoids are chemicals that act like vitamins. Mainly there are two types of vitamins: those that dissolve in fat (like A, D, and E) and those that dissolve in water (like B, C, and P). Nutraceuticals include things like herbal diets (Sharma et al., 2020; Rane et al., 2020a–c), natural products, biofortified crops, and genetically modified and processed food products (Keservani et al., 2010a, b; Skrovankova, 2011). Beyond basic nutrients, nutraceuticals (Keservani et al., 2017, 2020) can improve health, boost immunity, and/or prevent and treat certain diseases. Functional foods are entire, fortified, enhanced, or improved foods that offer additional health advantages over mere nutrient provision. They are labeled into different groups based on the food group, the diseases they prevent or treat, their physiological effects, etc. Food components are things like antioxidants, food preservatives, food coloring agents, flavoring agents, anti-infective agents, excipients, and other similar things that are used to make or store food or feed for animals. Excipients don't have much of a healing effect, but they do help the active pharmaceutical ingredient (API) work better. They also help keep the quality, efficacy, safety, etc., of the ingredients. Excipients include solvents, diluting, suspending, and emulsifying agents, as well as anti-oxidants, preservatives, pharmaceuticals, coloring agents, flavoring agents, vehicles, excipients, ointment bases, etc. (Ottaway et al., 2008). Proteins and peptides (Keservani et al., 2015) make it possible to make antibodies, and special fermentations, purification processes, and recombination technology have made it possible to make protein drugs at the perfect price. These drugs can be used to treat a wide range of diseases through different routes, such as orally, transdermally, nasally, pulmonaryly, ocularly, buccally, and rectally. Multiple sclerosis, chronic lymphocytic leukemia, coronary artery thrombosis, and rheumatoid arthritis can all be treated with protein-based medications. Papain is an enzyme that comes from plants. It could be very helpful in preventing atherosclerosis and coronary heart disease in diabetics. People have employed natural painkillers like cocaine, methyl salicylate, capsaicin, piperine, opium, etc., since the dawn of time. Cosmetics and medications are combined to create cosmeceuticals. They are meant to improve the health and beauty of the skin by giving it a certain effect, like getting rid of acne or wrinkles or protecting the skin from the sun (Smith & Hong-Shum, 2011).

The discovery of vitamins is the result of research into vitamins and what they do in living things. In 1880, the Russian doctor N. I. Lunin was the first to show that, Beyond the well-known fundamental components (proteins, fats, carbohydrates, water, and minerals), the body also needs a few other accent parts to grow and stay healthy. In 1905, an English doctor named W. Fletcher was trying to figure out what caused Beriberi. He found that eating unpolished rice instead of polished rice kept people from getting Beriberi, so he thought that there must be some special nutrients in the rice husk. In 1912, a Polish scientist named C (Ball, 2004).

Funk called the first nutritional parts of food "vitamins" after the Latin word "vita," which means "life," and the "amines" he found in the thiamine he took out of rice bran. 'Vitamine' was shortened to 'vitamin' over time (Singh et al., 2017a). Vitamins are low-molecular-weight natural compounds that are essential for life. They are needed in small amounts for important metabolic reactions in the body, and a lack of them can cause specific signs of illness (Christianson et al., 2005). The word "diet" no longer includes important vitamins like nutritional minerals, important fatty acids, or important amino acids. It also doesn't include the many different vitamins that are good for your health. As well as giving cells structure and energy, nutrients either help make coenzymes or control how biochemical processes work. When your body doesn't get enough of a certain nutrient, it shows specific signs that might not go away, even if you take other vitamins. Vitamins in the animal world come from plants and microorganisms (Sinbad et al., 2019). Vitaminoids are "nutrient-like" compounds like flavonoids (Keservani & Sharma, 2014; Keservani et al., 2016a, b), inositol, carnitine, choline, lipoic acid, and the essential fatty acids. Except for the essential fatty acids, there isn't much evidence that any of them is a nutritional necessity. Except for vitamins B6 and B12, they are easily passed out of the body in urine without much storage, so they will need to be taken regularly. They are usually safe in amounts above what the body needs, but people who take a megadose of niacin, vitamin C, or pyridoxine (B6) have shown signs of sickness (Sazawal et al., 1997). All of the B vitamins work as coenzymes or cofactors, which help important enzymes do their jobs and keep energy-making reactions going normally. Overcooking makes it easy to lose nutrients that dissolve in water. Bacteria in the small intestine produce the vitamins K and B complex in the human body. When skin is exposed to sunshine, vitamin D can be produced. For some species, the same chemical can function as a vitamin and as a normal substance. For instance, since it is not produced in human or guinea pig tissues, ascorbic acid is a vitamin for both species. Since it is produced in their tissues, ascorbic acid is not a vitamin for rats, rabbits, or dogs. The two main sources of sustenance for humans are food and gut microbes.

15.2 VITAMINOSIS

Lack of vitamins for an extended period of time results in vitaminosis (beriberi, scurvy, rickets, and pellagra). Vitaminoses A Niacin (B3) deficit causes pellagra, thiamine (B1) deficiency results in Beri-Beri, megaloblastic anemia from vitamin B12 deficiency, scurvy from vitamin C deficiency, rickettsia from vitamin D deficiency, and blood clotting issues from vitamin K shortage. Hypovitaminosis refers to any illness marked by a nutritional deficit in one or more nutrients. Antivitamins are substances that inhibit the metabolism of vitamins or break them down (El Ati-Hellal & Hellal, 2021). Antivitamins are made up of enzymes that break down vitamins (thiaminase and ascorbase) and compounds that form inactive complexes with vitamins (avidin) or have structures that are similar to vitamins (sulfonamides, etc.). Hypervitaminosis, also called vitamin intoxication, is a condition caused by taking too many vitamins or vitamin supplements over an extended period

(nausea, diarrhea, and vomiting). Hypervitaminosis, also called vitamin toxicity, is shown by a number of common symptoms, such as loss of appetite, sickness in the motor function of the gastrointestinal tract, a strong headache, an overactive nervous system, hair loss, skin scaling, and other symptoms. Hypervitaminosis can also be fatal. Hypervitaminosis can be caused by eating too much food high in a fat-soluble vitamin (like the liver of a polar bear or whale, which is high in vitamin A) or by taking too much of a vitamin that is meant to be taken by mouth (Alamgir, 2017) (Table 15.1).

TABLE 15.1 The Information on Sources and Functions of Water-Soluble Vitamins

Name	Sources	Function
Vitamin B1 (Thiamine)	Pork, beans, nuts, whole-grain or fortified breads and cereals, seeds, and legumes all contain trace amounts of iron.	Part of an enzyme that is important for nerve function and is needed for energy metabolism.
Vitamin B2 (Riboflavin)	Leafy green vegetables, breads, milk and milk products, and cereals made with whole grains that have been fortified.	Part of an enzyme that helps turn food into energy; important for healthy eyes and skin.
Vitamin B3 (Niacin)	Specifically, leafy green veggies, asparagus, and mushrooms, whole-grain or enriched breads and cereals, as well as meat, poultry, and fish.	Component of an enzyme required for energy metabolism; significant for the health of the nervous system, gastrointestinal system, and skin.
Vitamin B5 (pantothenic acid)	Widespread in foods	A part of an enzyme responsible for energy metabolism.
Vitamin B6 (pyridoxine)	Vegetables, fruits, meat, fish, poultry	A component of an enzyme that helps red blood cells develop by metabolizing proteins.
Vitamin B7 (biotin)	Microorganisms are pervasive in food and can be found in the intestine.	A part of an enzyme involved in metabolizing energy.
Vitamin B9 (folic acid)	Leafy greens, orange juice, legumes, seeds, and liver used to be among the foods with the most refined grains.	A portion of an enzyme is necessary for the synthesis of new cells, including red blood cells and DNA.
Cobalamin (vitamin B12)	Meat, seafood, poultry, eggs, fish, milk, and milk products do not contain plant foods.	It is a part of an enzyme that aids in cell division and is essential for nerve function.
Ascorbic acid (vitamin C)	The only fruits and vegetables that contain this chemical are citrus fruits, cantaloupe, cabbage vegetables, strawberries, peppers, lettuce, papayas, tomatoes, potatoes, mangoes, and kiwifruit.	Antioxidant; part of an enzyme that metabolizes proteins; crucial for the immune system to operate; increases iron absorption.

15.3 ROLE OF VITAMINS

Vitamins are essential substances that cannot or can only be manufactured in very small amounts by humans; as a result, humans must consume them through their diet. Vitamin deficiency may be prompted now no longer only with the aid of using inadequate consumption of foodstuffs but additionally due to elevated requirements with the aid of using certain groups of humans (humans on unique diets, smokers), bad absorption, or insufficient utilization. Seaweeds are usually a great supply of a few B-group vitamins (B1, B2, and B12). There are other B-complex vitamins, however, only in low or hint amounts (niacin, B6, biotin, folates) (Croft et al., 2006). Several seaweeds contain enormous amounts of carotenoids, a provitamin form of vitamin A, and the antioxidant vitamins C and E. The hydrosoluble vitamins are wanted as enzyme cofactors. The vitamin will have one or some very specific roles or much greater extensive roles. A number of B-group vitamins function as coenzymes for enzymes with features withinside the catabolism of foodstuffs to provide strength for the body. Some of them are essential even for his or her antioxidant activity and different fitness benefits. Thus, low degrees of a few B institution vitamins (B2, B6, B12) can bring about decreased degrees of DNA methylation and consequently in a few styles of cancer (Hernandez et al., 2003).

Thiamin, riboflavin, cobalamin, and ascorbic acid are among the vitamins that are abundantly present in seaweeds. Thiamin (vitamin B1) is essential for many enzymes, including pyruvate dehydrogenase, pyruvate decarboxylase, and transketolase, and plays a significant role in the intermediary carbon metabolism. The usage of riboflavin (vitamin B2) is widespread across the entire cell. Methionine synthase and methylmalonyl CoA mutase are two biosynthetic enzymes that depend on cobalamin (vitamin B12) to function. Interestingly, even though vitamin B12 isn't determined in vascular plants, it's miles abundant in algae. Since only prokaryotes possess the cap potential to synthesize cobalamin, all the vitamin B12 determined in algae have to have originally been produced via way of means of bacteria (Croft et al., 2006). Ascorbic acid (vitamin C) is an essential antioxidant withinside the ascorbate–glutathione pathway. Along with violaxanthin deep oxidase, ascorbate oxidase, and ascorbate peroxidase, it is a cofactor of enzymes and protects those that have prosthetic transition metal ions. Vitamin E and provitamins A are two fat-soluble vitamins that can be found in seaweeds. The essential liposoluble antioxidant vitamin E (tocopherols and tocotrienols) is decisive in preventing the oxidation of dietary polyunsaturated fatty acids.

As particularly oxidatively altered LDL is thought to play a crucial role in the development of atherosclerosis, tocopherols help limit the oxidation of LDL and block the production of reactive oxygen species generated at some point in oxidation (Steinberg, 1991). Retinal vitamin A, which serves as the chromophore for visual pigments, is crucial for the development of vision (Blackwell, 2009). Vitamin A provides crucial systemic abilities inside the growth and reproductive efficiency in addition to maintaining epithelial tissue and preventing its keratinization. Algae-derived plant meals, however, no longer contain intrinsic vitamin A; instead, they now contain provitamins, carotenoids, and linear polyenes with cyclic shapes and b-rings. B-carotene is the most prevalent carotenoid with a provitamin component in seaweed. It may be cleaved with the aid of using a b-carotene-15, 150-dioxygenase, ensuing withinside the formation of retinal (DellaPenna & Pogson, 2006).

15.3.1 NUTRIFICATION

Nitrification is the process of adding nutrients to meals to make them more nutritious. Food enrichment is the process of restoring a food's natural nutritional value before it is processed. The addition of nutrients such as vitamins and minerals to a food at higher levels than it already had is known as fortification. Fortification processes such as adding iodine to salt, fluoride to drinking water, or vitamin D to milk are popular (Allen & Burgess, 1950).

15.4 ROLE OF VITAMINS AS A NUTRACEUTICALS

A dietary supplement is a product that is used orally and contains a "dietary ingredient" meant to enhance food intake, according to the US Food and Drug Administration (FDA). In the US, Canada, and some European nations, dietary supplements are frequently used (Ball, 2004; Sinbad et al., 2019). Approximately 50% of adults and a third of children use these supplements in economically developed cultures. You can use dietary supplements to make up for deficiencies or make sure you get enough of a certain nutrient. However, if ingested in high quantities, they can be harmful. Therefore, it's essential to monitor their levels to guarantee a balanced diet (Blackwell, 2009). In the United States, adults most frequently take vitamins and minerals as dietary supplements. The following 15 minerals have been demonstrated to have beneficial effects: calcium, phosphorus, potassium, sodium, chloride, magnesium, iron, zinc, iodine, chromium, copper, fluoride, molybdenum, manganese, and selenium—as well as 13 vitamins—A, B1, B2, B3, B5, B6, B8, B9, B12, C, D, and K—are crucial for human health. The first multivitamin/mineral (MVM) formula was developed in the 1930s, and today, the term is most commonly used to refer to a dietary supplement that contains three or more vitamins and minerals (Polcz & Barbul, 2019). MVM supplements are recommended for the prevention or treatment of viral diseases connected to nutrition, such as AIDS, which is brought on by the majority of cases of the human immunodeficiency virus (HIV) caused by all mortality in some developing nations (Gagner, 2012). Another persistent infectious condition associated with vitamin A levels in the body is tuberculosis. Indeed, numerous epidemiological studies have shown that healthy people have significantly greater blood levels of vitamin A than TB patients (McDowell, 2003). MVM-rich supplements are frequently utilized to support wellness and fend off cancer and chronic illnesses. The advantages of these supplements in terms of reducing cardiovascular diseases, however, have generated some controversy (Cowan et al., 2018). This chapter's objectives were to provide a general review of the most significant vitamins and minerals in our lives, as well as to identify the most typical consumers of MVM supplements, their usage patterns, and the illnesses linked to vitamin and mineral deficiencies.

Vitamins are chemicals that the body needs, but those humans are unable to synthesize them in large enough amounts (Allgeyer et al., 2010). Vitamins are only required in trace amounts for a healthy metabolism, in contrast to other nutrients that are ingested in considerable amounts and contribute to the creation of energy (micrograms or milligrams per day). A varied and balanced diet is a natural way to get vitamins, but they can also be added to meals. Overconsumption can have negative long-term effects, while a shortfall might result in health issues like cancer or cardiovascular disease (Joint, FAO, and World Health Organization, 1998).

The 20th century's early years saw the discovery of 13 vitamins, with vitamin B12 coming along in 1948 (Aluru et al., 2008). Antioxidants, coenzymes, hormones, and mediators of cell signaling are just a few of the biological functions performed by these substances. Both water-soluble vitamins C and E and fat-soluble vitamins A and D make up this group (e.g., vitamins B and C). Fat-soluble vitamins can be consumed less frequently than water-soluble vitamins due to their capacity to be stored in the liver and adipose tissue (Barak et al., 1993). Of the 13 known vitamins, six are water-soluble, and three are fat-soluble due to their high nutritional value and extensive use as food additives and dietary supplements.

15.4.1 VITAMIN A

In the early 1900s, McCollum and, separately, Osborne and Mendel recognized the need for vitamin A, a fat-soluble vitamin, as a dietary component for growth (Ball, 2004; Sinbad et al., 2019). Retinol (preformed vitamin A), retinal, retinoic acid, and retinyl esters are all forms of vitamin A, as are provitamin A carotenoids, principally -carotene, -carotene, and -cryptoxanthin. Retinol activity equivalents (RAEs), which are units of measurement for vitamin A, are defined as 1 g of preformed retinol, 12 g of carotene, and 24 g of either carotene or cryptoxanthin (Blackwell, 2009).

Preformed vitamin A is only found in products made from animals, including fish, dairy products, eggs, and foods like liver and fish liver oil. Additionally, it is utilized to increase the nutritional content of sauces, sweets, and cereals (Bender, 2009). Provitamin A carotenoids are mostly found in colorful fruits and vegetables, such as spinach, parsley, amaranth, lettuce, carrot, papaya, mango, and others (Polcz & Barbul, 2019).

The small intestine absorbs between 70% and 90% of preformed vitamin A that has been dissolved in lipid micelles. Carotenoids can enter the small intestine thanks to passive diffusion. These organisms have a biological availability that ranges from 5 to 60%. After absorption, chylomicrons and chylomicron remnants transport retinal esters and nonhydrolyzed carotenoids to the liver. Around 90% of retinol is kept in the liver as retinol palmitate. The remaining portion is transported to various adipose tissues via Retinol Binding Protein (RBP). A minor amount of vitamin A is eliminated in the bile, and the majority is done so through the urine or feces (Meyers et al., 2006).

Vitamin A is essential for healthy vision, reproduction, growth, gene expression, and immune system operation. The perception of low light in the visual system is correlated with the presence of rhodopsin, a photosensitive pigment produced in rod cells as a result of 11-cis-retinaldehyde binding to the opt-in protein (Gagner, 2012). Iodopsin pigments, which are produced in the cones when 11-cis-retinaldehyde binds to the photopsin protein in a similar manner, are present when forms and colors are perceived (Bieri & Evarts, 1974). Throughout embryonic development, retinoic acid and endogenous retinoids are essential for the anterior-posterior development of the central body axis and limb development. Their concentrations are strictly regulated both spatially and temporally. Due to its role in the formation of glycoproteins unique to spermatogenesis, vitamin A is also necessary for reproduction. Additionally, several cytosolic and nuclear receptor interactions with retinoic acid are required to control the expression of a number of genes (Block et al., 1992). Since these genes contain the growth hormone gene, a vitamin A shortage impacts children's normal growth and development. Finally, all-trans-retinoic acid, a vitamin A component, increases humoral and cellular immunity. It encourages the proliferation of lymphocytes and thymocytes as well as the synthesis of immunoglobulins.

15.4.2 VITAMIN B1 (THIAMIN)

The human disease "beriberi" has long been assumed to be treatable and preventable with vitamin B1. In 1936, its synthesis was finished, and its structure was established. The substituted pyrimidine and thiazole moieties of this water-soluble vitamin are linked by a methylene bridge. Thiamin monophosphate, thiamin diphosphate (the active coenzyme also known as thiamin pyrophosphate), and thiamin triphosphate are the three phosphorylated forms of thiamin that can be found in nature. Particularly dangerous substances include sulfites and polyphenols because they impair thiamin's biological action (Blackwell, 2009).

Yeast and yeast extract, whole grains, almonds, lean pork, wheat bran, heart, kidney, and liver, as well as fortified foods like bread and breakfast cereals, are some of the foods that are the most plentiful sources of vitamin B1. Fresh foods like fruits, vegetables, and dairy products (but not butter) may assist to prevent vitamin B1 deficiency if consumed regularly and in sufficient amounts (Bracco & Oral, 2011).

Dietary thiamin phosphates are hydrolyzed by intestinal phosphatases to release free thiamin. Then, free thiamin is absorbed by the duodenum and proximal jejunum. The two pathways that mediate thiamin absorption are saturable active transport at low physiological vitamin concentrations and passive diffusion at higher concentrations. Examples of biological variables that influence thiamin transport include age, diabetic status, and alcohol consumption. Thiamin monophosphate, which is associated to plasma proteins, circulates in the bloodstream together with free thiamin. In the intestinal mucosa, some thiamin is phosphorylated to thiamin monophosphate (Singh et al., 2017b; (Cheney, 1950). Around 30 mg of thiamin are present in the human body overall, with 80 mg of that being thiamin diphosphate, 10 mg being thiamin triphosphate, and the remaining 20 mg being free thiamin and thiamin monophosphate. Thiamin must be consumed often because it has a low capacity for storage and a moderately rapid turnover rate (Combs & McClung, 2016).

The oxidative decarboxylation of oxoacids is carried out by the three multienzyme complexes pyruvate dehydrogenase, -ketoglutarate dehydrogenase, and branched-chain ketoacid dehydrogenase, which all use thiamin diphosphate as a cofactor. Thiamin triphosphate is involved in the transport of salt and potassium via nerve transmission.

15.4.3 VITAMIN B2 (RIBOFLAVIN)

In 1935, Kuhn's and Karrer's groups separately synthesized the water-soluble vitamin riboflavin. This luminous, yellow crystalline substance was identified in the 1920s as a human "pellagra" and "beriberi" disease preventative factor. The flavin ring is connected to an alcohol similar to ribose in riboflavin (Fenech, 2012). Although it is a relatively heat-stable molecule, it is quickly inactivated when exposed to ultraviolet (UV) radiation.

Vitamin B2 is abundant in milk, dairy products, meat, and other animal items. Riboflavin can be found in green vegetables, including broccoli, turnip greens, and collard greens. Riboflavin content is low in natural grain products; however, supplementing them with the vitamin has raised riboflavin intake. Vitamin B2 is frequently utilized as a food coloring due to its vivid yellow hue (McDowell, 2003).

Alkaline phosphatase in the upper small intestine breaks down flavin coenzymes to liberate riboflavin, which is then absorbed. Absorption of riboflavin is enhanced when it is eaten with other meals and in the presence of bile salts. Most of the absorbed riboflavin is phosphorylated by the intestinal mucosa before it is released into the bloodstream as riboflavin phosphate. Around 50% of plasma riboflavin is free, with less than 10% of it being flavin mononucleotide (FMN) and less than 5% flavin adenine dinucleotide (FAD). Riboflavin typically makes up 0.03 M of plasma (Cowan et al., 2018). The liver is where vitamin B2 is largely kept. Other storage organs include the spleen, kidney, and heart muscle. The majority of vitamin B2 is eliminated in urine as free riboflavin, with a small amount also leaving the body as other glycosides and metabolites (Magoulas & El-Hattab, 2012).

The flavin coenzymes FMN and FAD, as well as covalently linked flavins, are all precursors to riboflavin. The mitochondrial electron transport chain is one of the metabolic routes that uses these coenzymes to catalyze oxidation-reduction reactions. The bulk of flavoproteins require FAD rather than FMN as the prosthetic group. Additionally, the metabolism of drugs, lipids, and steroids involves riboflavin (Ball, 2004; Sinbad et al., 2019).

15.4.4 VITAMIN B3 (NIACIN)

The two vitamins nicotinic acid and nicotinamide are collectively referred to as niacin. Huber identified nicotine oxidation as the source of nicotinic acid in 1867, but it wasn't until much later, in 1938, that researchers realized this substance could treat and even prevent the "pellagra" condition. Niacin is a crystalline substance that is white and water-soluble. It can be produced by the body from the necessary amino acid tryptophan, which is a key method of satisfying the body's niacin needs (Meyers et al., 2006).

The standard way to measure niacin needs is in mg niacin equivalents, where 1 mg niacin equivalent equals 1 mg preformed niacin plus 1/60 mg tryptophan. Foods high in proteins are significant sources of the vitamin due to the addition of tryptophan. Niacin and tryptophan are found in large quantities in poultry, fish, lean red meat, and liver. Ready-to-eat cereals containing nicotinic acid supplements are another source of niacin. Depending on dietary consumption, fruits and vegetables offer useful levels of the vitamin (Perlitz et al., 2019).

The two primary forms of niacin present in food are nicotinamide adenine dinucleotide (NAD) and nicotinamide adenine dinucleotide phosphate (NADP). In the intestinal lumen, these nucleotides are digested to release nicotinamide. A sodium-dependent enhanced diffusion mediates absorption from the small intestine at low doses. Passive diffusion is used for absorption at higher concentrations. Niacin molecules that enter the portal circulation are either taken up by erythrocytes for internalization or delivered to the liver. Nicotinamide and nicotinic acid are metabolized to tryptophan in the liver (NAD). The intracellular production of NAD and NADP is carried out by the niacin vitamers once they have reached the tissues. Niacin is prepared for urine excretion by the liver, which transforms excess niacin into methylated compounds.

Numerous oxidation-reduction reactions rely heavily on the nicotinamide nucleotides NAD and NADP. The NAD coenzyme is involved in catabolic activities, whereas NADP is more typically required in synthetic pathways, such as the synthesis of steroids and fatty acids. It is simple to convert the coenzyme NAD to NADP and vice versa. Both molecules can also change their oxidation state (Biesalski & Tinz, 2017). The energy-draining synthetic reactions and the energy-producing catabolic reactions are kept in balance by this conversion.

15.4.5 VITAMIN B6

First discovered by Lepkovsky in 1938, Harris and Folkers synthesized the pure crystalline water-soluble vitamin B6 in 1939. The three nutritionally active B6 vitamers are pyridoxine (PN), pyridoxal (PL), and pyridoxamine (PM), as well as their corresponding 5-phosphate esters pyridoxine phosphate (PNP), pyridoxal phosphate (PLP), and pyridoxamine phosphate (PMP). Aqueous vitamin B6 solutions are colorless, with the exception of PLP solutions, which are yellow and less stable in neutral or alkaline medium (Biesalski, 2017).

Significant levels of vitamin B6 are found in grain germs, yeast, liver, fortified cereals, and liver. Nuts, legumes, meat, seafood, avocado, bananas, and potatoes are other crucial sources. The vitamin is present in relatively small amounts in milk, fruit, and eggs.

Through a sodium-dependent carrier-mediated mechanism, vitamin B6 absorption takes place in the lumen of the intestine after the phosphorylated forms are hydrolyzed (Kocyowski et al., 2018). Following absorption, the various vitamin B6 vitamers are interconverted and delivered to the liver as free, unphosphorylated vitamers. Under the influence of the pyridoxal kinase enzyme, the vitamers are collected via diffusion in the liver and transformed into phosphorylated forms. Pyridoxine oxidase converts PNP and PMP to PLP. PLP that is linked to plasma albumin is discharged in part into the bloodstream. Pyridoxic acid, which enters the bloodstream, is, and eliminated in the urine, is created when the remaining component of PLP is dephosphorylated and oxidized (Combet & Buckton, 2015).

PLP, which is engaged in a wide range of amino acid processes, including transamination, transsulfuration, desulfurization, and decarboxylation, is the metabolically active vitamin. Additionally, PLP is necessary for the control of steroid hormone activities (Black, 1998). Additionally, PLP vitamer plays a crucial role in lipid metabolism and immunological function in addition to functioning as the cofactor of glycogen phosphorylase in muscle and liver.

15.4.6 VITAMIN B9 (FOLATES)

The water-soluble vitamin B9 is represented by the category of folates (from folium, the Latin word for leaf). In 1946, Angier's team was in charge of the synthesis, chemical structure analysis, and separation of vitamin B9. Since the early 1990s, researchers have been examining the link between folate intake and the likelihood of having a chronic illness or a poor birth outcome. Folic acid supplementation given daily during the periconceptional period has been linked to a lower risk of neural tube malformations in studies. Due to these important discoveries, mandatory folic acid fortification was implemented in North America as part of public health campaigns.

Fortified grain goods, orange juice, fresh dark green leafy vegetables, lentils, kidney beans, lima beans, avocado, peas, and peanut products are all excellent sources of folate. Meat doesn't contain a lot of folates, with the exception of liver (Bahl et al., 1998).

Around 80% of dietary folate is in the polyglutamate form, which is degraded to mono glutamate before being absorbed by enterocytes in the jejunum. A saturable, pH-dependent active transport mechanism transports mono glutamyl folate across the intestinal mucosa. Nonetheless, at high doses, nonsaturable passive diffusion is responsible for intestine uptake. Free folate and folate linked to albumin are the two principal types of plasma folate, which is mostly 5-methyl THF. High-affinity binders bind only a small percentage of plasma folate (less than 5%). The bulk of decreased mono glutamates entering from the gut is digested and stored in the liver rather than being released into the blood or bile (Lentjes, 2019). Folate is eliminated in the urine as folate derivatives, with just 1% to 2% of the vitamin remaining in the urine as intact folate.

Folates are important in the mobilization of one-carbon units in intermediate metabolism because of their chemical structure. Purines guanine and adenine, as well as the pyrimidine thymine, which are utilized to make the nucleoproteins deoxyribonucleic acid (DNA) and ribonucleic acid (RNA), require such processes (RNA). Folates also have a role in amino acid metabolism through THF derivatives, which act as one-carbon donors in a variety of synthetic processes.

15.4.7 VITAMIN B12

After numerous important contributions, vitamin B12 was found in several domains, such as medicine, chemistry, and microbiology, which resulted in Nobel Prizes being awarded. Dorothy Hodgkin, an X-ray crystallographer who won the Nobel Prize for science in 1964, deduced the molecular structure of vitamin B12. Robert Woodward, who won the Nobel Prize in Chemistry in 1965, led the whole chemical synthesis of vitamin B12, which took 11 years. Cobalamins, which have a structure identical to heme but with a cobalt atom in place of the central iron atom, are collectively referred to as vitamin B12. Cyanocobalamin, a water-soluble purplish-red powder, is the most stable of the cobalamin that are active forms of vitamin B12. It is a typical component of medications and dietary supplements. Nevertheless, it is a light-sensitive molecule (Miller et al., 2005).

Vitamin B12 is almost solely found in animal-based foods, with the liver being the most prevalent dietary source, followed by the kidney and heart. Milk, eggs, fish, shellfish, and muscle meat are also key sources. Adenosyl- and hydroxocobalamin are found in meat and fish, and sulfitocobalamin is small levels of cyancobalamin, which is also present in canned fish and pork, are found in egg white and cheeses (Kibirige & Mwebaze, 2013).

There are two ways to take vitamin B12: actively and passively. A small glycoprotein termed intrinsic factor, which is secreted by the parietal cells of the stomach mucosa, is where vitamin B12 binds before being absorbed primarily through the intestinal lumen. Vitamin B12 binds to the stomach protein cobalophilin, which is broken down in the duodenum, and then binds to the intrinsic factor. Transcobalamin I and II proteins, which vitamin B12 is connected to in the bloodstream, prevent it from being eliminated in the urine when it passes through the kidney. The liver contains the highest concentration of vitamin B12 in the body, making up almost 60% of the body's total vitamin content (Jenkins et al., 2018).

The metabolism of proteins, lipids, and carbohydrates depends on vitamin B12. Folic acid must be transformed into 5-methyl-folic acid in order to prevent its rapid excretion in the urine. Vitamin B12 is required for both myelin lipoprotein synthesis and the transport and storage of folic acid in cells. The right DNA synthesis, methionine regeneration for appropriate protein synthesis and methylation capacity, and prevention of homocysteine buildup, which can cause a number of degenerative disorders, are all dependent on vitamin B12 (Sangle et al., 2020).

15.4.8 VITAMIN C (ASCORBIC ACID)

Hippocrates originally recorded the condition of scurvy, which is brought on by a deficiency of vitamin C, in the 1500 B.C. Ebers papyrus. It was endemic in many places, particularly during the early expeditions of the New World, when over 2 million sailors perished of scurvy during the "Age of Sail." Walter Haworth and his colleagues at the University of Birmingham in England discovered the structure of vitamin C in 1933 (Burke, 2007). The same research team synthesized it in the same year. All molecules possessing the biological activity of L-ascorbic acid are referred to as vitamin C. It's a water-soluble white crystalline powder that's solid at room temperature and works well as a reducing agent (Bendich et al., 1986).

All living things, with the exception of humans, other primates, guinea pigs, fish, fruit-eating bats, and some exotic birds, practically manufacture vitamin C. Green vegetables, fresh fruit—especially citrus fruits and blackberries—and animal organs like the liver, kidney, and brain all contain considerable levels of it. The following foods also contain a lot of vitamin C: potatoes, tomatoes, strawberries, and cabbage. Wheat grains and muscle meat have subpar vitamin B12 evaluations. Cooking causes high vitamin C losses as a result of leaking into the cooking water and air oxidation. Ascorbic acid and dehydroascorbic acid are the forms of vitamin C that are physiologically active. Both vitamins are absorbed passively and through carriers across the buccal mucosa (Camarena & Wang, 2016). Intestinal absorption of vitamin C is mediated by active transport at physiological levels, but at excessive doses, it is mediated by a significantly less effective passive diffusion that happens extremely slowly. With undetectable quantities of dehydroascorbic acid, vitamin C is mostly present in plasma as free ascorbate. The liver has the best supply of vitamin C in the body due to its special property of size. Among the organs that ascorbate is found in include the kidney, pancreas, and brain. Ascorbic acid or its catabolites are only minimally excreted in feces, and vitamin C is largely excreted in urine (Hallberg et al., 1989).

Many hydroxylation reactions that are catalyzed by oxygenases require vitamin C as a cofactor. For instance, vitamin C is necessary for the production of collagen and catecholamines. Additionally, it contributes to the liver's production of carnitine, which is made from the amino acid lysine. The catabolism of phenylanaline and thyrosine enzymes, which is hindered by a vitamin C shortage, requires copper and vitamin C as cofactors. Additionally, the presence of copper, oxygen, and ascorbate activates peptide hormones like peptidylglycine (Carr & McCall, 2017). By encouraging the integration of iron into ferritin, vitamin C affects how iron is distributed throughout the body. Additionally, it is essential for the metabolism of nitrosamine and histamine. Vitamin C also makes leukocytes more mobile and guards against oxidative damage on their membranes. Due to its strong reducing capacity, vitamin C has an important biochemical feature of antioxidants. Due to its potent antioxidant effects, vitamin C can shield the eye from free radical damage as well as sperm from oxidative stress (Beaton et al., 1992).

15.4.9 VITAMIN D

A vitamin D deficiency-related illness called rickets was first noted approximately 50,000 B.C. Due to air pollution and a lack of sunlight during the Industrial Revolution, rickets spread over northern Europe, England, and the United States. Ergocalciferol (vitamin D2) and cholecalciferol (vitamin

D3) are the two different forms of vitamin D (vitamin D2). In Germany, in 1932 and 1936, respectively, Windaus and his coworkers identified the structures of vitamin D2 and vitamin D3 (DeRegil et al., 2016). The first three-dimensional model of vitamin D3 was created by Nobel laureate X-ray crystallographer Dorothy Hodgkin. Plants, fungi, and yeasts produce vitamin D2 by exposing ergosterol to sunlight, but humans produce vitamin D3 as a result of sunlight's influence on the skin (Pludowski et al., 2018).

Vitamin D has a modest number of reassessments. The most nutrient-dense fish liver oils are those made from halibut. Additionally rich in vitamin D are fatty fish, including herring, sardines, pilchards, and tuna. Vitamin D can be found in dairy products, eggs, and mammalian liver. Contrarily, vitamins are absent from grains, fruits, and vegetables. Examples of fortified items include milk, breakfast cereals, and margarine. The skin can also manufacture vitamin D after being exposed to sunlight. A much more significant source of vitamin D than diet is endogenous vitamin D production (Hsia et al., 2007).

Lipid micelles containing vitamin D are taken up by the lymphatic system and combined with chylomicrons. Immediately following intestinal absorption, vitamin D is swiftly absorbed by the liver, where it is hydroxylated to produce the 25-hydroxy derivative calcidiol before being released into the blood in combination with a vitamin D-binding globulin. When calcidiol enters the kidney, it either undergoes 1- or 24-hydroxylation to create the apparently inactive metabolite 24, 25-dihydroxyvitamin D (calcitriol) or the active metabolite 1, 25-dihydroxyvitamin D (calcitriol) (24-hydroxycalcidiol). These changes are influenced by the plasma's calcium and phosphorous mineral content. Vitamin D is catabolized by the liver into highly polar inactivation products that are primarily excreted in bile (Marya et al., 1981).

Maintaining the body's plasma concentrations of calcium and phosphorus is vitamin D's primary physiological role. Increased calcium absorption in the gut, reduced calcium excretion, and mobilization of calcium from bone are all effects of calcitriol (Lips, 2010). It is crucial for the health of the immune system, the neurological system, and cell differentiation. Nuclear receptors that control gene expression are activated; it also regulates the expression of more than 50 genes. 24-hydroxycalcidiol plays a physiologic role in the growth of bone or cartilage in knockout mice (El Ati-Hellal & Hellal, 2021).

15.5 CONCLUSION

The human body needs vitamins to develop and function properly. Among the 13 essential vitamins are vitamins B, A, C, D, E, and K (thiamine, riboflavin, niacin, pantothenic acid, biotin, B6, B12, and folate). Different functions of vitamins maintain the body functioning effectively. While some vitamins support healthy neurons and infection resistance, others may aid in correct blood clotting or food energy absorption. You can consume enough of the majority of these vitamins by following the dietary guidelines.

KEYWORDS

- **ascorbic acid**
- **food energy absorption**
- **human nutrition**
- **nutraceuticals**
- **nutrification**
- **vitaminosis**
- **vitamins**

REFERENCES

Alamgir, A. N. M., (2017). *Therapeutic Use of Medicinal Plants and Their Extracts* (Vol. 1). Springer International Publishing AG.

Allen, M. A., & Burgess, S. G., (1950). The losses of ascorbic acid during the large-scale cooking of green vegetables by different methods. *British Journal of Nutrition, 4*(2, 3), 95–100.

Allgeyer, L. C., Miller, M. J., & Lee, S. Y., (2010). Sensory and microbiological quality of yogurt drinks with prebiotics and probiotics. *Journal of Dairy Science, 93*(10), 4471–4479.

Aluru, M., Xu, Y., Guo, R., Wang, Z., Li, S., White, W., Wang, K., & Rodermel, S., (2008). Generation of transgenic maize with enhanced provitamin A content. *Journal of Experimental Botany, 59*(13), 3551–3562.

Bahl, R., Bhandari, N., Hambidge, K. M., & Bhan, M. K., (1998). Plasma zinc as a predictor of diarrheal and respiratory morbidity in children in an urban slum setting. *The American Journal of Clinical Nutrition, 68*(2), 414S–417S.

Ball, G. F. M., (2004). *Vitamins: Their Role in the Human Body.* [sl] Blackwell Publishing Ltd.

Barak, A. J., Beckenhauer, H. C., Junnila, M., & Tuma, D. J., (1993). Dietary betaine promotes the generation of hepatic S-adenosylmethionine and protects the liver from ethanol-induced fatty infiltration. *Alcoholism: Clinical and Experimental Research, 17*(3), 552–555.

Beaton, G. H., Martorell, R., L'Abbé, K. A., Edmonston, B., & McCabe, G., (1992). *Effectiveness of Vitamin A Supplementation in the Control of Young Child Morbidity and Mortality in Developing Countries: Summary Report.*

Bender, D. A., (2009). *A Dictionary of Food and Nutrition*. OUP Oxford.

Bendich, A., Machlin, L. J., Scandurra, O., Burton, G. W., & Wayner, D. D. M., (1986). The antioxidant role of vitamin C. *Advances in Free Radical Biology & Medicine*, *2*(2), 419–444.

Bieri, J. G., & Evarts, R. P., (1974). Gamma tocopherol: Metabolism, biological activity and significance in human vitamin E nutrition. *The American Journal of Clinical Nutrition*, *27*(9), 980–986.

Biesalski, H. K., & Tinz, J., (2017). Multivitamin/mineral supplements: Rationale and safety–A systematic review. *Nutrition*, *33*, 76–82.

Biesalski, H. K., (2017). Sustainable micronutrients in Europe: Is there cause for concern? In: *Sustainable Nutrition in a Changing World* (pp. 143–166). Springer, Cham.

Black, R. E., (1998). Therapeutic and preventive effects of zinc on serious childhood infectious diseases in developing countries. *The American Journal of Clinical Nutrition*, *68*(2), 476S-479S.

Block, G., Patterson, B., & Subar, A., (1992). Fruit, vegetables, and cancer prevention: A review of the epidemiological evidence. *Nutrition and Cancer*, *18*(1), 1–29.

Bracco, P., & Oral, E., (2011). Vitamin E-stabilized UHMWPE for total joint implants: A review. *Clinical Orthopedics and Related Research®*, *469*(8), 2286–2293.

Burke, K. E., (2007). Interaction of vitamins C and E as better cosmeceuticals. *Dermatologic Therapy*, *20*(5), 314–321.

Camarena, V., & Wang, G., (2016). The epigenetic role of vitamin C in health and disease. *Cellular and Molecular Life Sciences*, *73*(8), 1645–1658.

Carr, A. C., & McCall, C., (2017). The role of vitamin C in the treatment of pain: New insights. *Journal of Translational Medicine*, *15*(1), 1–14.

Cheney, G., (1950). Anti-peptic ulcer dietary factor (vitamin" U") in the treatment of peptic ulcer. *Journal of the American Dietetic Association*, *26*, 668–672.

Combet, E., & Buckton, C., (2015). Micronutrient deficiencies, vitamin pills, and nutritional supplements. *Medicine*, *43*(2), 66–72.

Combs, Jr. G. F., & McClung, J. P., (2016). *The Vitamins: Fundamental Aspects in Nutrition and Health*. Academic Press.

Cowan, A. E., Jun, S., Gahche, J. J., Tooze, J. A., Dwyer, J. T., Eicher-Miller, H. A., Bhadra, A., et al., (2018). Dietary supplement use differs by socioeconomic and health-related characteristics among US adults, NHANES 2011–2014. *Nutrients*, *10*(8), 1114.

Croft, M. T., Warren, M. J., & Smith, A. G., (2006). Algae need their vitamins. *Eukaryotic Cell*, *5*(8), 1175–1183.

Dai, L., Zhu, J., Liang, J., Wang, Y. P., Wang, H., & Mao, M. (2011). Birth defects surveillance in China. *World Journal of Pediatrics*, *7*, 302–310.

De Pee, S., Kraemer, K., Van, D. B. T., Boy, E., Grasset, C., Moench-Pfanner, R., Zlotkin, S., & Bloem, M. W., (2008). Quality criteria for micronutrient powder products: Report of a meeting organized by the world food program and sprinkles global health initiative. *Food and Nutrition Bulletin*, *29*(3), 232–241.

DellaPenna, D., & Pogson, B. J., (2006). Vitamin synthesis in plants: Tocopherols and carotenoids. *Annu. Rev. Plant Biol.*, *57*, 711–738.

De-Regil, L. M., Palacios, C., Lombardo, L. K., & Peña-Rosas, J. P., (2016). Vitamin D supplementation for women during pregnancy. *Cochrane Database of Systematic Reviews*, (1).

Harrison, T. J., Smith, J. A., Martin, G. R., Chamberlain, D. E., Bearhop, S., Robb, G. N., & Reynolds, S. J. (2010). Does food supplementation really enhance productivity of breeding birds? *Oecologia, 164*, 311–320.

Enghag, P., (2008). *Encyclopedia of the Elements: Technical Data-History-Processing-Applications*. John Wiley & Sons.

Fenech, M., (2012). Folate (vitamin B9) and vitamin B12 and their function in the maintenance of nuclear and mitochondrial genome integrity. *Mutation Research/Fundamental and Molecular Mechanisms of Mutagenesis*, *733*(1, 2), 21–33.

Food and Nutrition Board, Institute of Medicine, (2001). *Dietary Reference Intakes for Vitamin A, Vitamin K, Arsenic, Boron, Chromium, Copper, Iodine, Iron, Manganese, Molybdenum, Nickel, Silicon, Vanadium, and Zinc.* National Academy of Medicine.

Francis, E. C., Zhang, L., Witrick, B., & Chen, L. (2021). Health behaviors of American pregnant women: A cross-sectional analysis of NHANES 2007–2014. *Journal of Public Health, 43*(1), 131–138.

Gagner, J. J., (2012). Nutritional, herbal, and homeopathic supplements. *Evidence-Based Management of Low Back Pain*, 258–268.

Hallberg, L. E. I. F., Brune, M. A. T. S., & Rossander, L. E. N. A., (1989). The role of vitamin C in iron absorption. *International Journal for Vitamin and Nutrition Research. Supplement= Internationale Zeitschrift fur Vitamin-und Ernahrungsforschung. Supplement, 30*, 103–108.

Hernandez, B. Y., McDuffie, K., Wilkens, L. R., Kamemoto, L., & Goodman, M. T., (2003). Diet and premalignant lesions of the cervix: Evidence of a protective role for folate, riboflavin, thiamin, and vitamin B12. *Cancer Causes & Control, 14*(9), 859–870.

Hsia, J., Heiss, G., Ren, H., Allison, M., Dolan, N. C., Greenland, P., Heckbert, S. R., et al., (2007). Calcium/vitamin D supplementation and cardiovascular events. *Circulation, 115*(7), 846–854.

Indraccolo, U., Gentile, G., Pomili, G., Luzi, G., & Villani, C., (2005). Thiamine deficiency and beriberi features in a patient with hyperemesis gravidarum. *Nutrition, 21*(9), 967–968.

Institute of Medicine (US) Standing Committee on the Scientific Evaluation of Dietary Reference Intakes, (1997). Dietary reference intakes. In: *Dietary Reference Intakes for Calcium, Phosphorus, Magnesium, Vitamin D, and Fluoride*. National Academies Press (US).

Jenkins, D. J., Spence, J. D., Giovannucci, E. L., Kim, Y. I., Josse, R., Vieth, R., Blanco, M. S., et al., (2018). Supplemental vitamins and minerals for CVD prevention and treatment. *Journal of the American College of Cardiology, 71*(22), 2570–2584.

Joint F. A. O., & World Health Organization, (1998). *Carbohydrates in Human Nutrition: Report of a Joint FAO/WHO Expert Consultation, Rome*.

Keservani, R. K., & Sharma, A. K., (2014). Flavonoids: Emerging trends and potential health benefits. *Journal of Chinese Pharmaceutical Sciences, 23*(12), 815.

Keservani, R. K., Kesharwani, R. K., Sharma, A. K., Vyas, N., & Chadoker, A., (2010b). Nutritional supplements: An overview. *International Journal of Current Pharmaceutical Review and Research, 1*(*1*), 59–75.

Keservani, R. K., Kesharwani, R. K., Vyas, N., Jain, S., Raghuvanshi, R., & Sharma, A. K., (2010a). Nutraceutical and functional food as future food: A review. *Der Pharmacia Lettre, 2*(1), 106–116.

Keservani, R. K., Sharma, A. K., & Jarouliya, U. (2015). Protein and peptide in drug targeting and its therapeutic approach. *ArsPharmaceutica (Internet), 56*(3), 165–177.

Keservani, R. K., Sharma, A. K., & Kesharwani, R. K., (2016a). Nutraceutical and functional foods for cardiovascular health. In: *Food Process Engineering* (pp. 257–278, 291–312). Apple Academic Press, CRC Press. ISBN: 9781771884020.

Keservani, R. K., Sharma, A. K., & Kesharwani, R. K., (2016b). Medicinal effect of nutraceutical fruits for the cognition and brain health. *Scientifica*, 10. Article ID 3109254. doi:10.1155/2016/3109254.

Keservani, R. K., Sharma, A. K., & Kesharwani, R. K. (2017). An overview and therapeutic applications of nutraceutical and functional foods. *Recent Advances in Drug Delivery Technology*, 160–201. ISBN:9781522507543.

Keservani, R. K., Sharma, A. K., & Kesharwani, R. K. (2020). *Nutraceuticals and Dietary Supplements: Applications in Health Improvement and Disease Management*. CRC Press. ISBN: 9781771888738.

Kibirige, D., & Mwebaze, R., (2013). Vitamin B12 deficiency among patients with diabetes mellitus: Is routine screening and supplementation justified? *Journal of Diabetes & Metabolic Disorders*, *12*(1), 1–6.

Kocyłowski, R., Lewicka, I., Grzesiak, M., Gaj, Z., Sobańska, A., Poznaniak, J., Von, K. C., & Suliburska, J., (2018). Assessment of dietary intake and mineral status in pregnant women. *Archives of Gynecology and Obstetrics*, *297*(6), 1433–1440.

Lentjes, M. A., (2019). The balance between food and dietary supplements in the general population. *Proceedings of the Nutrition Society*, *78*(1), 97–109.

Lips, P. T. A. M., (2010). Worldwide status of vitamin D nutrition. *The Journal of Steroid Biochemistry and Molecular Biology*, *121*(1, 2), 297–300.

Magoulas, P. L., & El-Hattab, A. W., (2012). Systemic primary carnitine deficiency: An overview of clinical manifestations, diagnosis, and management. *Orphanet Journal of Rare Diseases*, *7*(1), 1–6.

Marya, R. K., Rathee, S., Lata, V., & Mudgil, S., (1981). Effects of vitamin D supplementation in pregnancy. *Gynecologic and Obstetric Investigation*, *12*(3), 155–161.

McDowell, L. R., (2003). *Minerals in Animal and Human Nutrition* (p. 644). Netherlands: Elsevier Science.

Meyers, L. D., Hellwig, J. P., & Otten, J. J., (2006). *Dietary Reference Intakes: The Essential Guide to Nutrient Requirements*. National Academies Press.

Miller, A., Korem, M., Almog, R., & Galboiz, Y., (2005). Vitamin B12, demyelination, remyelination and repair in multiple sclerosis. *Journal of the Neurological Sciences*, *233*(1, 2), 93–97.

Namazi, N., Kelishadi, R., Heshmat, R., Motlagh, M. E., Sanaei, M., Shafiee, G., Ziaodini, H. et al. (2019). Determinants of taking dietary supplements in Iranian children and adolescents: The CASPIAN-V study. *Journal of Diabetes & Metabolic Disorders*, *18*(2), 409–417.

Ottaway, P. B., (2008). *Food Fortification and Supplementation: Technological, Safety and Regulatory Aspects*. Elsevier.

Perlitz, H., Mensink, G., Lage, B. C., Richter, A., Brettschneider, A. K., Lehmann, F., Patelakis, E., et al., (2019). Use of vitamin and mineral supplements among adolescents living in Germany—Results from EsKiMo II. *Nutrients*, *11*(6), 1208.

Pludowski, P., Holick, M. F., Grant, W. B., Konstantynowicz, J., Mascarenhas, M. R., Haq, A., Povoroznyuk, V., et al., (2018). Vitamin D supplementation guidelines. *The Journal of Steroid Biochemistry and Molecular Biology*, *175*, 125–135.

Polcz, M. E., & Barbul, A., (2019). The role of vitamin A in wound healing. *Nutrition in Clinical Practice*, *34*(5), 695–700.

Rane, B. R., Bharath, M. S., Patil, R. R., Keservani, R. K., & Jain, A. S. (2020b). Novel approaches in nutraceuticals; Chapter 11. In: Rajesh, K. K., Raj, K. K., & Anil, K. S., (eds.), *Enhancing the Therapeutic Efficacy of Herbal Formulations Through Novel Drug Delivery Systems* (pp. 241–266). IGI Global International Publisher, Pennsylvania, USA. ISBN13: 9781799844532.

Rane, B. R., Patil, A. S., Keservani, R. K., & Jain, A. S., (2020a). Novel approaches in herbal formulation; Chapter 2. In: Rajesh, K. K., Raj, K. K., & Anil, K. S., (eds.), *Enhancing the Therapeutic Efficacy of Herbal Formulations Through Novel Drug Delivery Systems* (pp. 43–68). IGI Global International Publisher, Pennsylvania, USA. ISBN13: 9781799844532.

Rane, B. R., Tadavi, S. A., & Keservani, R. K., (2020c). Naturopathy; Chapter 12. In: Anil, K. S., Raj, K. K., & Surya, P. G., (eds.), *Herbal Product Development* (pp. 321–347). Apple Academic Press, CRC Press, Taylor & Francis Group. ISBN: 9781771888776.

Sangle, P., Sandhu, O., Aftab, Z., Anthony, A. T., & Khan, S., (2020). Vitamin B12 supplementation: Preventing onset and improving prognosis of depression. *Cureus*, *12*(10).

Sazawal, S., Black, R. E., Bhan, M. K., Jalla, S., Sinha, A., & Bhandari, N., (1997). Efficacy of zinc supplementation in reducing the incidence and prevalence of acute diarrhea–a community-based, double-blind, controlled trial. *The American Journal of Clinical Nutrition*, *66*(2), 413–418.

Sharma, A. K., Keservani, R. K., & Gautam, S. P., (2020). *Herbal Product Development.* Apple Academic Press, CRC Press, Taylor & Francis Group. ISBN: 9781771888776.

Sinbad, O. O., Folorunsho, A. A., Olabisi, O. L., Ayoola, O. A., & Temitope, E. J. (2019). Vitamins as antioxidants. *Journal of Food Science and Nutrition Research*, *2*(3), 214–235.

Singh, P., Kesharwani, R. K., & Keservani, R. K., (2017a). Antioxidants and vitamins: Roles in cellular function and metabolism. In: *Sustained Energy for Enhanced Human Functions and Activity* (pp. 385–407). Academic Press. ISBN:9780128054130.

Singh, P., Kesharwani, R. K., & Keservani, R. K., (2017b). Protein, carbohydrates, and fats: Energy metabolism. In: *Sustained Energy for Enhanced Human Functions and Activity* (pp. 103–115). Academic Press. ISBN:9780128054130.

Skrovankova, S., (2011). *Seaweed Vitamins Nutraceutical Marine Medicinal Foods: Implications and Applications, Macro and Microalgae: Advances in Food and Nutrition Research Series*, *64*, 357–369.

Smith, J., & Hong-Shum, L., (2011). *Food Additives Data Book.* 2nd Edition. John Wiley & Sons. ISBN: 978-1-405-19543-0.

Steinberg, D., (1991). Antioxidants and atherosclerosis. A current assessment. *Circulation*, *84*(3), 1420–1425.

Yadav, M., Verma, M. K., & Chauhan, N. S. (2018). A review of metabolic potential of human gut microbiome in human nutrition. *Archives of Microbiology*, *200*, 203–217.

Index

D

W

X

Y

Z